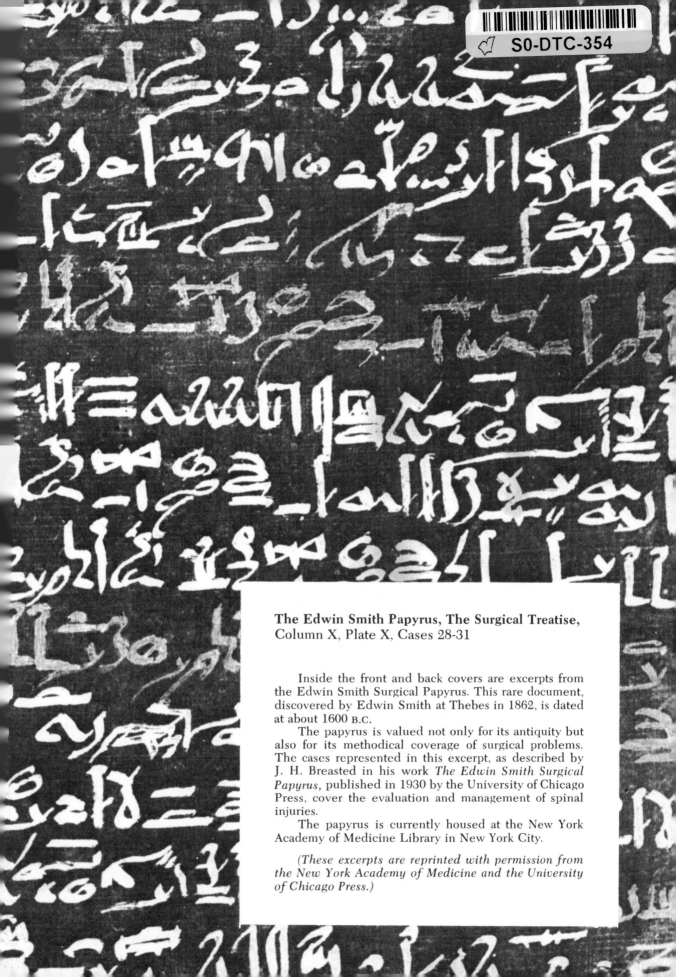

The Edwin Smith Papyrus, The Surgical Treatise, Column X, Plate X, Cases 28-31

Inside the front and back covers are excerpts from the Edwin Smith Surgical Papyrus. This rare document, discovered by Edwin Smith at Thebes in 1862, is dated at about 1600 B.C.

The papyrus is valued not only for its antiquity but also for its methodical coverage of surgical problems. The cases represented in this excerpt, as described by J. H. Breasted in his work *The Edwin Smith Surgical Papyrus,* published in 1930 by the University of Chicago Press, cover the evaluation and management of spinal injuries.

The papyrus is currently housed at the New York Academy of Medicine Library in New York City.

E. JAMES POTCHEN, M.D., *Consulting Editor*

Professor and Chairman
Department of Radiology
Michigan State University
East Lansing, Michigan

Published

Volume 16 in the Series
SAUNDERS
MONOGRAPHS
IN CLINICAL
RADIOLOGY

Forthcoming Monographs

ARTHROGRAPHY: PRINCIPLES AND TECHNIQUES
  Tom W. Staple, M.D.

XEROMAMMOGRAPHIC PATHOLOGY
  *Michael D. Lagios, M.D., H. Joachim Burhenne, M.D., and
  F. Margolin, M.D.*

CARDIAC IMAGING IN CHILDREN AND ADOLESCENTS
  *Michael J. Kelley, M.D., C. Carl Jaffe, M.D., and
  Charles S. Kleinman, M.D.*

THE
RADIOLOGY
OF
VERTEBRAL
TRAUMA

JOHN A. GEHWEILER, Jr., M.D.

Associate Professor of Radiology, Duke University
Medical Center, Durham, North Carolina

RAYMOND L. OSBORNE, Jr., M.D.

Attending Radiologist, Middlesex Memorial Hospital,
Middletown, Connecticut; Formerly Assistant Professor of
Radiology, Cornell University Medical Center, and
Assistant Attending Roentgenologist, Memorial Sloan-Kettering
Cancer Center, New York, New York

R. FREDERICK BECKER, Ph.D.

Emeritus Professor of Anatomy, East Carolina Medical School,
Greenville, North Carolina

1980
W. B. SAUNDERS COMPANY • Philadelphia • London • Toronto

W. B. Saunders Company: West Washington Square
Philadelphia, PA   19105

1 St. Anne's Road
Eastbourne, East Sussex BN21 3UN, England

1 Goldthorne Avenue
Toronto, Ontario M8Z 5T9, Canada

9 Waltham Street
Artarmon, N.S.W. 2064, Australia

Library of Congress Cataloging in Publication Data

Gehweiler, Jr., John A.

The radiology of vertebral trauma.

(Saunders monographs in clinical radiology; v. 16)

1. Spine—Wounds and injuries.   2. Spine—Radiography.
I. Osborne, Jr., Raymond L., joint author.   II. Becker,
Roland Frederick, 1912–   joint author.   III. Title.
[DNLM: 1. Spinal injuries—Radiology. WE725.G311r]

RD533.G45   617′.56   78–65376

ISBN 0–7216–4065–6

The Radiology of Vertebral Trauma   ISBN   0-7216-4065-6

Last digit is the print number: 9   8   7   6   5   4   3   2   1

TO OUR FAMILIES

PREFACE

This monograph is written for a select group of readers — namely, *you*, the physician. You obviously have a special interest in vertebral column injuries, and in this monograph we hope to provide answers to your basic questions in successfully diagnosing these injuries.

This monograph originated as a series of instructional courses dealing with vertebral trauma given by the senior authors at both local and national meetings. The task of assembling all of the available knowledge of vertebral column trauma for the radiologist and surgeon proved to be a far more arduous job than originally envisioned. We thank you for your patience and for your encouragement.

Since many physicians feel fallible when confronted by traumatic injuries of the vertebral column, we have tried to simplify the problems and provide a practical guide to diagnosis. To accomplish our goals, we have divided the monograph into *three major sections*. The first is a comprehensive review of anatomy, both gross and roentgenographic, providing a foundation upon which to build knowledge and understanding of vertebral trauma. The second section deals with injuries of the cervical vertebral column, and the third with injuries of the thoracolumbar and sacrococcygeal column. The latter two sections encompass clinical information, incidence, mechanisms of injury, roentgen diagnosis, and differential diagnosis.

This monograph is designed to instruct and to provide a broad base of concepts upon which to build additional knowledge from teachers, colleagues, and, of course, patients. We wish you well and we hope that we have fulfilled your requirements as a physician in relation to the exciting subject of vertebral column injuries.

ACKNOWLEDGMENTS

All teachers are deeply indebted to those persons, both living and dead, from whom they have learned and in particular to those who have stimulated and encouraged them. The teacher attempts to synthesize his own personal experience and knowledge and the knowledge of others from a variety of medical disciplines. We acknowledge with gratitude the aid and assistance of many persons.

Five authors of monographs on the cervical column deserve special mention—Drs. Martin Abel, R. Braakman, L. Penning, Detlef von Torklus, and Walter Gehle. These men, through their classic books, provided the stimulus to the senior author to pursue his study of cervical column injuries. Hundreds of other authors of both papers and books, too numerous to mention, also deserve our profound thanks by adding to our knowledge of vertebral column injuries and conditions simulating trauma.

Many colleagues in radiology and surgery helped in the preparation of papers—Oliver Charlton, William Clark, Richard Daffner, Denise Duff, Richard Kramer, Richard Laib, Salutario Martinez, Michael Miller, Carlisle Morgan, Barry Powers, Robert Schaaf, and Grady Stewart. Those papers form the major portion of Part II of this monograph.

Special gratitude belongs to five departmental chairmen—Charles E. Putman of the Duke University Medical Center, Richard G. Lester of the University of Texas at Houston, Robin C. Watson of Memorial Sloan-Kettering Cancer Center, Joseph P. Whalen of New York Hospital—Cornell University Medical Center, and Robert H. Freiberger of The Hospital for Special Surgery, New York, New York—for encouragement and aid.

Illustrations were provided by the Department of Audiovisual Education, Duke University Medical Center, and by Carlin Medical Photography, Westwood, N.J. The outstanding artwork is predominately the work of William E. Loechel of Wayne State University. Additional artwork was provided by Wayne Williams of East Carolina University, and David Bolinsky.

For the typing and retyping of the manuscript, we are indebted to many people but especially Jackie Wright, Faith Gehweiler, Gloria Vences, and Patricia Aranibar.

The University of Chicago Press granted permission to reproduce the many quotations from the translation of the *Edwin Smith Surgical Papyrus* by Dr. J. H. Breasted. Permission was also granted to use Plate X of the papyrus for the book folio.

To the staff at the W. B. Saunders Company in general and especially Mr. Jack Hanley, we are ever grateful for your many kindnesses, patience, and understanding. We also wish to thank Mary Cowell, Susan Hunter, and Carol Hoidra for editorial assistance.

ACKNOWLEDGMENTS
TO JOURNALS AND BOOKS

The following is a list of journal articles, books, and tape presentations published by the senior author, or by the senior author in coauthorship with colleagues, from which some of the illustrations in this book were derived. Our gratitude goes to the publishers and editors for granting permission to use these materials in Chapters 3, 4, and 5.

The American College of Radiology

Disorders of the Head and Neck (Second Series). Edited by L. F. Rogers. Chicago, American College of Radiology, 1978.

The American Roentgen Ray Society

Gehweiler, J. A., Martinez, S., Clark, W. M., Miller, M. D., and Stewart, G. C.: Spondylolisthesis of the axis vertebra. Am. J. Roentgenol. 128:682, 1977.

Congress of Neurological Surgeons

Powers, B., Miller, M. D., Kramer, R. S., Martinez, S., and Gehweiler, J. A.: Traumatic anterior antlanto-occipital dislocation. Neurosurg. 4:12, 1979.

Educational Reviews, Inc.

Practical Reviews Seminars in Radiology. II. Cervical spine trauma: a practical diagnosis (tape & illustrations by J. A. Gehweiler). Coordinating editor A. E. Robinson. Leeds, Alabama, Educational Reviews, 1978.

International Skeletal Society

Gehweiler, J. A., Duff, D. E., Martinez, S., Miller, M. D., and Clark, W. M.: Fractures of the atlas vertebra. Skeletal Radiol. 1:97, 1976.

Schaaf, R. E., Gehweiler, J. A., Miller, M. D., and Powers, B.: Lateral hyperflexion injuries of the cervical spine. Skeletal Radiol. 3:73, 1978.

Charlton, O. P., Gehweiler, J. A., Morgan, C. L., Martinez, S., and Daffner, R. H.: Spondylolysis and spondylolisthesis of the cervical spine. Skeletal Radiol. 3:79, 1978.

Clark, W. M., Gehweiler, J. A., and Laib, R.: Twelve significant signs of cervical spine trauma. Skeletal Radiol. 3:201, 1979.

Martinez, S., Morgan, C. L., Gehweiler, J. A., Powers, B., and Miller, M.D.: Unusual fractures and dislocations of the axis vertebra. Skeletal Radiol. 3:206, 1979.

Radiological Society of North America

Stewart, G. C., Gehweiler, J. A., Laib, R. H., and Martinez, S.: Horizontal fracture of the anterior arch of the atlas. Radiology 122:349, 1977.

Gehweiler, J. A., Clark, W. M., Schaaf, R. E., Powers, B., and Miller, M. D.: Cervical spine trauma: The common combined conditions. Radiology 130:77, 1979.

CONTENTS

Part I

GROSS ANATOMY OF THE VERTEBRAL COLUMN

Chapter 1

OSTEOLOGY

"...every follower of medical pursuits should be intelligent in the minutiae of anatomy, if he wishes to practice with ease to himself and to the benefit of the patient...."

John Morgan

INTRODUCTION

Thirty-three irregular bones, the *vertebrae*, form the human *vertebral column* (Fig. 1–1). It is anatomically correct to refer to this column of bones as the *vertebral column*, although the term *spine* enjoys such widespread medical usage that it will be retained where required by clinical and radiologic convention. The vertebrae, arranged in a series, extend from the base of the skull through the entire length of the neck and trunk. They are connected by muscles, ligaments, and intervertebral disks to form a strong, flexible support for the body. The vertebrae also afford protection to the spinal cord and its meninges.

Vertebrae are arranged regionally as seven *cervical*, twelve *thoracic*, five *lumbar*, five *sacral*, and four *coccygeal* segments. The upper 24 *presacral vertebrae* remain separate throughout life; they are the *true, or movable, vertebrae*. In the adult, the five sacral vertebrae fuse to form the *sacrum*, and the four coccygeal vertebrae fuse to form the *coccyx*. The sacrum and coccyx are the *false, or fixed, vertebrae* (Fig. 1–1).

THE MORPHOLOGY OF A "TYPICAL VERTEBRA"

Except for the atlas (C-1) and the axis (C-2), the movable presacral vertebrae have many common characteristics. We may analyze these structural characteristics and firmly establish the anatomic terminology to be used in this book by studying a model, or "typical vertebra." Where is such a specimen to be found? We will observe anatomic tradition and select the typical vertebra from the midthoracic region (Fig. 1–2 *A, B*).

The basic parts of a vertebra consist of the following: (1) the weight-bearing *body* located ventrally; and (2) a dorsal portion, the *vertebral arch*, which acts as a protective encasement for the spinal cord and its meningeal coverings and blood vessels.

The vertebral arch is composed of two *pedicles* and two *laminae*. The pedicles join the arch to the vertebral body; the laminae span the pedicles and form the dorsal boundary of the vertebral foramen (Fig. 1–2 *A, B*), through which passes the spinal cord.

Seven projections, or *processes*, are supported by the vertebral arch. Two *transverse processes* and one *spinous process* serve as levers on which muscles pull. Four *articular processes (zygapophyses)* determine the direction and degree of all movement in the vertebral column (Fig. 1–2 *A, B*).

In an isolated vertebra, the vertebral body and vertebral arch enclose the *vertebral foramen* (Fig. 1–2 *A*). When the vertebral column is articulated, a series of vertebral foramina collectively form the *vertebral canal*. This canal encloses and protects the spinal cord and its meninges and vessels.

The terms *vertebral body* and *centrum*, and *vertebral arch* and *neural arch*, are often used synonymously in medical writing. These terms will not be used interchangeably in this book, however, and the reason for this should be quite apparent after studying Figure 1–3.

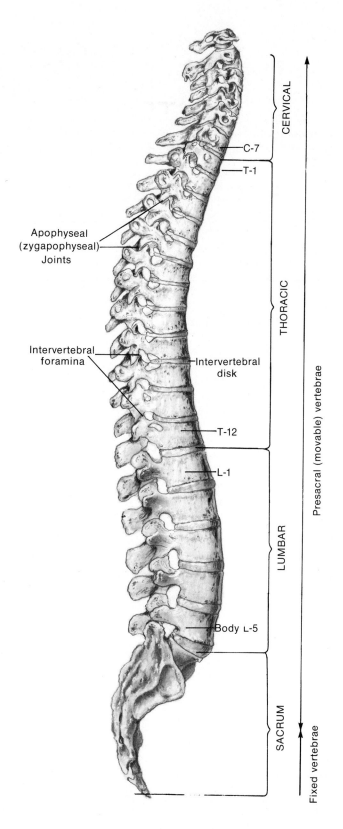

Apophyseal (zygapophyseal) Joints

Intervertebral foramina

Intervertebral disk

C-7

T-1

CERVICAL

THORACIC

T-12

L-1

LUMBAR

Body L-5

SACRUM

Presacral (movable) vertebrae

Fixed vertebrae

Figure 1–1. Lateral view of the articulated vertebral column.

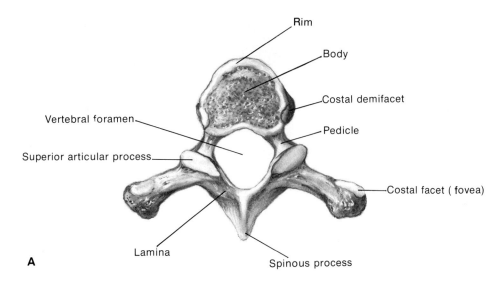

Rim

Body

Costal demifacet

Pedicle

Vertebral foramen

Superior articular process

Costal facet (fovea)

Lamina

Spinous process

A

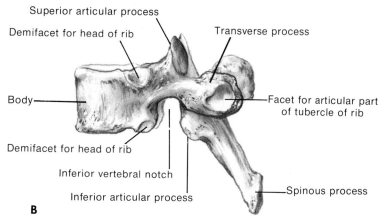

Superior articular process

Demifacet for head of rib

Transverse process

Body

Facet for articular part
of tubercle of rib

Demifacet for head of rib

Inferior vertebral notch

Inferior articular process

Spinous process

B

Figure 1–2. A "typical" thoracic vertebra. *A*, Cranial aspect. *B*, Lateral view.

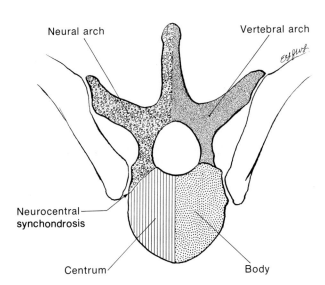

Neural arch

Vertebral arch

Neurocentral synchondrosis

Centrum

Body

A

B

Figure 1–3. Schematic drawing of the neural arch and centrum (*A*), and the vertebral arch and body (*B*). Note that these terms are not interchangeable (see text). It should be noted that the rib does not articulate with the centrum, but only with the neural arch.

At birth, a vertebra is composed of three ossification centers joined by cartilage — the centrum and the neural arch halves. The neurocentral synchondrosis unites the centrum to the neural arch. During the first year of life, the neural arch halves unite dorsally. This union occurs first in the lumbar region and proceeds cranially through the thoracic and cervical regions.

The neural arch fuses with the centrum in the cervical region at three years. This union proceeds caudally and is usually complete in the sacrum by age seven. As shown in Figure 1–3, the neural arch forms not only the vertebral arch but also contributes a tiny portion to the centrum on each side to form the vertebral body.[1] Thus, on radiographs, we may easily differentiate a vertebral arch from a neural arch, and a vertebral body from a centrum, depending upon the presence or absence of the neurocentral synchondrosis (Fig. 1–36 A, B, C).

THE VERTEBRAL BODY

The cranial and caudal surfaces, or *endplates,* of a vertebral body are flattened and roughened centrally (Fig. 1–2 A). The periphery of the cylindrically shaped bodies has an elevated rim of smooth cortical bone, formed from the fusion of the secondary ossification center of the vertebral end-plate to the body. These end-plates give strong attachment to the fibrocartilaginous intervertebral disks, which bind the vertebral bodies together. Between the disk and the end-plate there is a thin layer of hyaline cartilage that extends peripherally to the marginal rim, but does not cover it in the adult. The sides of the vertebral body are slightly concave ventrally and laterally, while dorsally they are relatively flat (Fig.

1–2 A, B). The ventral, lateral, and dorsal surfaces of a vertebral body are studded with many small holes that serve to transmit nutrient vessels to the bone. Those situated ventrally and laterally are much smaller than the foramina on the dorsal surface (Fig. 1–4). These *ventrolateral foramina* are the openings for small arteries and veins. Those situated dorsally transmit the basivertebral veins from the interior of the vertebral body, and some small arterial twigs to the body. The vascular supply in and about the vertebral column will be considered in detail later.

Structurally a vertebral body has an inner core of spongy (cancellous) bone containing red marrow, and a thin-shelled outer encasement of compact bone. A sagittally cut section of a vertebra shows the inner cancellous bone arranged in vertically aligned lamellae in order to resist compression (Fig. 1–4).

THE VERTEBRAL ARCH

Dorsal to the vertebral body is the *vertebral arch,* composed of paired pedicles and laminae. The arch supports seven processes.

The *pedicles* (L. *pediculus,* a little foot) are short, stout bars of bone that spring from the upper dorsolateral aspect of the vertebral body (Fig. 1–2 A, B). There is one pedicle on each side of the vertebra. They form the sides of the vertebral foramen. In the articulated spine, the pedicles are the only parts of the vertebrae that are not united by ligaments.

Observe in Figure 1–2 B that the pedicles are notched deeply on their inferior surfaces but only slightly superiorly. These notches are termed the *inferior and superi-*

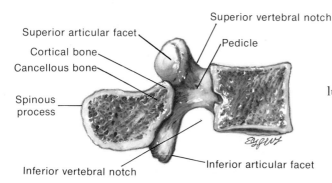

Superior vertebral notch

Superior articular facet

Cortical bone

Cancellous bone

Pedicle

Spinous process

Inferior vertebral notch

Inferior articular facet

Figure 1–4. Median sagittal section of a lumbar vertebra.

or vertebral notches (incisures). In the articulated vertebral column, the vertebral notches together with the intervening vertebral bodies, intervertebral disk, and articular processes form the boundaries of the intervertebral foramina (Fig. 1–1). These foramina serve for transmission of spinal nerves and their accompanying vascular supply.

Laminae (L. *lamina*, a thin plate; having a plate-like form) of the typical vertebra are broad, bony plates. One extends dorsomedially from each pedicle to fuse in the midline dorsally (Fig. 1–2 A, B). The laminae form the dorsal boundary of the vertebral foramen. They are joined together vertically by the ligamenta flava of adjacent articulated vertebrae.

The vertebral arch supports seven *processes* (L. *processus*, a projection). A single *spinous process* arises from the laminal junction (Fig. 1–2 A, B) and is directed dorsally or dorsally and caudally. These bony struts give attachment to the interspinous and supraspinous ligaments and paraspinal muscles.

The *articular processes* arise from the junction of the pedicles and the laminae (Fig. 1–2 A, B). Each side has a superior and inferior articular process. The *superior articular process* projects cranially, with a facet on its dorsal surface. In the case of many typical vertebrae, the *inferior articular process* projects caudally and its facet faces ventrally.

At this point we shall take a moment to generalize about the planes of facet facings in the presacral spine. In the cervical region, facet facings are in the obliquely horizontal plane (Fig. 1–1). In the thoracic region, facets are in the coronal (frontal) plane. In the lumbar region, facet facings are in the sagittal plane, with the lowest ones gradually becoming coronal again.

The *facets of the articular processes* are covered by a thin layer of hyaline cartilage. Between the articulating facets are diarthrodial synovial joints. While these synovial joints are best termed *facet joints*, they are also known as *apophyseal (zygapophyseal) joints* (Fig. 1–1); (G. *zygon*, yoke + apophysis; an offshoot or projection from bone — an articular process). In the German literature they are referred to as "the *small joints* of the spine."

On each side of the vertebra, a *transverse process* extends laterally from the region between the articular processes near the junction point of the lamina and pedicle (Fig. 1–2 A, B). Muscles and ligaments attach to the transverse processes and from the first through the tenth thoracic vertebrae; ribs articulate with them also.

REGIONAL CHARACTERISTICS OF THE VERTEBRAE

The Cervical Vertebrae

The distinguishing feature of the cervical vertebræ is the presence of a *transverse foramen* in each transverse process.

Since the atlas (C-1), axis (C-2), and the seventh cervical vertebra (C-7), have some special morphologic characteristics, they are considered separately.

"Typical" Cervical Vertebrae

The vertebral body is elliptical in shape, being wider from side to side than from front to back. Its ventral and dorsal surfaces are slightly concave, and are usually of equal height (Figs. 1–5 B, 1–6).

In viewing large series of radiographs of the cervical spine, the ventral surface of the sixth cervical vertebra (C-6) will often be decreased in vertical height. This seems to be a variation from the normal. In cases of trauma, this finding should not be mistaken for fracture (Fig. 1–6 A).

The upper surface of the typical cervical vertebra appears slightly convex from front to back and concave transversely owing to the laterally raised lips of the uncinate processes (Figs. 1–5, 1–6). The upper anterior surface is beveled and in the articulated spine overlapped by the protruding rim of the anterior inferior surface of the body above (Fig. 1–6 A). The remainder of the lower surface of the body is reciprocally concave anteroposteriorly and convex transversely. Laterally the lower surface is beveled to accommodate the uncinate processes of the vertebra below (Fig. 1–6 B).

Uncinate processes are not present at birth (Fig. 1–7). These structures grow and assume their full height in the adult (Fig. 1–6 A, B). They are thought to function as guide rails for the vertebral bodies to prevent lateral displacement during movement of the cervical spine. The uncinate processes are half-moon-shaped lips that project cranially from the upper lateral margins of the vertebral bodies of C-3 through C-6 and from the posterolateral upper margin of C-7 and T-1.

Within the substance of the intervertebral disks, between the uncinate processes and the laterally beveled lower surface of the vertebral body above, lie the *uncovertebral (uncinate) "joints" or fissures of Luschka* (Fig. 1–5 *C*). We will examine these so-called "joints" later (p. 74).

The short, stout *pedicles* (Fig. 1–5 *A*) spring from the dorsolateral aspects of the vertebral body, and are directed dorsally and laterally. In a typical cervical vertebra, the pedicles are notched to an equal depth both on superior and inferior surfaces (Fig. 1–5 *B*).

Cervical *laminae* are relatively narrow and thinned cranially (Fig. 1–5 *A*, *B*) but somewhat thicker caudally. When the arti-culated vertebral column is viewed on an oblique radiograph it can be seen that the caudal borders of the laminae slightly over-lap the cranial borders of the laminae below in the manner of tiles on a roof, or *imbrica-tion* (Fig. 1–6 *C*).

The *vertebral foramen* is large and trian-gular rather than oval (Fig. 1–5 *A*).

Spinous processes are short and directed dorsally and caudally. They are usually bifid in Caucasians, but not in Blacks.[2] The divisions of a bifid spinous process may be of unequal size (Fig. 1–5 *A*, *B*).

The superior and inferior articular proc-esses on each side and the bone between them form the rhomboid-shaped *articular pillars* (Fig. 1–5 *B*). These pillars project lat-erally from the junction of the lamina and pedicle. The *articular facets* are oval and flat — the superior facets face upward and dorsally; the inferior downward and ven-trally.

The distinguishing feature of all cervical vertebrae is the presence of a round to oval

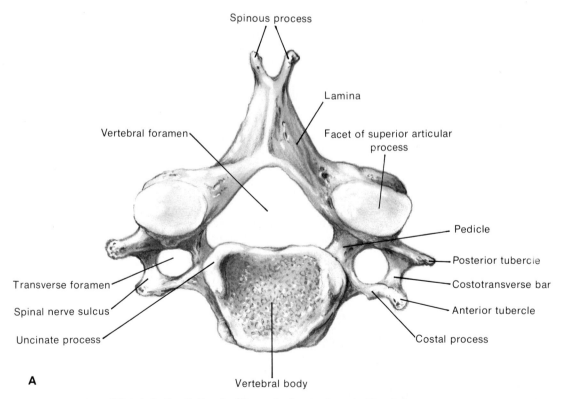

Spinous process

Lamina

Facet of superior articular process

Vertebral foramen

Pedicle

Posterior tubercle

Costotransverse bar

Anterior tubercle

Transverse foramen

Spinal nerve sulcus

Uncinate process

Costal process

Vertebral body

A

Figure 1–5. A "typical" cervical vertebra. A, Cranial aspect.

Illustration and legend continued on the opposite page

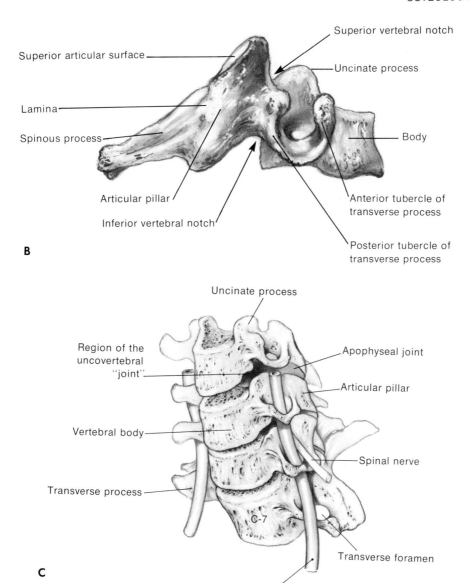

B, Superior articular surface, Superior vertebral notch, Uncinate process, Lamina, Spinous process, Body, Articular pillar, Inferior vertebral notch, Anterior tubercle of transverse process, Posterior tubercle of transverse process

C, Uncinate process, Region of the uncovertebral "joint", Apophyseal joint, Articular pillar, Vertebral body, Transverse process, Spinal nerve, C-7, Transverse foramen, Vertebral artery

Figure 1–5 Continued. B, Lateral view. C, Oblique view of lower four cervical vertebrae.

transverse foramen in each transverse process (Fig. 1–5 A). Although there are many variations, the upper six cervical vertebral transverse foramina usually transmit the vertebral artery and vein and a sympathetic plexus of nerves. In most anatomic specimens, the vertebral artery does not pass through the transverse foramen of the seventh cervical vertebra (Fig. 1–5 C). At times complete or partial division of one or more transverse foramina by a bony bar may be found. This is more frequently true of the

transverse foramen of C-7 than at other levels.

The *transverse process* consists of two roots: posterior and anterior. The *posterior root* springs from the junction of the pedicle and lamina. It is directed laterally and ventrally (Fig. 1–5 A, B). The tip of this posterior root is bulbous and is called the *posterior tubercle.* The *anterior root* of the transverse process is the costal process and it too ends in a tubercle, the *anterior tubercle.*

Text continued on page 13

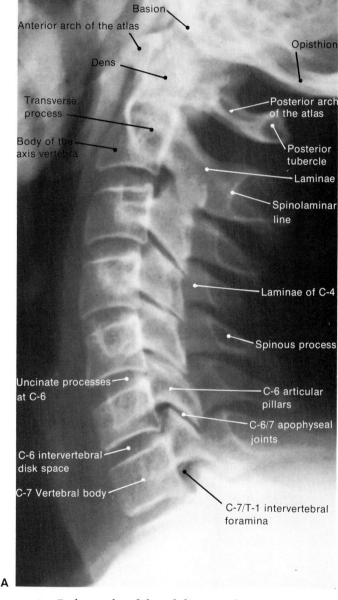

Figure 1–6. Radiographs of the adult cervical spine. *A*, Lateral view.

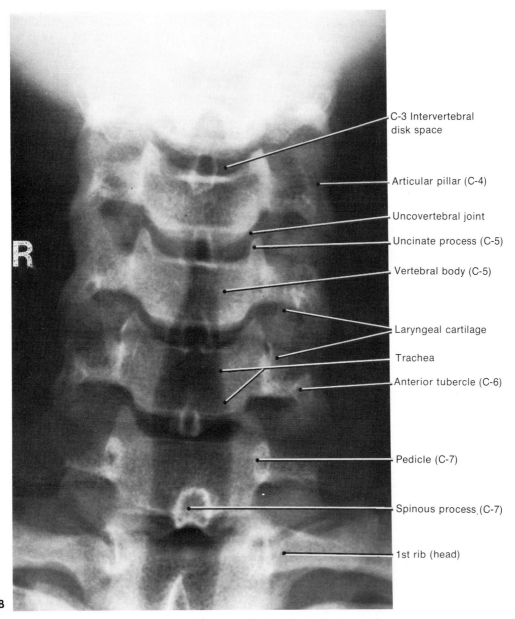

C-3 Intervertebral disk space

Articular pillar (C-4)

Uncovertebral joint

Uncinate process (C-5)

Vertebral body (C-5)

Laryngeal cartilage

Trachea

Anterior tubercle (C-6)

Pedicle (C-7)

Spinous process (C-7)

1st rib (head)

Figure 1–6 Continued. B, Frontal view.
Illustration and legend continued on the following page

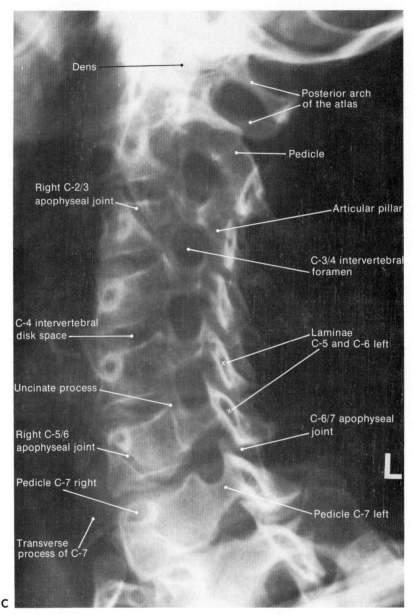

Dens

Posterior arch
of the atlas

Pedicle

Right C-2/3
apophyseal joint

Articular pillar

C-3/4 intervertebral
foramen

C-4 intervertebral
disk space

Laminae
C-5 and C-6 left

Uncinate process

Right C-5/6
apophyseal joint

C-6/7 apophyseal
joint

L

Pedicle C-7 right

Transverse
process of C-7

Pedicle C-7 left

C

Figure 1–6 Continued. C, 45 degree oblique view.

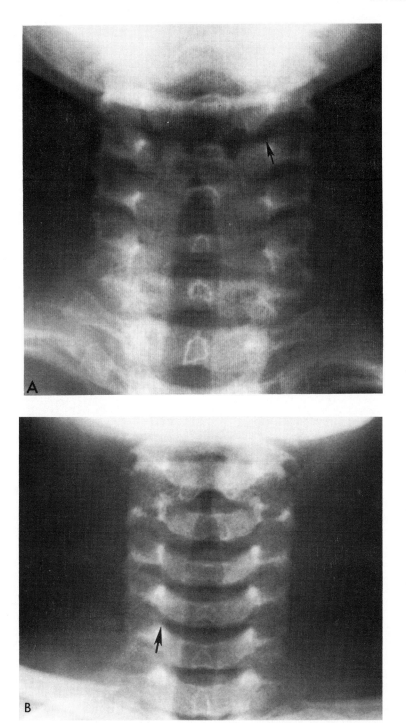

Figure 1-7. Frontal views of the cervical spine. *A*, Two year old. *B*, Five year old. Note that the uncinate processes (arrows) are not present in the two year old child; however, they are developing in the five year old. They are fully developed in the adult (Figure 1-6*B*).

During embryologic development all vertebrae have transverse and costal processes. In the thoracic region, the costal process gives rise to the rib (Fig. 1-8 *A*). In the cervical region, however, the transverse process represents a composite of the embryonic transverse and costal processes. The embryonic transverse process forms

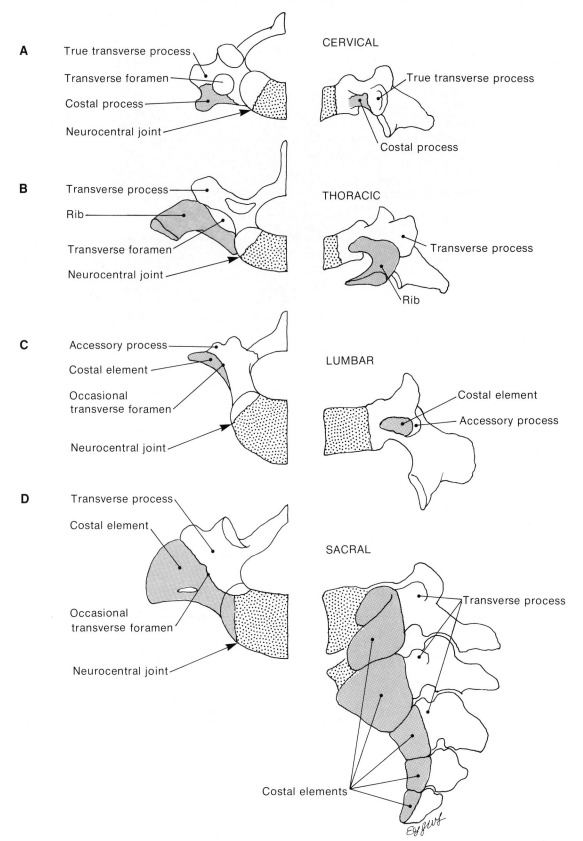

Figure 1-8. Schematic diagram of homologous parts of vertebrae. *A*, Cervical. *B*, Thoracic. *C*, Lumbar. *D*, Sacral. Vertebrae viewed from above on the left; from side on the right. (After Romanes[19]).

only the posterior boundary of the transverse foramen. The embryonic costal process, corresponding to the head and neck of a rib, fuses with the cervical vertebral body. It then forms the anterolateral boundary of the transverse process (Figs. 1–5 A, 1–8 A). However, overdevelopment of the costal process results in *cervical ribs*. In the lumbar region, the embryonic costal process forms the transverse process for the most part, while the embryonic transverse process gives rise to *accessory and mammillary processes* (Fig. 1–8 C). Lumbar ribs result from overdevelopment of the costal process, and usually occur at the level of L-1. The embryonic costal processes of the sacral region fuse with the transverse processes to form the lateral parts of the sacrum (Fig. 1–8 D).

At times, the *costal process of the sixth cervical vertebra* (C-6) is quite large and may be seen on lateral radiographs projecting ventral to the vertebral body (Fig. 5–9). This is an anatomic variation well known to anatomists. The *carotid artery* is situated immediately ventral to the C-6 costal process. The artery may be readily compressed against the enlarged costal process,

which is, therefore, called the *carotid tubercle* (Chassaignac's tubercle).

Situated between the anterior and posterior roots of the transverse process is the *transverse foramen*. The foramen is limited anterolaterally by a curved bar of bone, the *costotransverse bar (lamella)* (Fig. 1–5 A, C). Observe that the bar is deeply grooved on its upper surface; this sulcus is for the ventral ramus of the spinal nerve (Fig. 1–5 C).

Atypical Cervical Vertebrae

FIRST CERVICAL VERTEBRA (ATLAS). The *atlas* (C-1) differs from all other cervical vertebrae. It lacks a body and a spinous process.

For purposes of description, the ring-shaped atlas (Fig. 1–9 A–C) may be divided into five parts. The anterior one fifth is formed by the anterior arch; posteriorly, two fifths are made up by the posterior arch; and the remaining two fifths by the lateral masses.

The anterior arch (Fig. 1–9 A–C) is convex on its ventral surface. Centrally it has a tubercle, the *anterior tubercle,* to which the anterior longitudinal ligament attaches. The

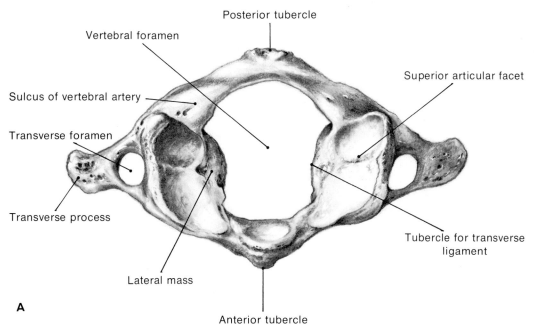

A

Figure 1–9. The first cervical, or atlas, vertebra. A, Cranial aspect.
Illustration and legend continued on the following page

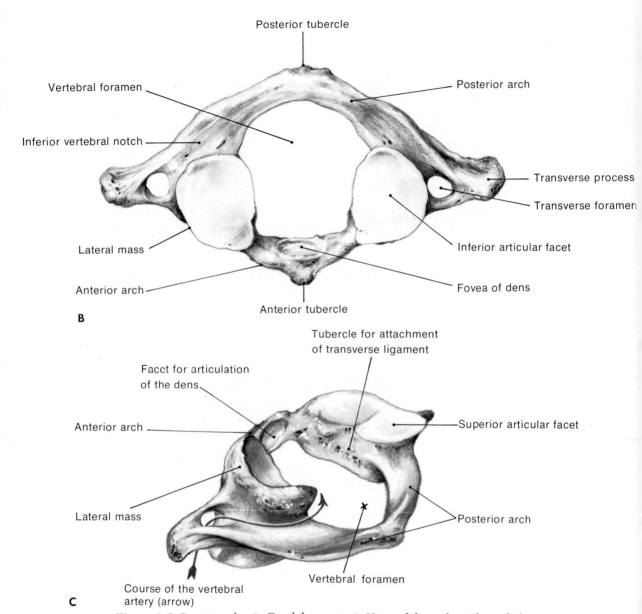

Posterior tubercle

Vertebral foramen

Inferior vertebral notch

Posterior arch

Transverse process

Transverse foramen

Lateral mass

Inferior articular facet

Anterior arch

Fovea of dens

Anterior tubercle

B

Facet for articulation of the dens

Tubercle for attachment of transverse ligament

Anterior arch

Superior articular facet

Lateral mass

Posterior arch

Vertebral foramen

Course of the vertebral artery (arrow)

C

Figure 1–9 Continued. B, Caudal aspect. C, Viewed from the side and above.

posterior surface of the anterior arch is slightly concave. In its midportion there is a smooth, oval to circular facet *(fovea)* for articulation with the dens (odontoid process) of the axis (C-2)

The curved posterior arch (Fig. 1–9 A–C) has a tiny, roughened tubercle, the *posterior tubercle,* instead of a spinous process. The posterior tubercle is usually tipped upward and gives attachment to the nuchal ligament and several muscles. Just behind the superior articular surface of the lateral mass on each side, the posterior arch is grooved on its cranial surface (Fig. 1–9 A, C). This *vertebral artery sulcus* is analogous to the superior vertebral notch of a "typical" cervical vertebra. Crossing this sulcus are the vertebral artery and the first cervical spinal (suboccipital) nerve. In Figure 1–9 C an arrow depicts the course of the vertebral artery. After passing out of the transverse foramen of the atlas, the vertebral artery courses around its lateral mass in a dorsomedial direction and across the sulcus before turning cranially to enter the cranial cavity through the foramen magnum. The first cervical spinal nerve lies between the vertebral artery and the bony sulcus of the vertebral artery (Fig. 1–23 A).

Below the sulcus of the vertebral artery on the caudal surface of the posterior arch and just behind the inferior articular facet of each lateral mass is a shallow groove, the *inferior vertebral notch* (Fig. 1–9 B).

The *lateral masses* of the atlas are quite large; they must bear the weight of the skull (Fig. 1–9 A, C). Each lateral mass carries two articular facets: superior and inferior.

The *superior articular facets* articulate with the occipital condyles. These facets are large, concave, and reniform. They tend to converge on each other anteriorly and diverge posteriorly (Fig. 1–9 A). Each facet faces superiorly, medially, and posteriorly to accommodate the articulating occipital condyles above. Some skeletal specimens may show one or both superior articular facets to be constricted or even completely divided in two by a bony ridge.

In Figure 1–9 B, the atlas is viewed from below to demonstrate *the inferior articular facet* on each lateral mass. These facets are slightly concave, circular and set obliquely so that they face downwards, medially and backwards. They articulate with the superior articular surface of the axis and permit rotation of the head at the atlantoaxial joint.

A small tubercle for the attachment of the strong *transverse ligament of the atlas* projects medially from each lateral mass (Figs. 1–9 A, 1–10 A). This transverse ligament divides the vertebral foramen of the atlas into two uneven compartments: a smaller anterior compartment accommodates the dens of the axis, while the posterior and larger compartment provides protection for the spinal cord and its meninges and blood vessels. Observe the synovial joints (middle atlantoaxial joints) situated anterior and posterior to the dens in the articulated atlas-axis (Fig. 1–10 A).

The strong *transverse processes* of the atlas are the longest in the cervical spine (Fig. 1–9 A–C). They extend laterally from the lateral masses and they are inclined slightly inferiorly. Muscles assisting in rotation of the head attach to these levers. Each transverse process, as with all cervical vertebrae, has a *transverse foramen* that is inclined cranially and dorsally.

SECOND CERVICAL VERTEBRA (AXIS). The *axis* is readily distinguished from all other vertebrae by its toothlike projection from the upper end of the body, the *dens* (Figs. 1–10 A, 1–11 A, B). Just above the junction of the dens with the body of the axis there is a distinct constriction of the dens in the form of a neck. Anteriorly the dens has an oval or circular facet for articulation with the corresponding facet on the innermost surface of the anterior arch of the atlas (Fig. 1–11 B). Posteriorly and posterolaterally, the neck of the dens is grooved by the *transverse ligament of the atlas* (Figs. 1–10 A, 1–11 A). The apex of the dens is pointed, and it is here that the *apical ligament* attaches. Just below the apex of the dens, its sides are flat and roughened for the attachment of the *alar ligaments*. The apical and alar ligaments (Fig. 2–12 A, B) join the dens to the anterior and lateral margins, respectively, of the foramen magnum.

The *pedicles of the axis* are both broad and strong (Fig. 1–11 A). The inferior vertebral notch is quite deep, while the superior vertebral notch is not discernible. Observe that the pedicles are covered in part by the superior articular surfaces (Fig. 1–11 A).

Strong, thick *laminae* — actually the thickest of all the cervical vertebrae — fuse dorsally with a very broad, short, bifid spinous process (Fig. 1–11 A).

Tiny *transverse processes* end in but a single tubercle (Fig. 1–11 A, B). Each transverse process is pierced by a transverse foramen that faces superolaterally (Fig. 1–10 B). Thus the vertebral artery, after passing through the transverse foramen of the axis, must take a more lateral course to reach the more widely separated transverse foramen of the atlas above (Fig. 1–23 A).

Figures 1–11 A, B show the large, oval, slightly convex *superior articular surfaces* of the axis, which are directed inferolaterally. Each extends laterally from the vertebral body and pedicle. There is no superior vertebral notch and, therefore, the second cervical spinal nerve passes dorsal to the superior articular surface over the lateral atlantoaxial joint (Fig. 1–23 A). On each side the superior articular surface overhangs the transverse foramen. The *inferior articular process*, which has an articular facet, is simi-

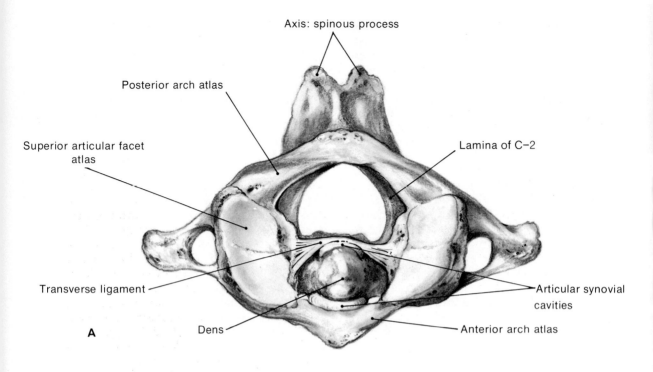

Axis: spinous process

Posterior arch atlas

Superior articular facet atlas

Lamina of C–2

Transverse ligament

Articular synovial cavities

A

Dens

Anterior arch atlas

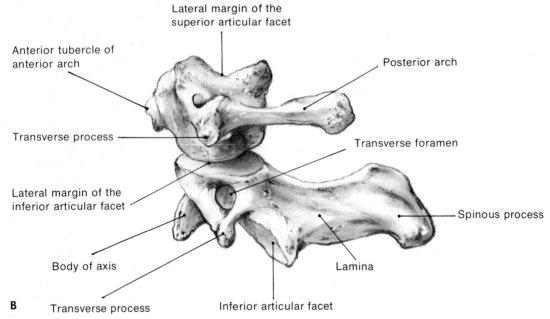

Lateral margin of the superior articular facet

Anterior tubercle of anterior arch

Posterior arch

Transverse process

Transverse foramen

Lateral margin of the inferior articular facet

Spinous process

Body of axis

Lamina

B

Transverse process

Inferior articular facet

Figure 1–10. The articulated first and second cervical vertebrae. *A,* From above showing the transverse ligament of the atlas and the middle atlantoaxial joints (articular synovial cavities). *B,* Lateral view.

lar to that of the "typical" cervical vertebrae. The axis does not have an articular pillar nor a lateral mass.

SEVENTH CERVICAL VERTEBRA. The presence of an elongated, thick, nonbifid, and nearly horizontal *spinous process* is the most distinctive feature of this vertebra. This may be easily palpated at the root of the neck. Therefore C-7 is often referred to as the *vertebra prominens*. The spinous process ends in a bulbous tubercle to which the nuchal ligament attaches (Fig. 1–12).

While its *transverse process* is large, it does not nearly equal that of the atlas in lateral extent (Fig. 1–21 *B, C*). The posterior root of the transverse process is quite prominent and extends as far laterally as the first thoracic transverse process, while the anterior root is quite small or absent (Fig. 1–12 *A*).

At times, the anterior root of the transverse process of C-7 may develop separately to form a *cervical rib*. About 2 per cent of skeletons have cervical ribs, more prevalent

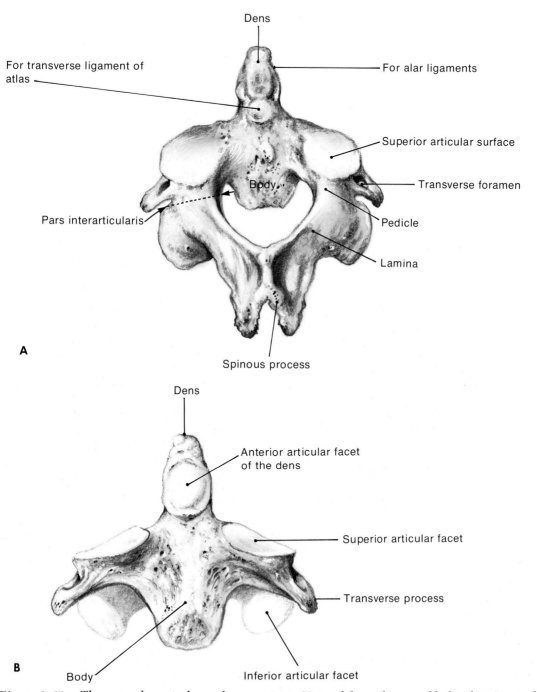

Figure 1–11. The second cervical vertebra or axis. *A*, Viewed from above and behind. *B*, Viewed from in front.

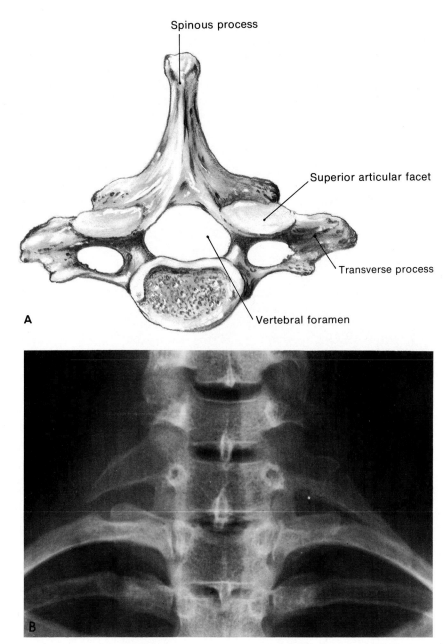

Spinous process

Superior articular facet

Transverse process

Vertebral foramen

A

B

Figure 1–12. *A,* The seventh cervical vertebra, cranial aspect. *B,* Frontal radiograph showing a cervical rib on the left and elongation of the transverse process of C-7 on the right. Note that the elongated transverse process extends more laterally than the transverse process of T-1 below.

on the right than the left[2] — Figure 1–12 *B.* Cervical ribs may be associated clinically with thoracic outlet neurovascular compression syndromes.

If the transverse process of C-7 extends beyond the lateral aspect of the transverse process of T-1, then it is said to be elongated and may have similar clinical consequences to cervical ribs. (Fig. 1–12 *B*).

Anatomic specimens show many variations in the *transverse foramina* of the seventh cervical vertebra. While they may rival the size of foramina in other cervical vertebrae, they are frequently smaller in size. Occasionally they are divided into two compartments by a bony spicule and, infrequently, they are entirely absent.

Occasionally the left vertebral artery

takes passage through the left seventh transverse foramen. More commonly the vertebral veins traverse them bilaterally. Usually the vertebral artery passes ventral to the transverse process rather than through the transverse foramen (Fig. 1–5 C).

The Thoracic Vertebrae

The 12 thoracic vertebrae are readily distinguished from all other vertebrae of the spinal column by their costal facets. They exhibit one pair of costal facets, superior and inferior, on each side of their bodies and another pair of costal facets on their transverse processes, for articulation with the heads and articular tubercles of the ribs respectively (Fig. 1–13 A, B). Usually the last two or three thoracic vertebrae lack facets on their transverse processes (Fig. 1–15).

The second through the eighth thoracic vertebrae (T-2–8) are "typical" of this region; all others are atypical. Each group will be considered separately.

"Typical" Thoracic Vertebrae

These vertebrae have a reniform body with a small waist dorsally (Fig. 1–13 A, B). Their transverse and anteroposterior dimensions are about equal; however, they are slightly taller dorsally than ventrally, resulting in the normal thoracic kyphotic curve. When searching for minimal compression fractures of the thoracic vertebrae it must be borne in mind that the vertical height ventrally is 1.5–2.0 mm less than the vertical height dorsally in the same vertebral body.

All of the vertebral body surfaces are slightly concave. On each side of the vertebral body, ventral to the root of the pedicle,

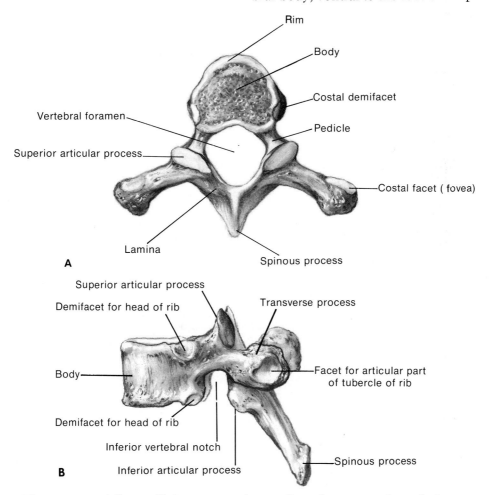

Figure 1–13. A "typical" thoracic vertebra. *A,* Cranial aspect. *B,* Lateral view.

there is a concave *superior costal demifacet* for articulation with a rib head. Lower down on the lateral aspect of the body, ventral to the inferior vertebral notch, is a small *inferior costal demifacet* (Fig. 1–13 *B*) for articulation with the head of the next lower rib.

In the articulated vertebral column, the larger superior costal demifacet together with the intervening intervertebral disk and suprajacent inferior costal demifacet form an oval, concave surface for the articulation of the rib head.

All typical *ribs* (Fig. 1–14) have two facets, cranial and caudal, at their rib heads. The head of any typical rib will articulate with the superior vertebral demifacet of its own numbered vertebra and the inferior vertebral demifacet of the next vertebra above. The articular facet of the neck of any typical rib always articulates with the facet on the transverse process of its own numbered vertebra. Ribs 1, 10, 11, and 12, of course, are exceptions to these rules. This implies that vertebrae T-1 and T-10–12 will be different in respect to vertebral and transverse facets in one or more ways.

Short, thin *pedicles* (Fig. 1–13 *A*, *B*) are directed dorsally and slightly cranially. They spring from the body of the vertebra near its posterosuperior aspect. The inferior vertebral notches are large and quite deep, whereas the superior notches are shallow.

Thick, broad *laminae* slope dorsally and inferiorly to overlap (imbricate) the laminae of the vertebra below (Fig. 1–21 *C*). The vertebral foramen (Fig. 1–13 *A*) is usually small and circular. These foramina enlarge in the first, second, and tenth through twelfth vertebrae because of the cervical and lumbar enlargements of the spinal cord in these regions.

The *spinous processes* (Fig. 1–13 *A*, *B*) of the thoracic vertebrae are long, slender projections that slope caudally and inferiorly to overlap the spine of the vertebra below. Figure 1–21 *A*, *C* shows that there is some variation in the slope of the spinous processes of the thoracic region. Those of T-5 to T-8 are nearly vertical. T-1 and T-2 as well as T-11 and T-12 are almost horizontal in position. The spinous processes of T-3,4,9, and 10 are directed inferiorly.

At the junction of the pedicle and lamina on each side, the thin *superior articular process* projects cranially (Fig. 1–13 *A*, *B*). These have flattened articular facets that face posterolaterally and slightly cranially. Similarly there are *inferior articular processes* that project caudally from the laminae. Their facets face ventromedially and caudally.

A *transverse process* on each side emerges between the articular processes. These long, stout, club-shaped levers are directed dorsolaterally and slightly cranially (Fig. 1–13 *A*, *B*). Transverse processes decrease in length from the level of T-1 to T-12 (Fig. 1–21 *B*, *C*). On the ventral surface of the transverse processes of the first ten thoracic vertebrae, there are oval, concave costal facets that articulate with facets on the articular tubercles of their numerically corresponding ribs.

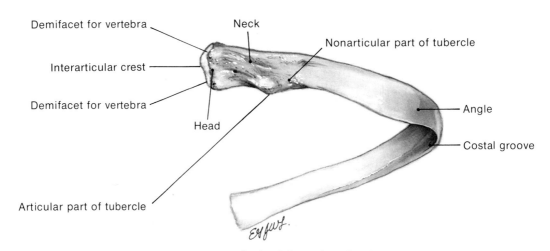

Demifacet for vertebra

Neck

Nonarticular part of tubercle

Interarticular crest

Demifacet for vertebra

Angle

Head

Costal groove

Articular part of tubercle

Figure 1–14.   A central rib of the right side, dorsal aspect.

Atypical Thoracic Vertebrae

FIRST THORACIC VERTEBRA (Fig. 1–15). The vertebral body is similar in shape to those of the cervical spine. On the dorsolateral upper surface of the body on each side are semilunar lips, the uncinate processes (Fig. 1–15). Uncinate processes are absent on other thoracic vertebrae.

The entire head of the first rib articulates in a full concave superior costal facet located laterally on the sides of the vertebral body at its dorsal superior aspect. The cranial demifacet of the head of the second rib articulates in the smaller, semilunar-shaped, inferior costal demifacet located on the posterior inferior portion of the body on each side. The first thoracic vertebra also has some other special features. These include a much elongated, thickened spinous process that is nearly horizontal in direction and rivals the spinous process of C-7 in prominence. It also has the deepest inferior vertebral notch of the entire thoracic region.

NINTH THORACIC VERTEBRA (Fig. 1–15). This vertebra usually has only a single superior costal demifacet on each side of its body for articulation with the caudal demifacet of the head of the ninth rib. Otherwise it shows all of the features of a typical thoracic vertebra.

Some anatomic specimens may have a small inferior costal facet for the cranial demifacet for the tenth rib. If this is the case, then it is usual to have a small superior costal demifacet on the tenth thoracic vertebra.

TENTH THORACIC VERTEBRA (Fig. 1–15). This vertebra usually has a single large costal facet for the articulation of the head of the tenth rib on each side. This costal facet is located on the posterolateral upper aspect of the body and may encroach upon the pedicle. It affords a relatively accurate point of reference for localization of vertebral levels in suspected transitional states.

At times, the transverse process does not have a facet for articulation with the articular tubercle of the tenth rib.

ELEVENTH THORACIC VERTEBRA (Fig. 1–15). The short transverse processes of this vertebra lack facets for rib articulation.

Costal facets for the eleventh rib heads, which have only a single facet, are large

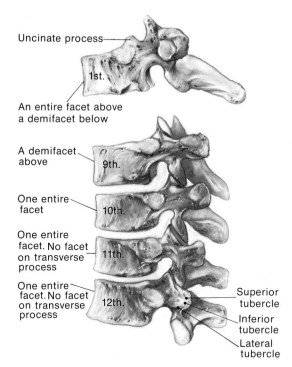

Figure 1–15. "Atypical" thoracic vertebrae.

circular concavities located mainly on the pedicles.

This vertebra resembles a lumbar vertebra in many respects, particularly in the shape of its body. The spinous process is short and almost horizontal in direction.

TWELFTH THORACIC VERTEBRA (Fig. 1–15). While this vertebra closely resembles T-11, it may be distinguished by the appearance of the inferior articular processes. These processes face laterally in order to articulate with the facets of the superior articular process of L-1, which are oriented in the sagittal plane rather than in the coronal plane.

Three tubercles replace the transverse process on each side of the vertebra. These are the cranially directed superior tubercle and the caudally directed inferior tubercle which are analogous to the mammillary and accessory processes of lumbar vertebrae (Fig. 1–16), and the lateral tubercle corresponding to the true transverse process. Careful examination of the skeleton may reveal similar traces of these tubercles on the tenth and eleventh thoracic vertebrae. However, it should be pointed out that there is great variation in respect to these

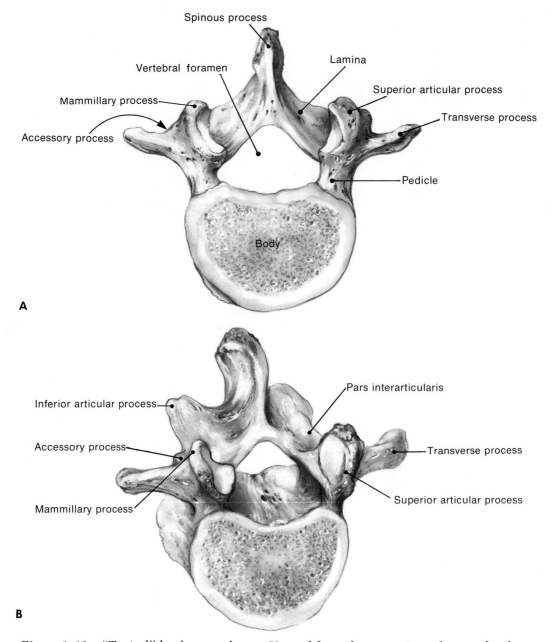

Spinous process

Vertebral foramen

Lamina

Mammillary process

Superior articular process

Accessory process

Transverse process

Pedicle

Body

A

Pars interarticularis

Inferior articular process

Accessory process

Transverse process

Mammillary process

Superior articular process

B

Figure 1–16. "Typical" lumbar vertebra. *A*, Viewed from above. *B*, From above and in front.

tubercles and they are often difficult to find. Indeed, the mammillary and, especially, the accessory tubercles are not always easy to observe on lumbar vertebrae. This is probably related to the strength and traction pull of the muscles attaching to them. The mammillary process gives origin to some fibers of the multifides muscles, and the accessory tubercle to a slip of the longissimus thoracis, the upward extension of the sacrospinalis (erector spinae) muscle complex.

The Lumbar Vertebrae

General Considerations

The largest and heaviest segments of the presacral part of the vertebral column are the lumbar vertebrae. As with the other regional vertebrae that we have thus far considered, lumbar vertebrae are readily distinguished from the others in the spinal column. The lumbar vertebrae lack costal facets on their bodies and they do not have transverse foramina in their transverse processes, but they do have large, thick rectangular spinous processes and thin transverse processes.

A lumbar vertebral body is large and kidney-shaped, with the shallow dorsal concavity facing the triangular vertebral foramen (Fig. 1–16 A). Viewed from above, we can see that the body is narrower from front to back than transversely. All of its surfaces are concave. The first and second lumbar vertebral bodies are taller dorsally than ventrally, but the reverse is true of the fourth and fifth lumbar vertebrae. The third lumbar body is variable and may simulate vertebral bodies above or below in height.

The *pedicles* are short, stout bars arising from the upper lateral margins of the vertebral body on each side (Fig. 1–16 A). The superior vertebral notches are noticeably shallower than the inferior notches.

While the lumbar vertebral *laminae* are large, sturdy structures, they are ofttimes asymmetric. They are not very broad and, therefore, between adjacent lumbar vertebrae, there is a convenient diamond-shaped space through which lumbar puncture may be performed (Fig. 1–21 C). That portion of the lamina situated between the superior and inferior articular processes on each side is known as the pars interarticularis, or isthmus (Fig. 1–16 B). This is the site of cleft formation in spondylolysis (spondyloschisis), to be considered later.

The *vertebral foramina* are triangular in shape and larger than those in the thoracic region but smaller than the foramina in the cervical vertebrae. Extending dorsally from the junction of the laminae is the thick, broad, rectangular (or rhomboid) spinous process. It is directed horizontally and ends in an uneven and frequently notched posterior border.

At the junction of the pedicle and lamina on each side, the superior and inferior *articular processes* arise (Fig. 1–16 A, B). The articular surfaces of the superior articular processes are slightly concave, and these face dorsally and medially. As one would expect, the articular surfaces of the inferior articular processes are convex; they face ventrally and laterally (Fig. 1–16 A, B). Observe in Figure 1–17 A that the superior articular processes are set wider apart as a rule than are the inferior articular processes,

since they must embrace the latter from without.

A noticeable hummock, the *mammillary process* (Fig. 1–16 A, B), protrudes from the dorsolateral tip of each superior articular process to afford attachment to certain slips of the postvertebral muscles. Recall that it corresponds to the superior tubercle of T-12.

Transverse processes are long, thin, and flattened anteroposteriorly. On the upper three lumbar vertebrae, they arise from the junction of the laminae and pedicles. On the last two lumbar vertebrae, they are situated more ventrally and spring from the junction point of the pedicles and body. The transverse processes of the upper three lumbar vertebrae are usually directed laterally; those of the last two lumbar vertebrae project laterally and cranially. By far the longest transverse processes are those of L-3. These processes decrease in length on the vertebrae above and below (Fig. 1–21 A, C).

Dorsally, at the base of the transverse process, there is a small rough tubercle, the *accessory process,* which is also for muscle attachment. If the accessory process exceeds 5 mm in length, then it is termed the *styloid process.*[3] On radiographs (Fig. 1–17 B), the styloid process points dorsally, laterally, and inferiorly.

FIFTH LUMBAR VERTEBRA. This is the largest of the presacral vertebra. It is wedge-shaped and noticeably taller ventrally than dorsally (Fig. 1–17 C). This shape contributes to the prominence of the lumbosacral angle (which will be discussed later) and to the normal lumbar lordotic curve.

The transverse processes are thick and of a conical shape. They arise from the junction of the body and pedicle. The spinous process is the smallest of any in the lumbar region. The articular surfaces (facets) of the inferior articular processes are often flattened, asymmetric, and usually face ventrally. From L-3 down, there is a gradual trend for articular facets to move from a typical lumbar sagittal orientation to the coronal, or frontal, plane, most prominently displayed at L-5.

The Sacrum

The five sacral vertebrae fuse in the adult to form this wedge-shaped bone that is lo-

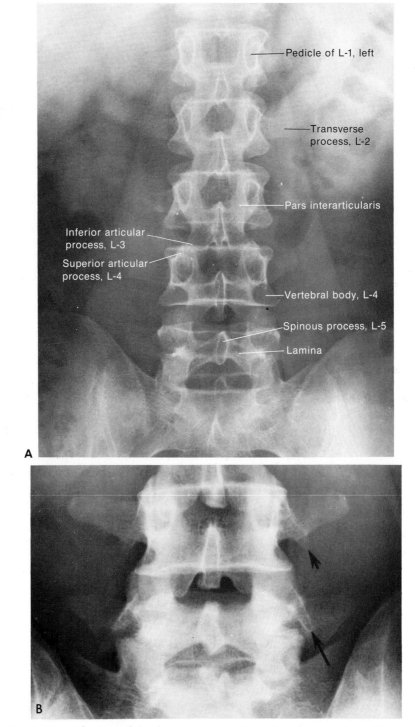

Pedicle of L-1, left

Transverse process, L-2

Pars interarticularis

Inferior articular process, L-3

Superior articular process, L-4

Vertebral body, L-4

Spinous process, L-5

Lamina

A

B

Figure 1–17. A, Frontal view of the lumbar spine. Note that the superior articular processes are set wider apart as a rule than the inferior articular processes. *B*, Styloid processes (arrows) in the lower lumbar spine. *C*, Lateral radiograph of the lumbosacral junction and sacrum. The fifth lumbar vertebra is wedge-shaped and noticeably taller ventrally then dorsally.

See illustration on the opposite page

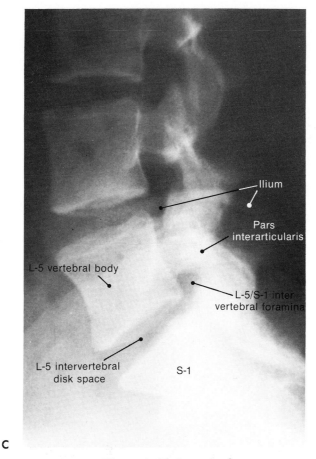

Ilium

Pars
interarticularis

L-5 vertebral body

L-5/S-1 inter
vertebral foramina

L-5 intervertebral
disk space

S-1

C

Figure 1–17 Continued.

cated between the *ossa coxae* (innominate; hip bones). The sacrum articulates with the ilia laterally, its base articulates with the last lumbar vertebra, and its apex with the coccyx.

The pelvic surface of the sacrum (Fig. 1–18 A) is concave and it faces downward and forward. Crossing its median part are four raised transverse ridges corresponding to the position of the intervertebral disks that separated the original five vertebral bodies. A sagittal section of the sacrum clearly shows these disk remnants (Fig. 1–18 D); they are also well demonstrated on lateral radiographs (Fig. 1–18 F). The smooth bone situated between the transverse ridges represents the bodies of the sacral vertebrae. The first sacral segment has many characteristics of a lumbar vertebra. It is the largest of the five sacral segments, each subsequent one gradually diminishing in size.

Aligned vertically on each side of the four raised transverse ridges on the pelvic surface of the sacrum are the *pelvic (anterior) sacral foramina* (Fig. 1–18 A). These foramina decrease in size from the cranial to the caudal end of the sacrum. They communicate with the sacral canal through intervertebral foramina. The costal elements, transverse processes, and the vertebral bodies fuse together to the lateral mass (pars lateralis, ala) of the sacrum, which lies lateral to the pelvic sacral foramina. *Only the atlas (C-1) and the sacrum have lateral masses.* Extending laterally to each side from the pelvic sacral foramina are broad, smooth grooves for the ventral divisions of the first four sacral spinal nerves that exit through the pelvic sacral foramina.

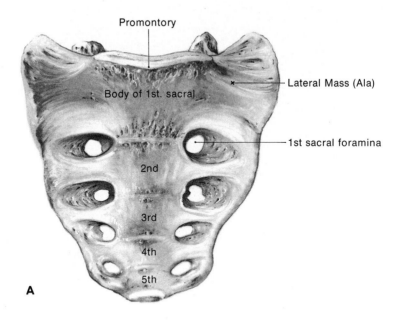

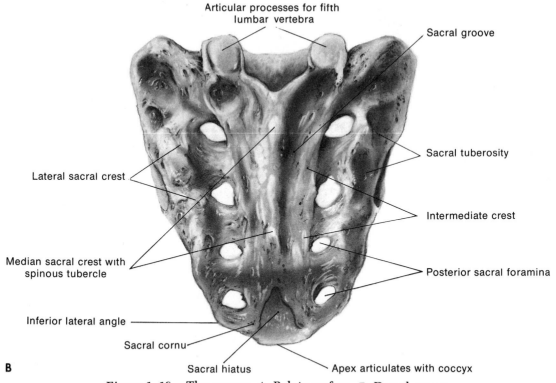

Figure 1–18. The sacrum. *A*, Pelvic surface. *B*, Dorsal aspect.

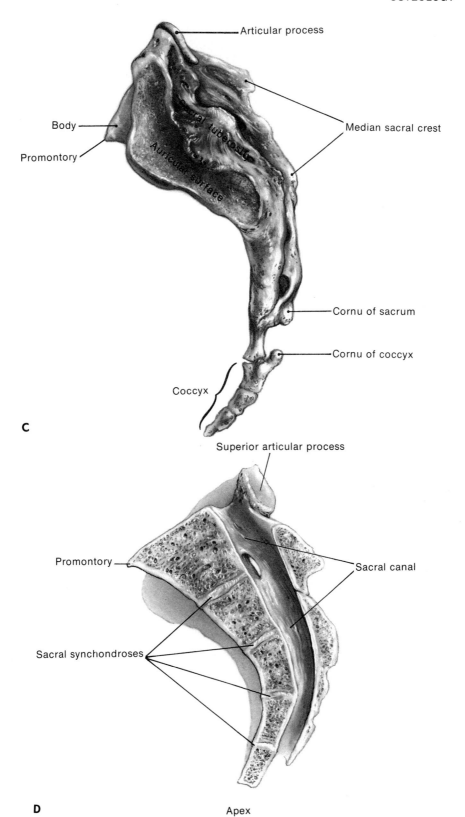

Articular process

Body

Promontory

Median sacral crest

Auricular surface

Cornu of sacrum

Cornu of coccyx

Coccyx

C

Superior articular process

Promontory

Sacral canal

Sacral synchondroses

D   Apex

Figure 1–18 Continued.   C, Lateral surfaces. D, Median sagittal section.
Illustration and legend continued on the following page

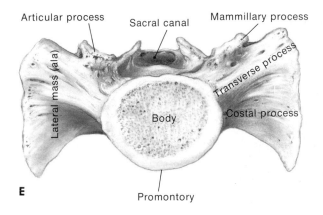

Articular process   Sacral canal   Mammillary process

Lateral mass (ala)

Transverse process

Body   Costal process

E

Promontory

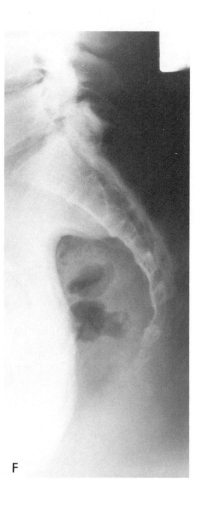

F

Figure 1–18 Continued.   E, Cranial aspect of the base. *F*, Lateral radiograph showing disk remnants between sacral segments; compare with *D*.

The dorsal surface (Fig. 1–18 *B*) is convex backward and upward. It is roughened and distinctly narrower than the pelvic surface of the sacrum. In the midline, there is a *median sacral crest* that is extremely variable in prominence. The crest bears three or four spinous tubercles, and it represents the fused spinous processes of the upper three or four sacral vertebrae. The upper spinous tubercle is the largest. The next two may be separate or fused and the fourth is frequently rudimentary. On either side of the median sacral crest is a shallow sacral groove formed by the fused laminae of the sacral vertebrae (Fig. 1–18 *B*). Since the laminae of the fifth sacral vertebra do not fuse dorsally in the midline, an inverted V-shaped defect, the *sacral hiatus,* is left, which opens into the terminal portion of the sacral canal. It is common to see the sacral hiatus extending more cranially than described here.

Lateral to each sacral groove and aligned vertically below the superior articular process of the first sacral segment is an indistinct series of tubercles, the *intermediate (articular) crest* (Fig. 1–18 *B*), formed by the fusion of the articular processes. While the superior articular processes of the first sacral vertebra are large and not unlike those of lumbar vertebrae, the inferior articular processes of the last sacral vertebra are reduced to small tubercles located on either side of the sacral hiatus and projecting caudally as the sacral cornua. These cornua articulate with the coccygeal cornua and are connected by the intercornual ligaments.

Lateral to each intermediate (articular) crest lie the four *dorsal (posterior) sacral foramina* (Fig. 1–18 *B*). These are much smaller in size and not as regularly formed as the anterior pelvic sacral foramina. Like the pelvic sacral foramina, these dorsal sacral foramina communicate with the sacral canal through intervertebral foramina. The dorsal sacral foramina transmit the small posterior rami of the sacral nerves as well as tiny blood vessels. The fused transverse processes of the sacral vertebra are seen in Fig. 1–18 B as yet another series of indistinct tubercles (transverse tubercles) forming the lateral sacral crest located just lateral to the dorsal sacral foramina.

When the sacrum is viewed from the side (Fig. 1–18 C), the lateral mass presents at its upper aspect a large, irregular, ear-shaped *auricular surface*. The auricular surface is covered by fibrocartilage in life, and forms a synovial articulation with the ilium. The articular surface of the ilium is chiefly covered by hyaline cartilage. Dorsally on each lateral mass and lateral to the lateral sacral crest is a roughened, raised area, the sacral tuberosity, which serves as partial attachment for the posterior sacroiliac ligament. The remaining lateral surface of the sacrum caudally is thin and ends below the last sacral foramen as a projection, the inferior lateral angle. Caudal to each sacral cornu is a notch that is converted to a foramen for the dorsal ramus of the fifth sacral spinal nerve when the coccyx is articulated with the sacrum and bridged by an intercornual ligament.

The middle of the base of the sacrum, displayed from above in Figure 1–18 E, shows the large body of the first sacral vertebra with its imposing ventral border, the *sacral promontory*. The promontory marks the third and shortest part of a curved line (the other portions consisting of the long arcuate line of the iliac fossa and the pubic pecten of the superior pubic ramus), which separates the true from the false pelvis. This curved line between true and false pelvis is designated the *terminal line* (often misdesignated as the "arcuate line"). The arcuate (or white) line does not involve the sacrum and is a fascial thickening over the obturator internus muscle for origin of the levator ani.

Dorsal to the body, the triangular *sacral canal* is usually roofed over by the laminae and the midline median sacral crest. About 12 per cent of anatomic specimens will be defective dorsally (Fig. 1–18 E) — a so-called *spina bifida occulta*.

On either side are the large dorsomedially directed *superior articular processes*. The facets of these articular processes usually lie in a near coronal plane, although asymmetry is quite common. The superior articular processes of the first sacral vertebra articulate with the inferior articular processes of the last lumbar vertebra. They are attached to the lateral masses and to the body of S-1 by stout, short pedicles. These pedicles are notched superiorly and form the caudal part of the intervertebral foramen between the last lumbar and first sacral vertebrae.

Each superior articular process bears a prominent mammillary process laterally (Fig. 1–18 E). At the caudal extremity of the sacrum is the *apex* (Fig. 1–18 D), an oval facet for articulation with the coccyx. An intervertebral disk usually separates the apex of the sacrum from the coccyx; however, this may completely ossify to fuse the first coccygeal segment to the distal sacrum.

The vertebral foramina of the sacral vertebrae make up the *sacral canal* (Fig. 1–18 D), which is open caudally at the sacral hiatus. The lateral wall of the sacral canal contains four intervertebral foramina permitting communication with the pelvic and dorsal sacral foramina.

Contained within the sacral canal are the cauda equina, spinal meninges, and the external portion of the filum terminale. The external filum exits through the sacral hiatus across the last sacral segment and the sacrococcygeal articulation, and attaches caudally on the coccyx.

The Coccyx

This wedge-shaped bone has a base, apex, pelvic and dorsal surfaces, and two lateral borders similar to the sacrum (Fig. 1–19 A, B). It is usually formed by four rudimentary vertebrae, although this number may vary from three to five.

The first three segments have diminutive bodies, articular and transverse processes, but they are devoid of pedicles, laminae and spinous processes. The first coccygeal segment is not only the largest but also the broadest. Its transverse processes are joined to the sacrum by ligaments that frequently ossify, thereby completing a bony foramen for the transmission of the ventral division of the fifth sacral nerve. The last three coccygeal segments are small and often fused. The base of the coccyx articulates with the apex of the sacrum by means of a small intervertebral disk.

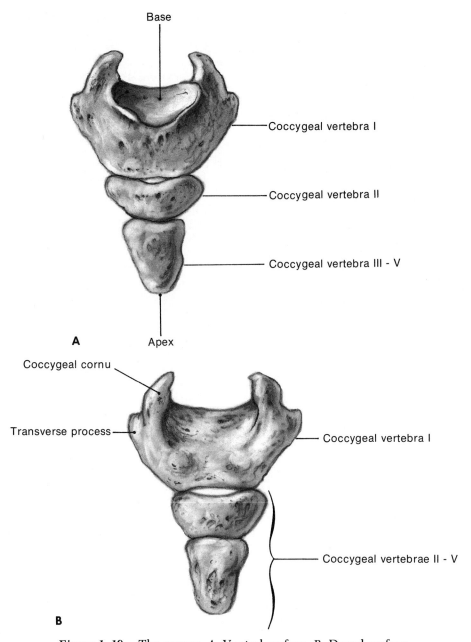

Base

Coccygeal vertebra I

Coccygeal vertebra II

Coccygeal vertebra III - V

A

Apex

Coccygeal cornu

Transverse process

Coccygeal vertebra I

Coccygeal vertebrae II - V

B

Figure 1–19. The coccyx. *A*, Ventral surface. *B*, Dorsal surface.

On the dorsal surface (Fig. 1–19 *B*), the rudimentary articular processes form a series of tubercles that are not always distinct on the lower coccygeal segments. These tubercles are largest on the first segment and are termed the coccygeal cornua. Coccygeal cornua articulate with the sacral cornua, which together provide a foramen for the transmission of the dorsal division of the fifth sacral nerve. Figure 1–19 *A* shows the pelvic surface of the coccyx and the transverse grooves marking the junctions of the segments.

THE ARTICULATED VERTEBRAL COLUMN

Now that we have examined the morphologic characteristics of the regional vertebrae, let us examine the articulated vertebral column. This will permit us to review the highlights of each region and to compare these features with the spine assembled as a structural unit (Figs. 1–6, 1–20, 1–21).

Numerical Variations in the Vertebral Column

About one-third of human vertebral columns show some variation from the "norm."

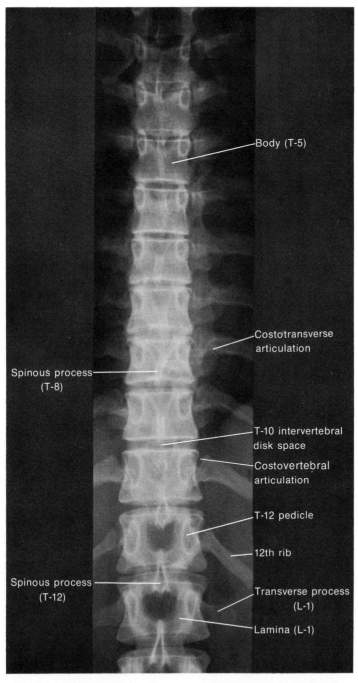

A

Figure 1–20. Normal roentgenograph of the articulated vertebral column. *A,* Thoracic vertebral column, frontal view.

Illustration and legend continued on the following page

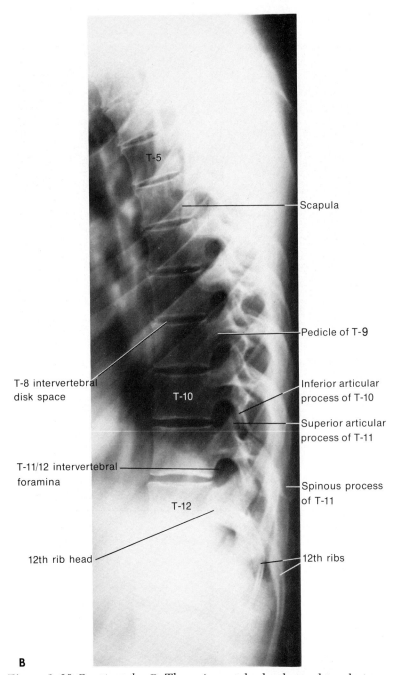

B

Figure 1–20 *Continued.* B, Thoracic vertebral column, lateral view.

Illustration and legend continued on the following page

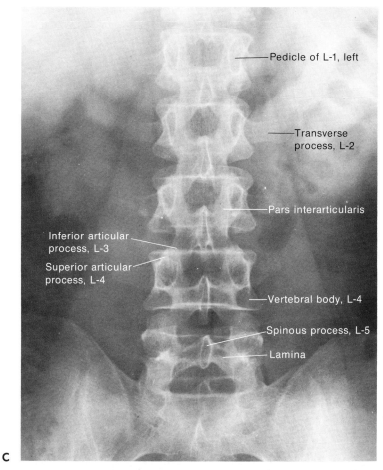

Pedicle of L-1, left

Transverse process, L-2

Pars interarticularis

Inferior articular process, L-3

Superior articular process, L-4

Vertebral body, L-4

Spinous process, L-5

Lamina

C

Figure 1–20 Continued. C, Frontal view of the lumbar region.

Illustration and legend continued on the following page

This may be reflected in an increase or decrease in the total number of vertebrae (32 or 34 rather than the "normal" 33) or a shift in the number of vertebrae in a particular region of the column. The latter change is more common than the former.[4]

Curvatures

The adult vertebral column in the male measures about 70 cm in length. The female column is 60 cm long. Of this total length, three-fourths is made up by the vertebral bodies and the remaining one-fourth by the 23 intervening intervertebral disks.

Viewed laterally, the adult vertebral column has four ventrodorsal curves: cervical, thoracic, lumbar, and pelvic (Fig. 1–22 D).

Early in fetal life, the vertebral column is uniformly curved ventrally (Fig. 1–22 A). By the third or fourth fetal month, the pelvic (sacrococcygeal) curvature appears as the body accommodates the pelvic viscera (Fig. 1–22 B). The thoracic concavity is retained after birth (Fig. 1–22 C). The two ventrally concave curves formed in utero, the thoracic and pelvic, are therefore referred to as the *primary curvatures* of the vertebral column (kyphoses).

The cervical and lumbar curvatures are secondary or compensatory, and they are convex ventrally (lordoses) (Fig. 1–22 D). While the cervical curve begins quite late in intrauterine life, it does not fully develop until the third or fourth postnatal month, when the infant holds his head erect and begins to support it. The lumbar curve is acquired at 12 to 18 months of age, as the infant begins to walk and assume an upright posture.

Vertebral Bodies

Vertebral bodies in the thoracic region and in most of the sacral region are taller dorsally than ventrally (Fig. 1–21 A). Since these regions have the least range of motion between their vertebrae, the intervertebral disks are the thinnest. In the adult, the disks between sacral vertebrae have ossified and fused to form the composite sacrum. The most mobile portions of the vertebral column, the cervical and lumbar regions, have the thickest intervertebral disks. These disks are wedge-shaped and are taller ventrally than dorsally.

Intervertebral disks are numbered by the vertebra above; for example, the seventh thoracic disk lies below the T-7 vertebral body.

Since the cervical vertebrae are of equal height front and back, the disks contribute to the curvature of the region. In the lumbar region, the vertebral bodies are not of uniform height. The first and second lumbar bodies, like those of the thoracic region, are slightly taller dorsally than ventrally; the third lumbar vertebral body is variable; while the fourth and fifth vertebral bodies are typically deeper ventrally (Fig. 1–21 A). Thus, both the vertebral bodies and the intervertebral disks contribute to the curvature of the lumbar spine.

In the articulated vertebral column (Fig. 1–21 A), the vertical height of the vertebral

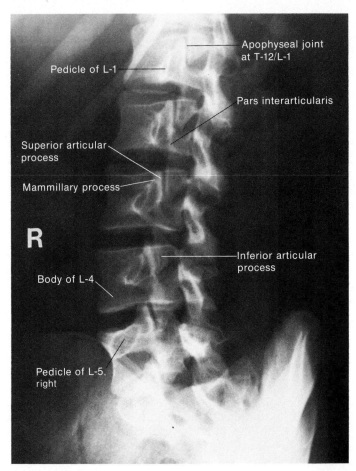

Figure 1–20 Continued. D, 45 Degree oblique view of the lumbar region.

Illustration and legend continued on the following page

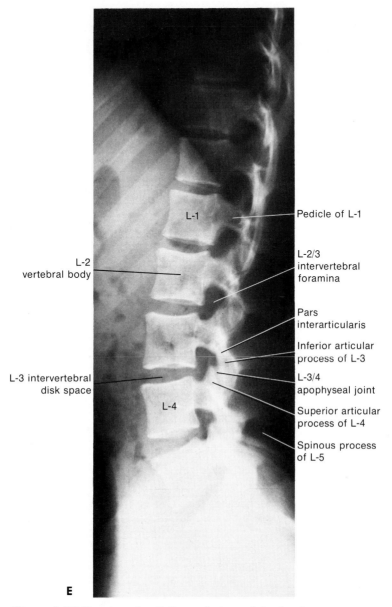

L-1

L-2
vertebral body

L-3 intervertebral
disk space

L-4

Pedicle of L-1

L-2/3
intervertebral
foramina

Pars
interarticularis

Inferior articular
process of L-3

L-3/4
apophyseal joint

Superior articular
process of L-4

Spinous process
of L-5

E

Figure 1-20 Continued. E, Lateral view of the lumbar region.

Illustration and legend continued on the following page

bodies increases progressively from the lower cervical region to the level of the fifth lumbar vertebra.

In the frontal view (Fig. 1–21 B), the column appears to be made up of four pyramids:[5] cervical, upper thoracic, thoracolumbar, and sacrococcygeal. The upper pyramid has its apex at the tip of the dens and vertebral body width progressively increases from the axis (C-2) to the cervico-thoracic junction, or the C-7 disk. At this point, the base of the cervical pyramid meets the base of the upper thoracic pyramid. The apices of the upper thoracic and thoracolumbar pyramid meet at the T-4 disk space. The diminished width of the upper four thoracic vertebrae is attributed to shifting of the weight of the upper limbs to the thoracic cage and subsequently to the lower thoracic region. The lower two pyramids

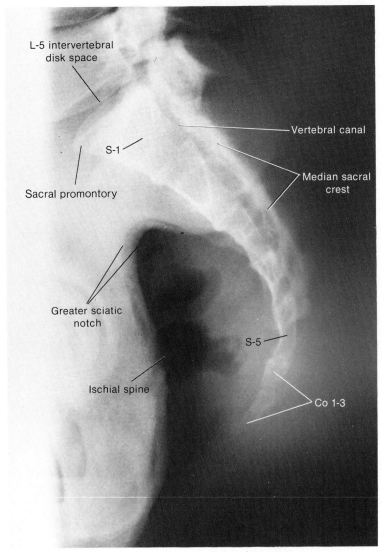

Figure 1–20 *Continued.* *F*, Lateral view of the sacrum and coccyx. (See Figure 1–6 for the cervical vertebral column.)

meet at the lumbosacral junction. The shift of body weight at this site to the pelvis and lower limbs results in the diminished width of the sacrum and coccyx.

Apophyseal (Zygapophyseal) Joints

The vertebral arch articulations are diarthrotic synovial joints, referred to as apophyseal, zygapophyseal, or facet joints. Their articular surfaces are covered in hyaline cartilage. They are surrounded by a loose articular capsule having a synovial lining and a synovial disk, or meniscus.

Viewed laterally, the apophyseal joints in the cervical region are inclined obliquely downward from ventral to dorsal aspect of the spine (Fig. 1–21 A). They are also tipped laterally (Fig. 1–6) just enough to prevent clear visualization on lateral radiographs (Fig. 1–6 A).

The apophyseal joints of typical thoracic vertebrae are oriented in the coronal (frontal) plane. Viewed in Figures 1–21 A, C, the thoracic apophyseal joints are inclined laterally as in the arc of a circle whose center is situated within the vertebral body.

In the upper lumbar spine, the apophyseal joints are oriented in a sagittal plane,

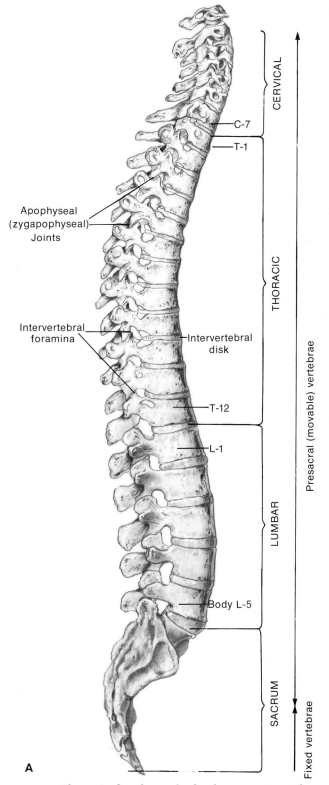

Figure 1–21. The articulated vertebral column. A, Lateral aspect.

Illustration and legend continued on following page

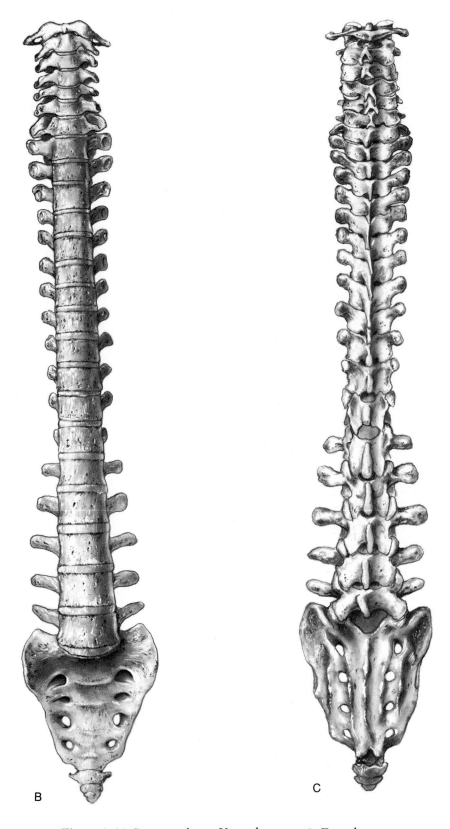

Figure 1–21 *Continued.* *B*, Ventral aspect. *C*, Dorsal aspect.

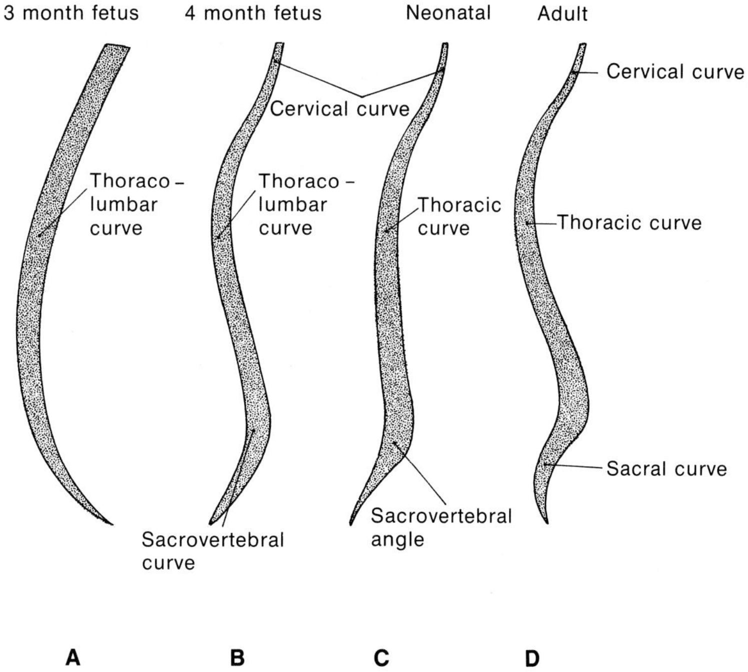

3 month fetus   4 month fetus   Neonatal   Adult

Figure 1-22. Evolution of the spinal curvatures. *A*, Three month fetus with C-shaped curve. *B*, Four month fetus. *C*, Neonate. *D*, Adult with normal cervical lordosis, thoracic kyphosis, and lumbar lordosis.

while the lower ones gradually tend to the coronal plane (Fig. 1–20 *C*; 1–21 *A*, *C*).

Intervertebral Foramina

Cervical intervertebral foramina are bounded by the pedicles above and below, posterolaterally by the articular processes, and anteromedially by the intervertebral disk (Fig. 1–21 *A*). Observe the relation of the uncovertebral "joints" or fissures to the intervertebral foramina in Figure 1–5 *C*.

There are eight pairs of cervical nerves, seven cervical vertebrae, but only six pairs of cervical intervertebral foramina. The presence of eight cervical nerves and only seven vertebrae is due to a rearrangement of somites during embryologic development (see p. 52).

There are no intervertebral foramina between the skull and atlas nor between the atlas and axis. The first cervical spinal nerve exits from the vertebral canal between the skull base and atlas, on the cranial surface of the posterior arch of the atlas in the sulcus of the vertebral artery (Fig. 1–23 *A*).

The second cervical spinal nerve leaves the vertebral canal between the posterior arch of the atlas and the pedicle of the axis. It crosses the dorsal aspect of the lateral atlantoaxial joint, ventral to the ligamenta flava (Fig. 1–23 *A*).

The next succeeding five cervical spinal nerves exit the vertebral canal through intervertebral foramina above the level of their corresponding vertebral foramina; for example, the fifth cervical nerve exits above C-5. The eighth cervical spinal nerve, however, exits between C-7 and T-1. Therefore all other spinal nerves will exit from the vertebral canal below the level of their respective vertebral bodies; for example, the fifth thoracic nerve exits below T-5 vertebra (Fig. 1–23 *A*, *C*).

The oval intervertebral foramina in the cervical region increase in size progressively from C-2/C-3 caudally. These short "canals" are directed anterolaterally and inferiorly.

Spinal nerves in the cervical intervertebral foramina largely fill their anteroposterior diameter. Therefore any pathologic process that narrows this AP width of the foramen, such as osteophytes about the apophyseal joints or the uncovertebral "joint" region, posterolateral protrusion or herniation of an intervertebral disk, or tissue edema, will compromise the spinal nerve at that level. A decrease in vertical height of an intervertebral foramen, however, usually does not affect the nerve.

In view of these facts, how does a posterolateral protrusion or herniation of the C-6 disk affect the C-7 cervical spinal nerve? Recall that the disks are numbered by the vertebra above them — thus the C-6 disk lies below the C-6 vertebral body. Cervical nerves, however, are numbered according to the vertebra *above* which each lies —the C-7 cervical spinal nerve exits the vertebral canal above the C-7 vertebra (Fig. 1–23 A). Therefore, a herniated C-6 disk will compress spinal nerve C-7.

The pear-shaped intervertebral foramina *in the thoracic region* (Fig. 1–21 A), on the contrary, are more than ample to accommodate the spinal nerves. They, too, are bounded by pedicles above and below, dorsally by the apophyseal joints and articular processes, and ventrally by an intervertebral disk. Observe, however, that there is a difference. The inferior vertebral notch of the pedicle above is quite deep while the superior vertebral notch below is quite shallow. As a result the more cranial vertebral body and the intervertebral disk form most of the ventral foraminal boundary. Only a small portion of the more caudal vertebral body contributes to the foramen boundary (Fig. 1–21 A). This same description of boundaries may be applied to the bean- (or kidney-) shaped lumbar intervertebral foramina (Fig. 1–21 A), although the lumbar foramina are larger.

Spinal nerves *in the lumbar region* exit from the vertebral canal under the pedicles of their corresponding numbered vertebra

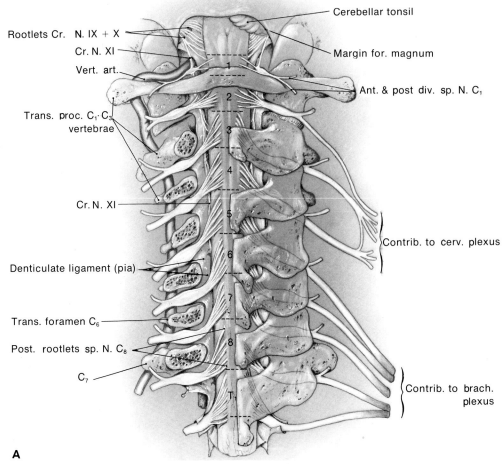

A

Figure 1–23. A, Dorsal view of cervical cord after laminectomy. The anterior division of the first cervical spinal nerve is seen crossing the dorsal arch of the atlas while the second crosses the atlanto-axial joint capsule. The eighth cervical emerges below C-7 vertebra while the seventh emerges above C-7. The vertebral artery is seen entering the transverse foramen at C-6. Observe the course of the eleventh *cranial nerve* (between dorsal and ventral rootlets) on the dorsal aspect of the pia denticulate ligament. It follows the last "tooth" of this "ligament" into the foramen magnum. (Numbers 1–8 and T_1 mark spinal cord segments.)

(Fig. 1–23 C). Because of the relatively large size of these foramina, it takes an extensive protrusion or herniation of disk tissue to affect the nerve exiting at the same disk level. Therefore, a posterolateral protrusion of the L-4 disk (below the L-4 vertebral body) does not usually affect the L-4 spinal nerve. It will usually encroach upon the dural sac and compress the most laterally placed nerve roots. These are the roots of the nerve that will exit one intervertebral foramen below (in this case the L-5 nerve). In similar fashion a protruded L-5 disk may compress the S-1 root (Fig. 1–23 C).

A central or midline disk protrusion may exert pressure on many nerve roots in the dural sac. For instance, a centrally herniated L-4 disk may not affect the L-4 nerve at all, but rather may press upon the L-5, S-1, and other sacral nerve roots.

Laminae

The *laminae* slightly overlap in the cervical spine (Fig. 1–21 C). This overlap becomes more exaggerated in the thoracic region. In the lumbar region, however, there is no overlapping of the laminae at all and, indeed, there are rather wide interlaminal gaps (Fig. 1–21 C). Other gaps may be found between the occiput and the atlas, the atlas and axis and, of course, at the lumbosacral junction.

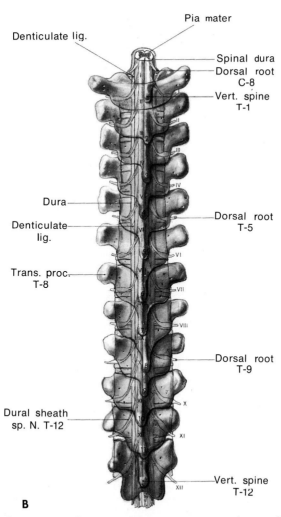

B

Figure 1–23 (Continued). B, Dorsal aspect of thoracic region with spinal cord in vertebral canal as seen "looking through" the translucent wall of bone. (Adapted from E. Pernkopf.)

Illustration and legend continued on the following page

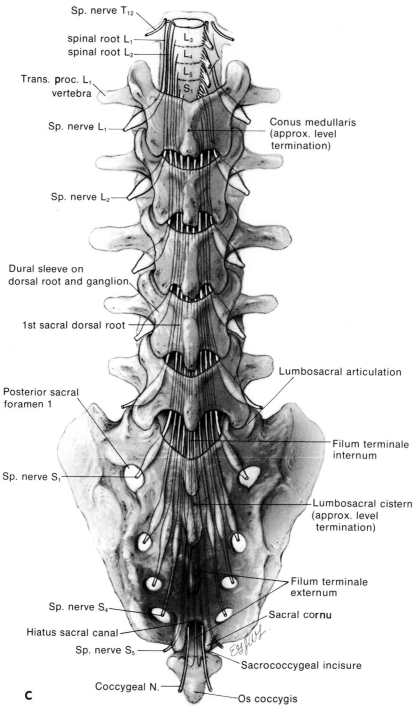

Sp. nerve T₁₂

spinal root L₁

spinal root L₂

L₃
L₄
L₅
S₁

Trans. proc. L₁ vertebra

Sp. nerve L₁

Conus medullaris (approx. level termination)

Sp. nerve L₂

Dural sleeve on dorsal root and ganglion

1st sacral dorsal root

Lumbosacral articulation

Posterior sacral foramen 1

Filum terminale internum

Sp. nerve S₁

Lumbosacral cistern (approx. level termination)

Filum terminale externum

Sp. nerve S₄

Sacral cornu

Hiatus sacral canal

Sp. nerve S₅

Sacrococcygeal incisure

C

Coccygeal N.

Os coccygis

Figure 1–23 (Continued). C, Terminal part of cord and cauda equina in lumbosacral region of vertebral column, dorsal view. Spines and laminae shown as if translucent. L₃, L₄, L₅, and S₁ are spinal cord segments.

Spinous Processes

As the spinous processes are compared in Fig. 1–21 A, C from cranial to caudal levels of the vertebral column, it is apparent that the spinous processes become more massive caudally and are directed caudalward.

The atlas (C-1) does not have a spinous process but, rather, a posterior tubercle. While the spinous processes from C-2 through C-6 are typically bifid in Caucasians, they are usually nonbifid in Blacks. The dorsal divisions of the bifid spinous processes are often unequal in size. Despite its name, vertebra prominens, the spinous process of the seventh cervical vertebra is frequently not as prominent posteriorly as that of the first thoracic vertebra.

While the midthoracic spinous processes (T-5 to T-8) overlap markedly, the spines of T-1, T-2, T-11, and T-12 are less steeply inclined caudalward.

Spinous processes in the lumbar region are large, thick quadrilateral plates. The spinous process of L-5 is the smallest in the lumbar region.

It is of great importance to note the alignment of spinous processes on radiographs, particularly in cases of injury. Displacement may indicate a fracture of the spinous process or locked articular facets unilaterally.

Transverse Processes

Each transverse process of the cervical spine has a transverse foramen. The upper six foramina transmit the vertebral artery and vein, while C-7 usually only transmits a vein. All transmit a plexus of sympathetic autonomic nerves.

Observe that the *cervical transverse processes* are located ventral to the articular surfaces (Fig. 1–21 A), lateral to the pedicles, and that they bend inferiorly and ventrally to overlap the intervertebral foramina. The breadth of the transverse processes of the atlas is the greatest. There is little variation in the transverse processes from the second through the sixth cervical vertebra. The transverse process of C-7 is not as long as that of the atlas. It should not normally exceed the lateral extent of the first thoracic transverse process. When it does, it may be associated with clinical findings suggestive of cervical ribs.

The stout, strong *transverse processes of the thoracic spine*, acting as muscle levers and fulcra for the ribs, are situated more dorsally than those of the cervical or lumbar spine (Fig. 1–21 A). They arise dorsal to the pedicles, articular processes, and intervertebral foramina. The upper ten thoracic transverse processes have articular facets for the articulation of the upper ten ribs on each side. The last articular tubercle usually occurs on the tenth rib. This is a very useful landmark in roentgenography when localizing vertebral levels, as the last rib-bearing vertebra (T-12) shows considerable variation.

The transverse processes at T-1 have the greatest breadth and these decrease caudally until, at T-12, they are mere vestiges (Fig. 1–21 A, C).

Lumbar transverse processes are thin, flat projections that extend dorsolaterally at L-1 but progressively seek a more ventrolateral position at L-5. At L-5 they overlap the vertebral body. Transverse processes are longest at L-3 and become progressively shorter on vertebrae above and below (Fig. 1–21 B, C).

BLOOD SUPPLY OF THE VERTEBRAE

Arteries

In embryologic growth, each vertebra develops a blood supply from paired segmental (spinal) arteries to the midportion of the vertebral body. In the cervical region, these segmental arteries are branches from the vertebral arteries. In the thoracic and lumbar regions, these arteries arise from the intercostal and lumbar arteries coming from the aorta. The sacral spinal arteries arise from the lateral sacral arteries. Each segmental artery provides twigs that enter the vertebral body through numerous foramina distributed over the anterolateral aspect of the body (Fig. 1–24).

Dorsal branches of the segmental arteries, which also supply the muscles of the back, give off spinal branches near the intervertebral foramina. As these spinal branches pass through the intervertebral foramina and enter the vertebral canal, they divide into three terminal branches: dorsal, intermediate, and ventral (Fig. 1–24). *Terminal dor-*

sal branches supply the osseous structures of the vertebral arch as well as supplying the spinal dura mater and the tissues lying within the extradural (epidural) space. They also form anastomoses with similar vessels cranially and caudally that accompany the posterior internal venous plexus. *Terminal intermediate branches* supply the spinal dura and nerve roots. They have inconstant radicular arteries, which accompany the nerve roots intradurally and aid in supplying the spinal cord. Supplying the vertebral bodies are the *terminal ventral branches,* which anastomose with those twigs that enter anterolaterally (Fig. 1–24). These terminal ventral branches of the dorsal blood supply to the vertebral body divide on each side into ascending and descending twigs, which pass beneath the posterior longitudinal ligament and course cranially and caudally to pierce the dorsal surfaces of two adjacent vertebral bodies. In this fashion each vertebral body will receive blood dorsally from an ascending and a descending artery on each side, four arteries supplying each body dorsally. These terminal ventral branches, like the terminal dorsal branches to the vertebral arch, also supply the spinal dura mater and the extradural space, form-

ing anastomotic channels that accompany the anterior internal venous plexus.

There is no arterial supply to the intervertebral disks in the adult. In the fetus and child, vessels from the vertebral body pierce the cartilaginous plate to reach the disk; however, these vessels degenerate during the first decade of life, leaving the tissues of the intervertebral disk to derive nourishment by imbibition of tissue fluid from adjacent vascular structures.

Veins

The vertebral venous system, or the venous plexus (Batson's plexus) is a valveless system isolated from the thoracoabdominal cavity. It provides a separate venous system that is composed of veins of the head and neck, the body wall and the valveless veins of the limbs, as well as the true vertebral veins.

We will concern ourselves here with that portion of the system in and about the vertebral column (Fig. 1–25).

The plexuses of veins that we will consider are those lying within the vertebral canal (internal vertebral venous plexuses) and

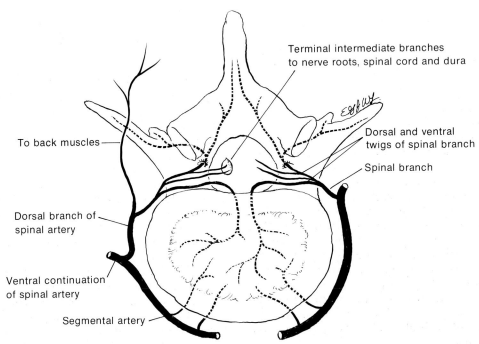

Terminal intermediate branches
to nerve roots, spinal cord and dura

To back muscles

Dorsal and ventral
twigs of spinal branch

Spinal branch

Dorsal branch of
spinal artery

Ventral continuation
of spinal artery

Segmental artery

Figure 1-24. Schematic diagram of the blood supply to a vertebra from above.

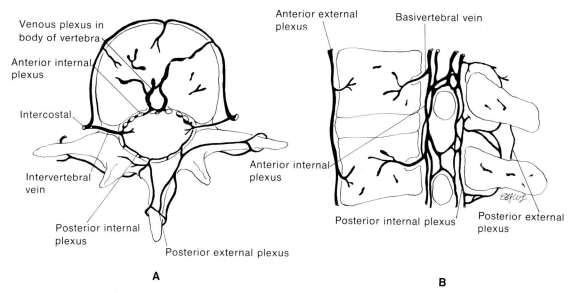

Figure 1-25. Vertebral venous plexus. *A,* Viewed in transverse section. *B,* Viewed in midsagittal section.

those outside (external vertebral venous plexuses).

The *internal vertebral venous plexuses* lie between the spinal dura mater and the vertebrae in the extradural space. As shown in Figure 1–25, there are the *anterior internal plexuses,* large plexuses of veins situated beneath the posterior longitudinal ligament, which receive tributaries from the basivertebral veins of the vertebral body. There are also longitudinal channels of the *posterior internal plexuses* coursing along the dorsal and dorsolateral margins of the vertebral canal in the extradural space. Venous rings connect the anterior and posterior internal vertebral plexuses.

The *external vertebral venous plexuses* also consist of anterior and posterior plexuses, situated outside the vertebral column, which are most evident in the cervical region of the column. The *anterior plexus* lies ventral to the vertebral bodies and receives tributaries from the basivertebral veins through tiny foramina on the anterolateral surface of the bodies. The *posterior external plexuses* lie on the dorsal aspect of the vertebral arches and their processes (Fig. 1–24).

Basivertebral veins (Fig. 1–25) form sinuous channels within the vertebral bodies. They communicate with the anterior external and internal venous plexuses.

Leaving the intervertebral foramina with the spinal nerves are the *intervertebral veins* (Fig. 1–25). These veins receive blood from the veins of the spinal cord and the internal vertebral plexuses. They terminate in the vertebral, intercostal, lumbar, and lateral sacral veins.

DEVELOPMENTAL ANATOMY

"Typical" Vertebral Development

This brief review of vertebral column development is necessary to the understanding of gross morphology, the borderlines of the normal and some of the pathologic changes found in the spine. Vertebral development is quite complex, and much of the story is beyond the scope of this book.

Except for certain special regions of the vertebral column, development follows a typical sequence of events. Therefore, in this section, we will follow development of a vertebra in the thoracic region and comment upon other regions later.

There are three stages of development: mesenchymal origin, chondrification, and ossification.

Mesenchymal Origin

Toward the end of the third week of life, the paraxial mesoderm of the embryonic germinal disk, situated on each side of a *notochord,* begins to segment into paired cellular masses called *somites* (Fig. 1–26). By this time, a *neural tube* has formed above the notochord — the midline, mesenchymal, rod-shaped, primitive "back bone" of the early developing embryo. It will be the fate of a part of each somite to incorporate the notochord and to fashion a bony vertebral column, intervertebral disks, and ribs. The fate of the column is to envelop and protect the hindmost part of the delicate, developing neural tube.

In the human embryo, each of these mesodermal somites has a somewhat indistinct cranial and caudal limit, soon to be demarcated by the appearance of *intersegmental arteries* between them, at about the time tissue cells begin to migrate from the somites to form vertebrae and other structures (Fig. 1–27 *B*).

The first pair of somites are formed near the caudal hindbrain, for the notochord, in man at least, does not extend cephalad beyond this point (Fig. 1–26).

By the end of the fifth week, 42 to 44 somite pairs have become organized: four occipital, eight cervical, twelve thoracic,

five lumbar, five sacral and eight to ten coccygeal. Not all of them remain to participate fully in embryonic development, especially the first occipital and five to seven of the coccygeal somites, which are evanescent and either fuse with other parts or disappear entirely.

Nor is paraxial mesoderm static. Shortly after somites form, a rearrangement of their cells begins. A schema of a transverse section through a somite shows that cells, in an early stage, align radially around a cavity or *myocele* (Fig. 1–27 *A*). This gives the early somite a somewhat triangular form, with a lateral, medial, and ventral wall.

Cells proliferate and differentiate as they migrate in different directions from each of these walls, some even filling in the myocele, which is short-lived and disappears within a week (Fig. 1–27 *C*).

The lateral wall, or *dermatomic* portion, of the somite is mainly concerned with adding to the developing dermis, or skin. These cells migrate laterad; and the peripheral processes of developing dorsal root

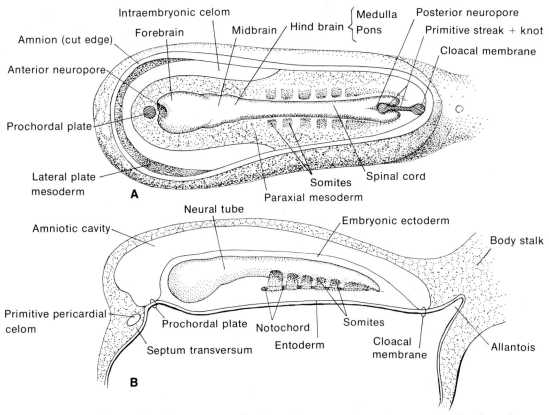

Figure 1–26. Schema of embryonic neural tube and somites. *A*, surface view and *B*, lateral view.

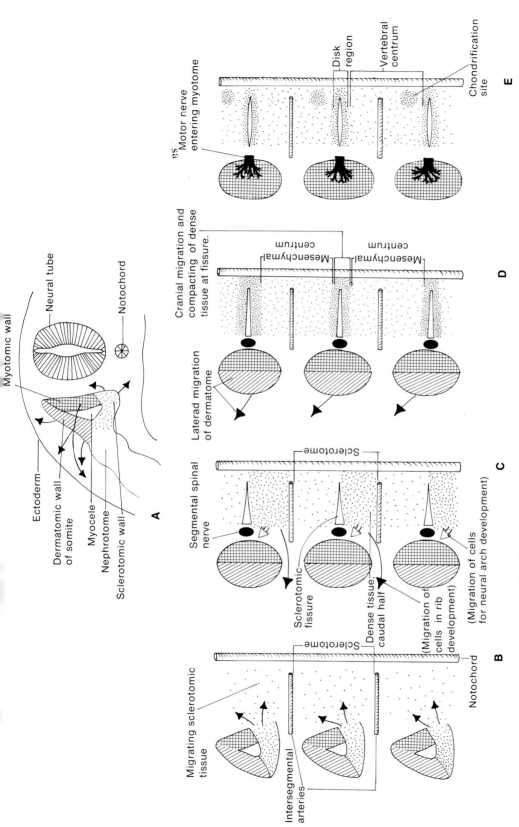

Figure 1–27. The development of vertebrae and intervertebral disks from the sclerotomal portion of embryonic somites. A, schematic transverse section through germinal plate and somite; arrows indicate direction of cellular migration from somite walls (nephrotome is an intermediate portion of paraxial mesoderm that becomes involved in development of urinary and reproductive tracts). B–E, schematic frontal sections through same region as A in three to six week embryos, diagraming the transformation of sclerotomes into vertebral bodies and disks. Sclerotomes organize *bilaterally* around the notochord. Changes are followed here on one side only. In E, chondrification centers have begun to appear in one side of the vertebral bodies. They will fuse with similar centers developing on the opposite side of these bodies. See text for discussion of events depicted in B–E.

ganglion cells follow them as a segmental, cutaneous nerve supply develops (Fig. 1–27 A, D).

The medial wall cells also migrate laterally and ventrolaterally as this myotomic portion of each somite develops into segmental muscle masses. The masses will be followed by emerging segmental motor axons from the developing segmented spinal cord (Fig. 1–27 A, E).

To follow the osseous and cartilaginous stages of development of a vertebral column, it is necessary to focus upon the ventral wall of the early somite — the *sclerotome*.

Between the fourth and fifth weeks of embryonic life, cells here migrate out of the somite in three main directions:

1. *Ventromedialward,* to surround the notochord (Fig. 1–27 B). Since somites are bilateral structures, this is a bilateral, mesiad migration toward the notochord, though Figure 1–27 shows it occurring on one side only. These cells are involved in the development of vertebral centra and intervertebral disks.

2. *Dorsalward,* around the sides of the neural tube to form the neural arches of vertebrae and, thus, to envelop the developing spinal cord situated dorsal to the notochord (Fig. 1–27 A, B).

3. *Ventrolaterad,* to form the costal processes of vertebrae that will develop into ribs (Fig. 1–27 C).

As sclerotomal mesoderm condenses about the notochord, it forms as segments separated by the appearance of *intersegmental arteries* (Fig. 1–27 B). These vessels lie at the cranial and caudal ends of adjacent sclerotomal segments.

A secondary structure soon appears, the *sclerotomal fissure,* another evanescent structure, which serves momentarily to subdivide each sclerotome into a cranial and caudal half. The fissure appears shortly after myocele closure and sclerotomal migration toward the notochord (Fig. 1–27 C).

A more rapid division of cells soon takes place in the caudal half of each sclerotomal segment, resulting in a more dense congregation of tissue cells there than in the cranial halves (Fig. 1–27 C). There then occurs a cranialward migration of this dense tissue toward, and partly into, the looser tissue of the cranial half of each segment. Its destination is the sclerotomal fissure about which it compacts (Fig. 1–27 D). Here, in this region

of a fast-disappearing sclerotomal fissure, the bilateral migration of dense tissue will have incorporated a segment of the notochord. The tissue will become involved in the formation of a fibrocartilaginous intervertebral disk, or, at least, in the anulus of such a disk. The softer tissue of the incorporated notochord eventually becomes the nucleus pulposus of the disk. Some secondary mucilaginous degeneration of the fibrocartilaginous anulus also adds to the definitive nucleus pulposus. Certain cells of this dense mass will also take part in the formation of the tough, ligamentous connective tissues of the vertebral column.

The cranialward migration of dense tissue from the caudal sclerotomal segment leaves behind a dispersement of tissue components as loosely organized as those tissue components of its cranial half (Fig. 1–27 D). It is the fusion of this looser tissue from the caudal half of one segment with similar tissue in the cranial half of the segment next below that will account for the development of vertebral bodies. Vertebral bodies, therefore, *arise from adjacent parts of sclerotomal segments,* not from their original segments, as was the case for intervertebral disks. This fusion of loose tissue from adjacent segments also incorporates the notochord next to it. However, as ossification develops in this tissue, all trace of a notochordal remnant is usually lost. Notochordal tissue merely persists in the disk segments.

As a result of such migration and secondary fusion of adjacent segment parts, an apparent, but not a real, shifting in position of segmental arteries and nerves has taken place. Originally, segmental nerves related to the midpoint of the sclerotomal mass or segment — site of the sclerotomal fissure — (Fig. 1–27 C, D). Intersegmental arteries related to the cranial and caudal ends of the sclerotomal segment. Afterward, nerves relate to disk areas between vertebral bodies (or to the cranial and caudal ends of bodies), while intersegmental arteries relate to the midpoint of the newly formed vertebral body (Fig. 1–27 E). Of course, the arteries and nerves have not moved. They remained where they always were as the sclerotomal tissue migrated; for example, the locus of the nerve next to the fast-disappearing sclerotomal fissure (Fig. 1–27 E) is now a disk area.

Thus, myotomes, as skeletal muscle,

come to bridge adjacent vertebrae. Spinal nerves come to lie close to disks and leave the vertebral canal via intervertebral foramina; and intersegmental arteries pass across vertebral bodies.

A dorsalward migration of sclerotomal cells forms segmental, mesenchymal (blastemal) condensations between forming spinal ganglia to circle dorsally around the sides of the neural tube (Fig. 1–28 A). Thus, a primitive neural arch, with a faint suggestion of a spinous process, is laid down by mesodermal connective tissue cells of the embryo. Later, the various processes of the arch take shape.

Everywhere, but especially in the thoracic region, ventrolateral migration from the sclerotomal part of somites begins to outline costal processes. These cellular concentrations come to lie just lateral to the level of the intersegmental arteries in the early embryo. They are contributed to by the tissue from cranial and caudal halves of adjacent sclerotomal segments, though contributions from the caudal halves tend to predominate. Thus ribs, as do vertebrae, develop from their own segment (caudal half) and the cranial half of the subjacent segment.

Costal processes attempt rib development at every vertebral level of the embryo, but, as a rule, only those in the thoracic region persist. Ribs, then, are integral parts of mesenchymal vertebrae.

In the definitive column, ribs commonly articulate with two adjacent vertebral bodies, and they gain an attachment to an intervening disk by means of an *intraarticular* ligament. Such an attachment subdivides the capsule of a typical costovertebral joint into two synovial cavities.

Chondrification

Chondrification of a mesenchymatous vertebra begins during the sixth week of development (Fig. 1–28 A). Intercellular chondroid material appears in the loose cells around the notochord in the primary centrum.[7] Some investigators,[4, 7] state that only one chondrification center appears in the centrum, while the majority,[8, 9] favor the formation of two chondrification centers laterally in the regions surrounding the notochord, which rapidly fuse.

A short time later chondrification centers appear in the neural arches and in the costal processes (Fig. 1–28 A). These chondrification centers in the neural arches extend ventrally into the pedicles and dorsally into the laminae. The latter meet in the midline dorsally by the fourth month in utero.

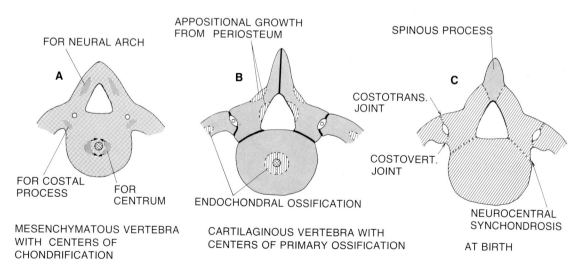

Figure 1–28. Schema illustrating further stages of vertebral development. *A*, Chondrification centers appearing in the mesenchymatous outline of a vertebra (sixth embryonic week). *B*, Primary ossification centers in the cartilaginous vertebra (third month). *C*, The vertebra at birth, consisting of three bony parts (centrum and halves of the neural arches). The spinous process is still undergoing ossification in its cartilaginous matrix. Note also the absorption of cartilage at the neurocentral joints, soon to become a synostotic union with the pedicles; and at costotransverse and costovertebral joint areas, where transformation to joint cavities, capsules, and ligaments is occurring.

Transverse and articular processes chondrify in continuity with the neural arches. The costal processes extend ventrally and, in the thoracic region, form the ribs. (Other homologues of the costal processes are shown in Figure 1–8 *A–D*.) Mesenchymal zones that do not form cartilage mark the sites of the neurocentral, costovertebral, and costotransverse joints (Fig. 1–28 *B, C*).

THE CRANIOVERTEBRAL REGION. The development of the *craniovertebral* (occipito-atlanto-axial) *region* has always been of interest to anatomists and physicians. A great number of variations and malformations occur there. Often the abnormalities are first observed following an episode of trauma to the head or neck. Therefore, they become of differential diagnostic significance.

It will be recalled that in the human embryo, near the end of the third week of development, somites (primitive segments) form (Fig. 1–26 *B*). These develop initially in the occipital region, and this differentiation of the paraxial mesoderm proceeds caudally. This section will be concerned with the fate of the four occipital and the first three cervical somites (Fig. 1–29).

The first occipital somite (Occ. #1 — see Fig. 1–29) is quite small, and disappears soon after its formation.[10] The fate of this first occipital somite is unknown.

The second occipital somite (Occ. #2) is also small, while the third and fourth somites (Occ. #3 and 4) are equal in size to those in the cervical region.

While sclerotomic and myotomic areas may be identified in the second to fourth occipital somites, these somites do not differentiate in the ordinary manner. However, there is some indication of segmentation of the fourth occipital somite by its relationship to the primitive hypoglossal artery at its cranial boundary, and to the first cervical artery at its caudal boundary.

In order to picture clearly the somites and their respective names, refer to Figure 1–29. The last, or fourth, occipital segment is designated Occ. #4 or the *anteproatlantal segment*. Since the first occipital segment is evanescent, some authors[5, 11] refer to the last occipital somite as the third occipital or the

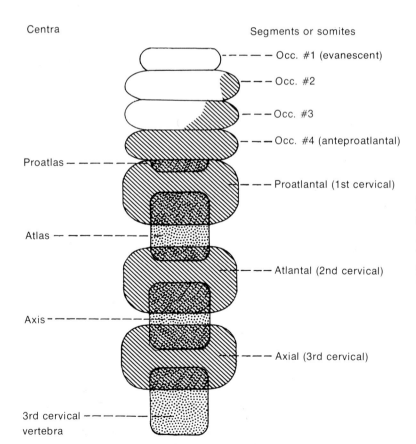

Centra

Segments or somites

— — — — Occ. #1 (evanescent)

— — Occ. #2

— — Occ. #3

— — Occ. #4 (anteproatlantal)

Proatlas — — — — —

— — Proatlantal (1st cervical)

Atlas — — — — — — —

— — Atlantal (2nd cervical)

Axis - — - — - — - —

— — Axial (3rd cervical)

3rd cervical — — — — —
vertebra

Figure 1–29. The fate of the four occipital and the upper three cervical somites. The shaded portions of Occ. #2 to 4 represent the relative contributions of the somites in the adult. (After Keith.)

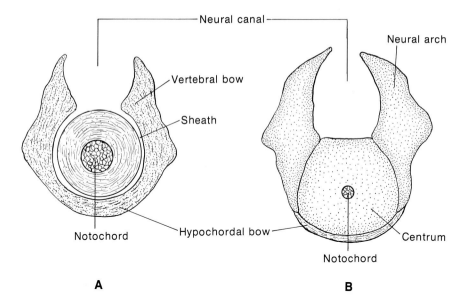

Figure 1–30. Stages in the development of a vertebra. *A*, Membranous stage. *B*, Cartilaginous stage.

third hypoglossal somite. Figure 1–29 shows the first cervical somite to be the *proatlantal* or *suboccipital,* the second cervical somite to be the *atlantal,* and the third cervical somite to be the *axial* segment.

The *atlas* (C-1) forms from a fusion of the caudal sclerotome-half of the proatlantal (first cervical) segment and the cranial sclerotome-half of the succeeding segment, that is, from the atlantal or second cervical segment (Fig. 1–29).

In turn, then, *the axis* (C-2) forms from the caudal sclerotome-half of the atlantal (second cervical) segment and the cranial sclerotome-half of the axial (third cervical) segment (Fig. 1–29).

Now the cervical spinal nerves have a segmental position. The first cervical, or suboccipital, nerve passes over the cranial end of the developing atlas, while the second cervical spinal nerve passes below it. We can now understand the presence of eight cervical nerves on each side in the cervical spine, but only seven cervical vertebrae.

The rearrangement of cervical sclerotomes that we have just described leaves one extra-sclerotome-half, namely the cranial sclerotome-half of the proatlantal (first primitive cervical) segment (Fig. 1–29). This sclerotome-half is referred to in the literature,[5, 7] as the *proatlas.* In some animals, such as the reptile, the cranial

sclerotome-half of the proatlantal segment joins with the last occipital sclerotome-half to form a bone called, appropriately, the proatlas. Despite some theoretical objections[11] to its use in man, this term has become established.

In man the proatlas (cranial sclerotome-half of the proatlantal or first primitive cervical segment) is thought to give rise to several structures. The centrum of the proatlas is thought to form the terminal ossicle of the dens. The neural arch of the proatlas contributes to the formation of the occipital condyles and the ligaments about the atlanto-occipital joint.

In the upper cervical region, a structure called the *hypochordal bow or arch* spans the ventral surface of the developing centrum. Although present in the mesenchymatous vertebra, it becomes more clearly defined during chondrification. The hypochordal arch joins the two neural arches (Fig. 1–30) ventral to the centrum. These hypochordal arches are transitory structures except in the developing atlas, where they persist.

In the atlas (C-1), the hypochordal arch chondrifies late and separates from the primitive centrum. The arch forms the anterior arch and the ventral portions of the lateral masses of the atlas, while the neural arch forms the posterior arch and the dorsal portions of the lateral masses.

The axis (C-2), while developing in a pattern similar to all typical vertebrae, has one exceptional feature: the centrum of the axis joins with the centrum of the atlas and the proatlas to form the dens.

The dens is derived from one and one-half primitive cervical segments. The terminal ossicle (Fig. 1–35) is derived from the proatlas or the cranial sclerotome-half of the primitive first cervical (proatlantal) segment. The remainder of the dens (Fig. 1–29) arises from the caudal sclerotome-half of the proatlantal segment and the cranial sclerotome-half of the atlantal (second cervical) segment.

The last occipital caudal sclerotome-half has identifiable neural arches, chordal processes and rib rudiments. There are also rib rudiments on the primitive atlas. In both instances, these rib rudiments may be the embryologic anlagen of the paracondylic and epitransverse processes.

If the caudal sclerotome-half of the last occipital segment (anteproatlantal segment) is incompletely incorporated into the other occipital somites, then the resulting bony abnormalities are referred to as a *"manifestation of occipital vertebra"* or *vertebralization of the occiput.*

Ossification

"TYPICAL VERTEBRA." Each cartilaginous vertebra (Fig. 1–28 *B*) is ossified from three primary centers: one for the centrum and one for each neural arch (Fig. 1–31 *A*).

These ossification centers appear at different times in the various portions of the vertebral column. The centrum ossifies endochondrally, the neural arches by appositional growth from the developing periosteum.

At about the seventh intrauterine week, a primary ossification center appears in each neural arch in the upper cervical region. These centers appear at the junction of the pedicle and the lamina. Ossification spreads into the seven developing processes (spinous, two transverse, and four articular). Since the pars interarticularis region is completely ossified from a single center, it is difficult to argue for a congenital basis of spondylolysis (see p. 401 — Spondylolysis). Ossification gradually proceeds in a caudal direction in the vertebral column. By the fourth month of intrauterine life, ossification has reached the sacral neural arches.

The primary ossification centers of the centrum appear about the eighth to the tenth intrauterine week in the lower thoracic and upper lumbar regions. Ossification spreads rapidly craniad and more slowly caudad, and by the fourth month all of the vertebral centra, with the exception of the coccyx, have centers.

At birth, vertebrae consist of three parts (Fig. 1–31 *A*): a centrum and two neural arches, all joined by cartilage. The *neurocentral synchondrosis* unites the centrum to the neural arch. The ends of the centrum are covered by plates of hyaline cartilage, which are histologically analogous to the epiphyseal plates of long bones. These car-

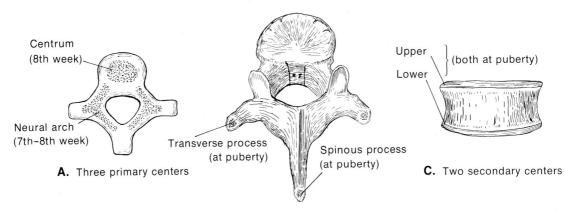

Centrum
(8th week)

Neural arch
(7th–8th week)

Transverse process
(at puberty)

Spinous process
(at puberty)

A. Three primary centers

B. Three secondary centers

Upper
Lower } (both at puberty)

C. Two secondary centers

Figure 1–31. Ossification of the vertebral column. *A*, Typical vertebra. *B*, A typical vertebra at puberty. *C*, Body of a typical vertebra at puberty. (After Gray[16]).

tilaginous plates are responsible for longitudinal growth of the vertebrae through endochondral ossification. Therefore they are the epiphyseal cartilages of the growth period.[2] Growth proceeds from the deep surfaces of these cartilaginous plates.[2, 3]

At birth the oval-shaped centrum has ventral and dorsal clefts, which are vascular channels (Fig. 1–32 A). The vertical height of the centrum is twice that of the intervertebral disk space.

During the first year of life, the neural arch halves unite dorsally. This union first occurs in the lumbar region shortly after birth, and extends cranialward into the thoracic and cervical regions by the second year.

Fusion of the neural arch to the centrum begins first in the cervical region at three years. This process proceeds caudalward and is completed in the sacrum by about age seven. The neural arch forms the vertebral arch and also contributes to the centrum to form the vertebral body (Fig. 1–3 A, B).

In the young child, the cranial and caudal surfaces of the vertebral body are covered by the thin cartilaginous plate. Peripherally, the cartilage is thickened, and this cartilage ring (cartilaginous marginal ridge) is set in a groove. Between the seventh and ninth year, foci of endochondral ossification appear in these cartilaginous marginal ridges (Fig. 1–32 B). These foci are usually triangular and they are easily mistaken for fracture, since they may not develop simultaneously in the same vertebral body on its upper and lower surfaces. With the appearance of the focal ossifications, the secondary centers of ossification of the vertebral body are established. Individual foci enlarge, fuse, and then form continuous ridges around the upper and lower vertebral body margins by about the twelfth year (Figs. 1–31 C, 1–32 C). These osseous marginal ridges are separated from the vertebral body proper by a thin layer of cartilage for several years.

By age 15, the osseous marginal ridge begins to fuse with the vertebral body. This fusion does not take place at all levels of the vertebral column simultaneously. It occurs last in the lumbar region before the age of 25.

Unlike the cartilaginous plates of the long bones, those at the ends of the vertebral body never completely disappear. They persist as thin, hyaline cartilaginous plates on the upper and lower surfaces of the body. Thus the deep portion of the cartilaginous plate functions as an epiphyseal plate during the period of growth, while its surface persists — the equivalent of an articular cartilage.

At puberty, three other secondary ossification centers begin to appear at the tips of the spinous, transverse, and articular processes. They fuse to the main mass of the vertebral arch at approximately 25 years.

The secondary centers of ossification are sometimes referred to as epiphyses. Clinicians object to this designation stating that they play no part in growth and are more nearly like traction apophyses.

THE ATLAS. Ossification of the atlas begins about the seventh week of intrauterine life in the lateral masses. One ossification center in each lateral mass arises from the perichondrium and extends dorsally.

At birth, the neural arches are separated by cartilage in the midline dorsally (Fig. 1–33). The arches fuse about the third or fourth year either directly or through another separate ossification center that develops in the cartilage.

The anterior arch is usually cartilaginous at birth, although about 20 per cent of newborns will have an ossification center here. Ossification of the anterior arch is quite variable and may proceed in a number of ways. A single center may appear in the anterior arch during the first year, or two centers may form. Rarely there is total absence of an ossification center, and the anterior arch forms from ventral extensions of the lateral mass centers. In any case, fusion of the anterior arch to the lateral masses is completed by the sixth to eighth year of life. Figure 1–33 shows the lines of separation of the various component parts of the atlas.

THE AXIS. Ossification of the axis is from five primary and two secondary centers (Fig. 1–34).

At about the seventh month of intrauterine life, one ossification center appears in each neural arch. These fuse dorsally at about the second year of life. Ossification of the centrum from one or, occasionally, two centers starts during the fourth or fifth prenatal month.

The dens ossifies from two laterally placed centers in the fifth or sixth prenatal

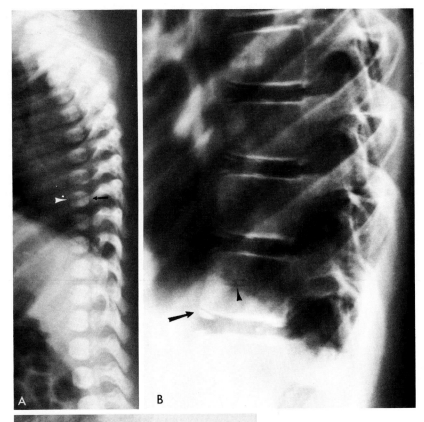

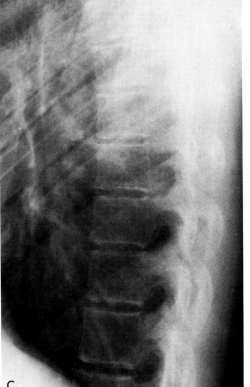

Figure 1–32. A, Lateral radiograph of a newborn. Note the ovoid-shaped vertebral bodies, the open neurocentral synchondroses (arrow), and the prominent vascular channels anteriorly and posteriorly (Hahn clefts) (arrow head). B, Ten year old child. Foci of endochondral ossification are present in the cartilaginous marginal ridges (arrow). Hahn clefts are less prominent (arrow head). C, Fifteen year old boy. The osseous marginal ridges (secondary ossification centers or apophyses) are complete around the upper and lower margins of the vertebral bodies.

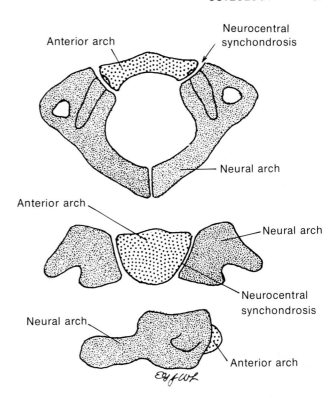

Figure 1-33. The first cervical vertebra (atlas); developmental components. The anterior arch may ossify during the last fetal months or the early postnatal months. Ossification of the neural arches begins about the seventh week of intra-uterine life. The dorsal synchondrosis between the neural arches fuses about the third or fourth year of life. Fusion of the anterior arch to the lateral masses occurs by the sixth to eighth year of life. (After Bailey, D. K.: The normal cervical spine in infants and children. Radiology 59:712, 1952.)

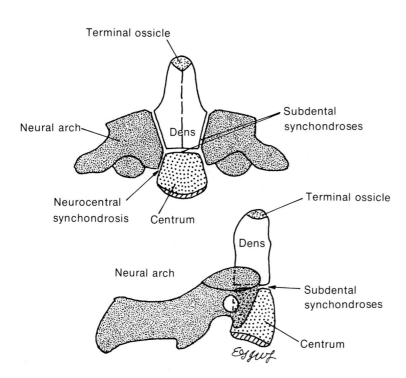

Figure 1-34. Developmental components of the second cervical vertebra (axis). A single ossification center (occasionally two) appears in the centrum in the fourth or fifth fetal month. At about the seventh month of fetal life, one ossification center appears in each neural arch, and fuses dorsally about the second or third year. The subdental and neurocentral synchondroses fuse between four and seven years of age. At puberty, the inferior epiphyseal ring appears and it fuses during early life. The terminal ossicle of the dens appears at about age two, and fuses with the dens by age 12. Two separate centers of ossification for the dens appear about the fifth or sixth prenatal months and they fuse before birth. (After Bailey, D. K.: The normal cervical spine in infants and children. Radiology 59:712, 1952).

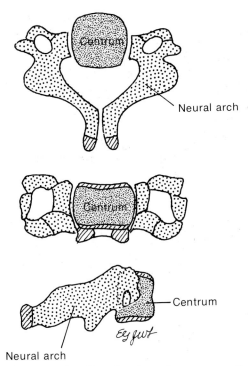

Figure 1–35. Developmental portions of a typical cervical vertebra. The ossification center for the centrum appears by the fifth fetal month. The anterior (costal) portion of the transverse process may develop from a separate ossification center that appears by the sixth fetal month and fuses with the arch by the sixth year. Ossification centers for the neural arches appear by the third fetal month, and fuse dorsally by the second or third year of life. The neurocentral synchondroses fuse at three to six years. At puberty, the superior and inferior epiphyseal rings appear and unite with the body at about 25 years. (After Bailey, D. K.: Radiology, 59:712, 1952.)

month. These two centers fuse before birth, forming the conically shaped bony mass seen in Figure 1–34. The cleft at the apex of the dens is filled by cartilage. In about 25 per cent of children, an inconstant ossification center, the *terminal ossicle*, appears at about age two. The terminal ossicle unites with the main portion of the dens by age twelve. It will be recalled that the terminal ossicle arises from the proatlas (Fig. 1–36 A).

The dens is separated from the centrum of the axis by cartilage, the *subdental synchondrosis* (Figs. 1–34, 1–36). This synchondrosis closes between four and seven years of age. A remnant of this synchondrosis may persist in the adult and should not be mistaken for a fracture.

"TYPICAL" CERVICAL VERTEBRA (Figs. 1–35, 1–36). The anterior (costal) portion of the transverse process may develop from a separate ossification center, which joins the arch by the sixth year. The synchondrosis between the neural arches posteriorly unites by the second or third year of life. Secondary ossification centers (apophyses) for bifid spinous processes appear at puberty and fuse with the spinous process at about 25 years.

The neurocentral synchondrosis unites at three to six years of age.

LUMBAR VERTEBRAE. Two additional secondary ossification centers (apophyses) appear in the lumbar vertebrae. These are for the mammillary processes (Fig. 1–37).

THE SACRUM. Ossification of the centrum of the first sacral vertebra begins at about the eighth prenatal month. This ossification of the sacral centra is not completed in the most caudal segments until the fifth to eighth month of fetal life.

Ossification of the neural arches and costal elements takes place between the sixth and eighth month of intrauterine life. The costal elements and the neural arches join about the second to the fifth years of age. In turn, these lateral parts unite with the centrum at about the eighth year.

Sacral vertebrae are separated by intervertebral disks as in other regions of the vertebral column. These disks ossify between the last two sacral vertebrae in about the eighteenth year. The union of sacral vertebrae then moves cranially, and is completed late in the third decade.

About puberty, centers appear for the auricular surfaces on each side of the sacrum and another for each lateral thin edge (Fig. 1–38 D).

The sacrum is depicted schematically at various stages in Figure 1–38.

THE COCCYX. Each coccygeal segment ossifies from a separate center. The first segment ossifies at about the first year of life. Ossification progresses slowly through the last three segments and is completed at about age 20. At the end of the third decade, union between the first and second segments occurs.

VERTEBRAL CANAL AND CONTENTS

The spinal cord, its meninges, and other related structures lie within the vertebral

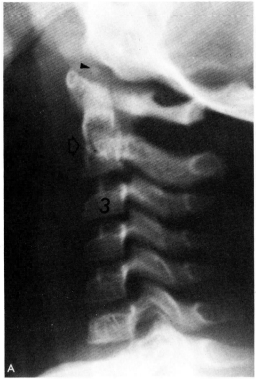

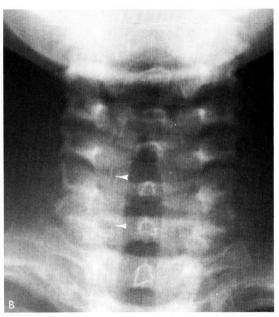

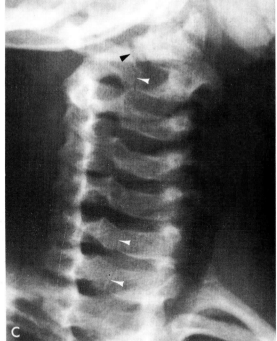

Figure 1–36. Cervical spine in a two year old. *A,* Lateral radiograph. The *open arrow* indicates the subdental synchondrosis, which simulates a low dens fracture. Note the terminal ossicle of the dens (arrow head). *B,* Frontal view showing the neurocentral synchondroses (white arrow heads). *C,* Oblique view showing the neurocentral synchondroses (white arrow heads) and the subdental synchondrosis (black arrow head).

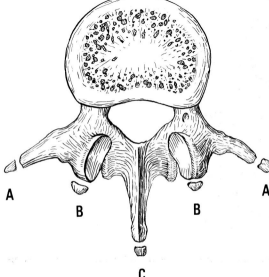

Figure 1–37. Lumbar vertebra showing secondary ossification centers (apophyses) of the transverse (A,A), mammillary (B,B), and spinous (C) processes.

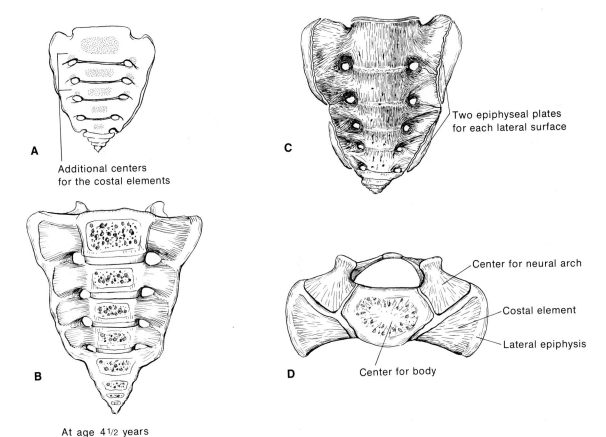

A Additional centers for the costal elements

C Two epiphyseal plates for each lateral surface

D Center for neural arch
Costal element
Lateral epiphysis
Center for body

B At age 4½ years

Figure 1–38. Ossification of the sacrum. *A*, At birth. *B*, At 4½ years. *C*, At age 25 years. *D*, Base of a young sacrum. (After Gray, H.: Anatomy of the Human Body. Goss, C. M., editor. Philadelphia, Lea & Febiger, 1966.)

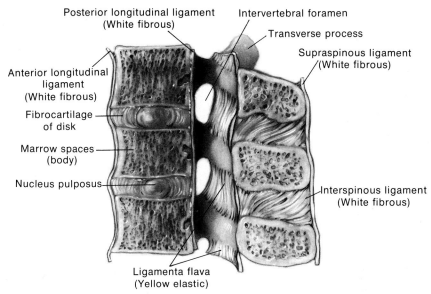

Posterior longitudinal ligament (White fibrous)
Intervertebral foramen
Transverse process
Supraspinous ligament (White fibrous)
Anterior longitudinal ligament (White fibrous)
Fibrocartilage of disk
Marrow spaces (body)
Nucleus pulposus
Interspinous ligament (White fibrous)
Ligamenta flava (Yellow elastic)

Figure 1–39. Sagittal section through part of vertebral column and vertebral canal to show associated ligaments.

canal. This canal is formed by the vertebral foramina of successive vertebrae of the articulated spine.

The boundaries of the vertebral canal are as follows: ventrally, the vertebral bodies with their intervening intervertebral disks and the posterior longitudinal ligament; laterally, the pedicles and intervertebral foramina; and dorsolaterally, the articulated articular processes, the laminae, and the ligamenta flava (Fig. 1–39).

The size and shape of the vertebral canal is not constant throughout the spinal column. There are regional differences that are directly related to the size and shape of the spinal cord. In the thoracic region, the vertebral canal is typically small and circular, while in those regions of the cervical and lumbar enlargements of the spinal cord (Fig. 1–40 A, B), the vertebral canal is large and triangular. Despite these differences in size and shape of the vertebral canal and the

spinal cord, the spinal cord occupies only about half of the available cross-sectional space of the canal.

In cases of trauma or disk herniation, the relation of the vertebral canal to the spinal cord becomes important. For the most part, the spinal cord is oval in shape with a greater lateral than anteroposterior dimension.

In the thickest portion of the cervical spinal cord enlargement, Elliott[12] found the average diameters to be 13.2 mm in width, 7.7 mm in AP depth. In the smallest cross-sectional region of the thoracic cord, these dimensions averaged 8.0 mm in width and 6.5 mm in depth. The average measurements in the lumbosacral enlargement were 9.6 mm and 8.0 mm respectively.

Aeby[13] gives the following dimensions for the vertebral canal: cervical region — width 24.5 mm, depth 14.7 mm; thoracic region — width 17.2 mm and depth 16.8 mm; and in

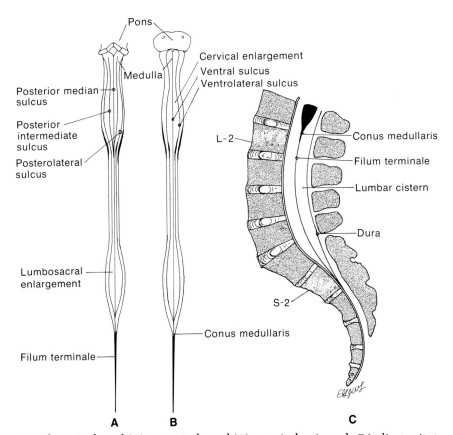

Figure 1–40. The spinal cord (*A*) posteriorly and (*B*) anteriorly viewed. *C* indicates its termination at the upper part of L-2 in the vertebral canal. The sac of dura-arachnoid continues beyond to terminate at S-2.

the lumbar region — width 23.4 mm and depth 17.4 mm.

While the cord would appear to occupy only about one-half of the available space of the vertebral canal in each dimension, these figures become critical in the cervical region, particularly in the patient with spondylosis deformans.

The figures given for the dimensions of the vertebral canal are an average and do not apply to individuals with constricted canals.

Spinal Cord

The spinal cord is continuous with the medulla oblongata at the level of the foramen magnum (Fig. 1–40). Until the third month of fetal life, the spinal cord and the vertebral canal are equal in length. The 31 pairs of spinal (segmental) nerves — eight cervical, twelve thoracic, five lumbar, five sacral, and one coccygeal — pass directly from their respective level of origin in the cord laterally through their specific intervertebral foramina. However, during continued fetal development, the vertebral column lengthens more rapidly than the neural tube, resulting in an apparent ascent of the spinal cord. At birth the terminal extremity of the cord is at the third lumbar vertebra. The result of this disproportionate growth between the vertebral column and the spinal cord is that the spinal nerves must take an oblique course from their segmental origin in the cord downward in order to reach their respective intervertebral foramina (Fig. 1–41 A, B). By age five, the spinal cord reaches its usual termination opposite the L-1 intervertebral disk (Fig. 1–41 B). In the adult male the spinal cord average length is 45 cm, while the vertebral column averages 70 cm in length. In the adult female the cord averages 42 cm, while the vertebral column is about 60 cm.

The cervical and lumbar enlargements of

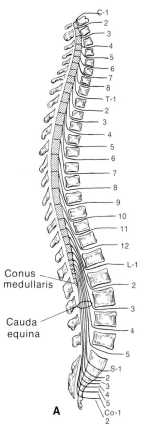

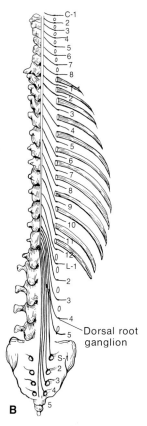

Figure 1–41. Relation of vertebral segments to emergence of cord rootlets. *A,* Lateral view. *B,* Dorsal view.

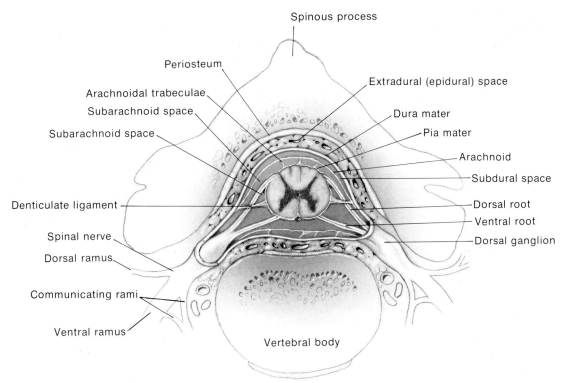

Figure 1–42. Relationship of the spinal cord and rootlets to their meningeal coverings. A cross-sectional view at the midthoracic level.

the spinal cord (Fig. 1–40 A, B) correspond to the origin of spinal nerves that supply the upper and lower limbs respectively. The terminal conical part of the spinal cord is the *conus medullaris,* which usually ends at the L-1 level but may, on occasion, be found as high as T-12 or as low as L-3.

From the apex of the conus medullaris, a thin, glistening, pial fibrous strand, the internal terminal film (filum of the spinal cord) continues caudally through the vertebral canal. The internal filum extends through the subarachnoid space to the level of S-3, where the arachnoid and dural sacs (lumbar cistern) terminate. Here the dura mater joins the pia mater, the former as the external terminal filum (filum of the dura). The newly reinforced *filum terminale* continues caudally in the vertebral canal and finally terminates on the coccyx, where it blends with the posterior longitudinal ligament.

The conus medullaris and filum terminale are surrounded in the subarachnoid space by the longitudinally directed dorsal and ventral roots of the caudal spinal nerves.

Since this configuration resembles a horse's tail, it is called the *cauda equina.*

Along the posterolateral sulcus of the spinal cord, a series of nerve filaments emerge (Figs. 1–42, 1–44) and join to form a *dorsal (posterior) sensory root* of a spinal nerve. In similar fashion the *ventral (anterior) motor roots* arise from nerve filaments located anterolaterally on the cord (Fig. 1–43).

The *spinal cord segment* is the part of the spinal cord from which a spinal nerve arises. Grossly, it is the distance between the most cranial filament of one root and the highest filament of the root below. These rather arbitrary spinal cord segments do not correspond to similarly numbered vertebrae, since we have already learned that the spinal cord is considerably shorter than the vertebral column. Indeed, the spinal cord segments are not of uniform length; for example, eight spinal segments in the cervical region extend over a shorter distance than the seven cervical vertebrae, and the lowest spinal cord segments are packed quite closely in the conus. We can get a general idea of the relationship of these spinal cord segments to the numbered vertebral bodies from Figure 1–41A,B.

Within the subarachnoid space, the separate dorsal and ventral nerve roots are immersed in cerebrospinal fluid and intimately covered by pia mater. We have seen how these roots are obliquely inclined (Fig. 1–41 A, B) to varying degrees according to the differences in the level of origin from the spinal cord and their exit through their respective intervertebral foramina. At the intervertebral foramina, the roots turn laterally, where they are enclosed by an arachnoid dural sheath.

The dorsal (sensory) and ventral (motor) roots unite just beyond the dorsal root ganglion forming a *mixed spinal nerve trunk*. Except for the sacral nerves, whose ganglia lie within the sacral canal, most dorsal root ganglia lie in the intervertebral foramina.

Two exceptions should also be noted. Since there are no intervertebral foramina between the occiput and atlas nor between the atlas and axis, the first cervical nerve, which commonly lacks a ganglion, exits between the skull and atlas in the sulcus of the vertebral artery on the posterior arch of C-1 (Fig. 1–44). The second cervical nerve lies dorsal to the lateral atlantoaxial joint (Fig. 1–44) and the dorsal root ganglion lies medial to the nerve.

Meninges and Spaces

The spinal cord is enclosed and protected by three membranes (meninges): the outermost meninx is the tough spinal *dura mater*; an intermediate delicate, spiderweb-like *arachnoid mater*; and an inner delicate vascular meninx, the spinal *pia mater* (Figs. 1–42, 1–43).

Spinal Dura Mater

The outermost investment of the spinal cord, the spinal dura mater, is formed by a dense, tough, fibrous connective tissue. This sheath extends from the foramen magnum to approximately the level of the middle of the second sacral vertebra.

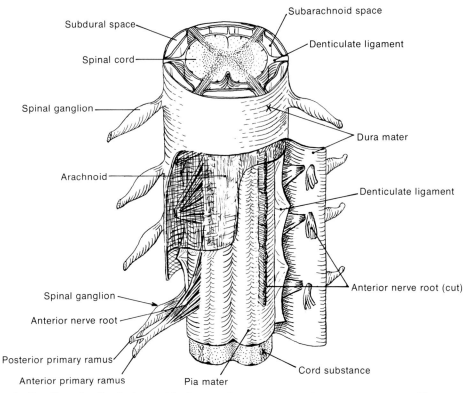

Figure 1–43. Longitudinal view with the meninges cut away in stages to expose filamentous rootlets and the pial denticulate ligament.

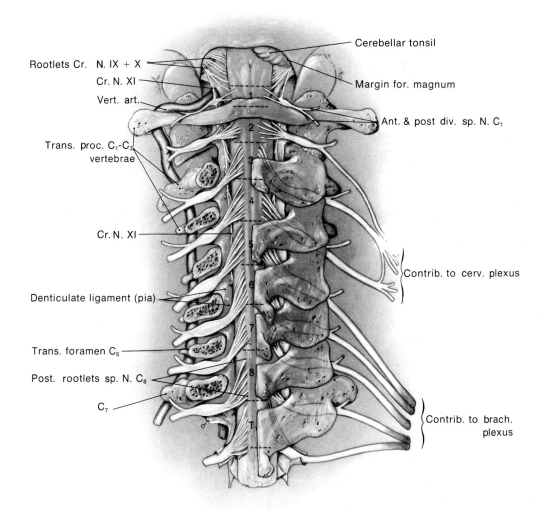

Figure 1–44. Dorsal view of cervical cord after laminectomy. The anterior division of the first cervical spinal nerve is seen crossing the dorsal arch of the atlas while the second crosses the atlanto-axial joint capsule. The eighth cervical emerges below C-7 while the seventh emerges above C-7. The vertebral artery is seen entering the transverse foramen at C-6. Observe the course of the eleventh *cranial nerve* (between dorsal and ventral rootlets) on the dorsal aspect of the pia denticulate ligament. It follows the last "tooth" of this "ligament" into the foramen magnum. (Numbers 1–8 and T_1 mark spinal cord segments.)

It corresponds with the inner meningeal layer of the cranial dura mater. The outer periosteal layer of the cranial dura is represented below the foramen magnum as the periosteum lining the vertebral canal. The inner and outer layers of cranial dura are tightly fused except at intervals for venous sinuses, or where the inner layer dips down between cerebral convolutions. However, there is a space, the extradural space, between the spinal dura mater and the periosteum of the vertebrae (Fig. 1–42). Connective tissue trabeculae bridging this space partially anchor the dura to the vertebral canal walls.

At the foramen magnum, the spinal dura mater is attached to its circumference and below it is firmly attached to the bodies of the axis and the third cervical vertebra and to the posterior longitudinal ligament.

Spinal nerves passing through intervertebral foramina are sheathed by prolongations of the spinal dura mater (Fig. 1–43). These dural sheaths are anchored to the walls of the intervertebral foramen.

The spinal dural sac terminates at about the middle of the second sacral vertebra; however, the dura continues caudally, invested over the filum terminale as the external terminal filum (Fig. 1–40 C). It descends to attach to the back of the coccyx.

Extradural (Epidural) Space

Between the walls of the vertebral canal and the spinal dura mater lies the extradural (epidural) space. The space contains areolar connective tissue, portions of the internal vertebral venous plexuses, and some branches of spinal arteries.

The extradural space is extended for a short distance with the spinal nerves to the intervertebral foramina.

The schematic diagrams, Figures 1–42 and 1–43, show this space to be about equal in size ventrally and dorsally. It is merely a slit-like space in life and, indeed, the ventral and dorsal parts of this space are related to the degree of filling of the vertebral venous plexuses. The extradural space increases ventrally in the lumbosacral region and may occupy more than half of the cross-sectional area of the vertebral canal.

Subdural Space

The subdural space (Fig. 1–43) is a potential space situated between the smooth inner surface of the spinal dura mater and the arachnoid mater. This potential space contains a thin film of serous fluid to keep its surfaces moist. It is penetrated by an occasional trabecula of connective tissue and some small veins (Fig. 1–42).

Cranially the subdural space is continuous with a similar space within the cranium. Caudally it becomes totally obliterated where the dura and arachnoid fuse at the external terminal filum.

Spinal Arachnoid Mater

Situated between the spinal dura mater and the innermost meninx, the pia mater, is the spinal arachnoid mater (Figs. 1–42, 1–43). This thin, avascular, transparent membrane is as loose and as delicate as a spider's web. It is separated from the spinal dura mater by the subdural space and from the pia mater by the cerebrospinal-fluid-filled subarachnoid space. This space is crossed by numerous filamentous arachnoidal trabeculae.

Cranially the arachnoid mater is continuous with the cranial arachnoid, investing the brain through the foramen magnum. Caudally it surrounds the cauda equina and terminates with the dura at the second sacral vertebra where it is pierced by the internal terminal filum. Laterally on each side, it is prolonged as arachnoidal pouches within the dural sheaths for a short distance over the spinal roots (Fig. 1–43).

Subarachnoid Space

The subarachnoid space (Fig. 1–43), situated between the spinal arachnoid mater and spinal pia mater, deserves our special attention. It contains the circulating cerebrospinal fluid, and it is in direct communication with the subarachnoid space in the cranium.

Depending upon the configuration of the spinal cord at its various levels, the subarachnoid space varies in size and shape. It is particularly small in the midthoracic region, where the spinal cord is also small, enlarging in those regions of the cervical and lumbar enlargements.

Laterally, the subarachnoid space accompanies the spinal nerve roots in dural sleeves as far as the inner margins of the intervertebral foramina. Below the conus medullaris, the subarachnoid space is large as it surrounds the cauda equina. This region, the lumbar cistern (Fig. 1–40 C), is the favored site to perform a spinal tap.

The *caudal sac* of the subarachnoid space usually ends at about the second sacral vertebra but this is variable. The sac assumes many shapes — wide, conical, and blunted.

Denticulate ligaments incompletely divide the subarachnoid space into anterior and posterior compartments (Figs. 1–42, 1–43). As we will see shortly, these denticulate ligaments arise from the pia mater on either side of the cord and fuse with the arachnoid and dura mater to hold the spinal cord in position within the vertebral canal.

The anterior subarachnoid space is uniform in caliber except for two locations. It is widest at the level of the atlas (C-1) and it is smallest at the level of the lumbar enlargement of the spinal cord.

Dividing the posterior subarachnoid space is an incomplete longitudinal subarachnoid septum that connects the pia and arachnoid along the medial sulcus of the spinal cord.

It should be noted that blood vessels that will supply the substance of the spinal cord and drain it lie within the subarachnoid space directly upon its next investment, the spinal pia mater.

Spinal Pia Mater

The spinal pia mater (Figs. 1–42, 1–43) is actually a two-layered membrane. The inner, circular, reticular layer tightly invests the spinal cord and nerve rootlets. It passes into the anterior median sulcus (fissure) of the spinal cord and ventrally forms the longitudinal median septum.

The outer layer of connective tissue is highly vascular and forms a network of longitudinal collagenous bands. Ventrally some of these bands form a glistening band, the linea splendens, which invests the anterior spinal artery along the median plane. Below, it continues as the internal terminal filum (Fig. 1–40 C). A few strands of collagenous fibers cross the subarachnoid space at intervals.

Laterally, on each side of the spinal cord, another group of pial collagenous bundles forms the denticulate ligament. The lateral edge of this ligament is free except at the 20 to 21 triangular processes (dentations) that continue further laterally to fuse with the arachnoid and dura, thereby anchoring the spinal cord and preventing its undue rotation.

Figure 1–44 shows the highest attachment of the denticulate ligament at the level of the foramen magnum situated between the hypoglossal nerve rootlets and the vertebral artery. The remaining processes are found anchored at intervals between. The dentations of the denticulate ligaments increase in size caudally. They are situated at short intervals in the cervical region, and the longest intervals are in the thoracic and lumbar regions. The last pair of dentations is situated either below the last thoracic nerve or between the last two thoracic nerves. Because of this variation, the last denticulation cannot be used as an absolute landmark. Further caudally, the denticulate ligament continues into the filum terminale.

The exact attachment of the denticulate ligament to the spinal cord is also variable. It attaches between the dorsal and ventral nerve roots but it may attach laterally or slightly dorsolaterally.

As a rule, the ligament anchors bilaterally by attaching to the dura between dorsal and ventral roots. Since there are only 20 to 21 dentations for lateral attachment, this cannot occur at every cord segment.

The posterior aspect of the longitudinal denticulate band is used by the fibers of the spinal portion of the spinal accessory nerve to reach the foramen magnum. This part of the eleventh cranial nerve is then conducted cranialward between dorsal and ventral rootlets, and it follows the uppermost "tooth" of the ligament into the cranium.

The anterior aspect of the denticulate ligament can be used to guide the scalpel to the lateral spinothalamic tract area in performing tractotomies for the relief of intractable pain (Fig. 1–45 A).

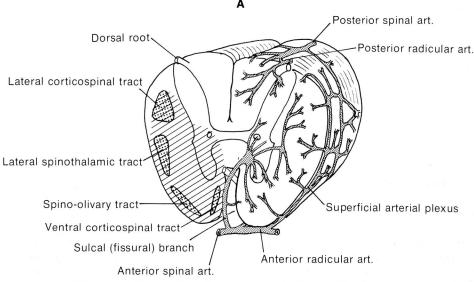

A

Dorsal root

Posterior spinal art.

Posterior radicular art.

Lateral corticospinal tract

Lateral spinothalamic tract

Spino-olivary tract

Ventral corticospinal tract

Sulcal (fissural) branch

Anterior spinal art.

Superficial arterial plexus

Anterior radicular art.

Figure 1–45. A, Schema of distribution of arteries to spinal cord. Shaded area represents distribution of anterior spinal artery. (Actually, lateral corticospinal tract lies lower and more medial in dorsolateral funiculus of white matter than sketched here.)

Illustration and legend continued on the following page.

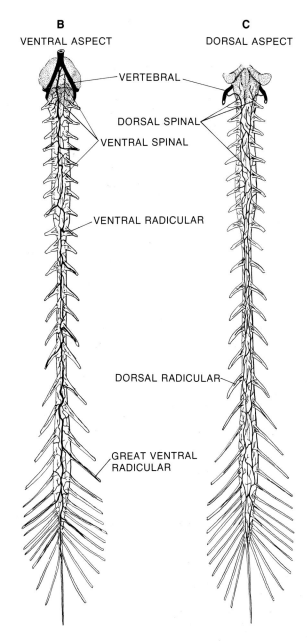

B
VENTRAL ASPECT

C
DORSAL ASPECT

—VERTEBRAL—

DORSAL SPINAL

VENTRAL SPINAL

VENTRAL RADICULAR

DORSAL RADICULAR—

GREAT VENTRAL
RADICULAR

Figure 1–45 Continued. B, C, Arterial supply of spinal cord from ventral (*B*) and dorsal aspects (*C*). Observe variation in size and frequent absence of radicular arteries at different levels.

BLOOD SUPPLY OF THE SPINAL CORD (SPINAL MEDULLA)

Arteries

The spinal cord is supplied in part by one anterior spinal artery and two posterior spinal arteries (Fig. 1–45 *A, B*). The *anterior spinal artery,* descending in the anterior median fissure (sulcus) of the spinal cord, arises from the vertebral arteries after they have entered the foramen magnum.

The smaller *posterior spinal arteries* coursing downward along the posterolateral sulci of the spinal cord arise either from the vertebral arteries or from the posterior inferior cerebellar arteries.

Since the anterior and posterior spinal arteries of the cord are not large and may often be irregular and incomplete, they are reinforced at irregular intervals by *radicular arteries,* branches of the intermediate (middle) division of the topographically nearest spinal arteries outside of the vertebral col-

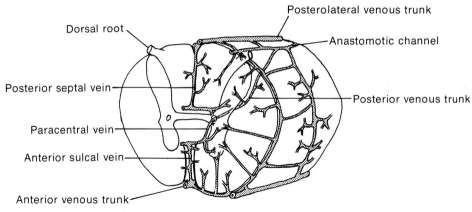

Dorsal root

Posterolateral venous trunk

Anastomotic channel

Posterior septal vein

Posterior venous trunk

Paracentral vein

Anterior sulcal vein

Anterior venous trunk

A

B
VENTRAL ASPECT

C
DORSAL ASPECT

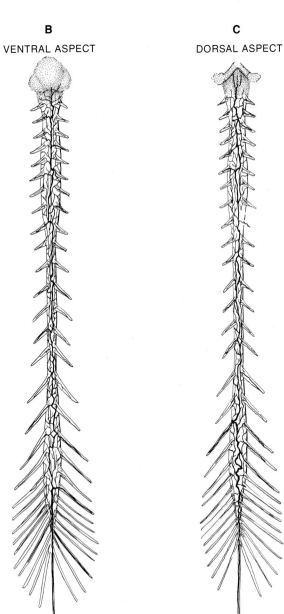

Figure 1–46. A, Schema of venous supply of spinal cord. B, C, Veins of the spinal cord in ventral and dorsal aspect. Observe extreme variation in size of radicular veins. Some common sites of emergence of the larger venous twigs are shown in respect to laterality.

umn (Fig. 1–45 *C*). About six to eight anterior radicular arteries[2] reinforce the anterior spinal artery of the spinal cord. The largest is the great radicular artery (of Adamkiewicz), which usually arises from the intercostal or lumbar arteries somewhere between T-10 and L-2 and usually on the left side of the body. Five to eight posterior radicular arteries aid the posterior spinal arteries of the cord. Anastomotic channels between the anterior and posterior spinal arteries of the spinal cord are greater in the cervical and lumbar regions than in the thoracic area.

Veins

The veins of the spinal cord are located within the pia mater. This venous plexus has six longitudinal channels: one near the anterior median fissure (sulcus), another behind the posterior median fissure of the cord, and four longitudinal veins running dorsal to the nerve roots (Fig. 1–46 *A, B*). These spinal cord veins drain into the intervertebral veins, which in turn communicate with the internal and external vertebral plexuses.

REFERENCES

1. Gardner, E., Gray, D. J., and O'Rahilly. R.: Anatomy. Philadelphia, W. B. Saunders Co., 4th Ed., 1975.
2. Hollingshead, W. H.: Anatomy for Surgeons. Vol. 3, The Back and Limbs. New York, Harper & Row, 1969.
3. Köhler, A., and Zimmer, E. A.: Borderlands of the Normal and Early Pathologic in Skeletal Roentgenology. Translated and edited by S. P. Wilk. New York, Grune & Stratton, 1968.
4. Schmorl, G., and Junghanns, H.: The Human Spine in Health and Disease, 2nd Amer. Ed. Translated and edited by E. F. Besemann. New York, Grune & Stratton, 1971.
5. Keith, A.: Human Embryology and Morphology, 6th ed. Baltimore, Williams & Wilkins, 1948.
6. Batson, O. V.: The function of the vertebral veins and their role in the spread of metastases. Ann. Surg., *112*:138, 1940.
7. Sensenig, E. C.: The early development of the human vertebral column. Contr. Embryol. Carneg. Instn., *33*:21, 1949.
8. Arey, L. B.: Developmental Anatomy — A Textbook and Laboratory Manual of Embryology. Philadelphia, W. B. Saunders Co., Rev. 7th Ed., 1974.
9. Hamilton, W. J., Boyd, J. D., and Mossman, H. W.: Human Embryology, 3rd Ed. Baltimore, Williams & Wilkins, 1962.
10. Arey, H. B.: The history of the first somite in human embryos. Contr. Embryol. Carneg. Instn., *27*:235, 1938.
11. McRae, D. L.: Craniovertebral junction. *In* Radiology of the Skull and Brain. Edited by Newton, T. H., and Potts, D. G. St. Louis, C. V. Mosby Co., 1971.
12. Elliott, H. C.: Cross-sectional diameters and areas of the human spinal cord. Anat. Rec., *93*:287, 1945.
13. Aeby, C.: Die Ältersverschiedenheiten der menschlichen Wirbelsäule. Arch. f. Anat. u. Physiol. (Anat. Abt.), 1879.

GENERAL REFERENCES

14. Anson, B. J. (Ed.): Morris' Human Anatomy, 12th Ed., New York, McGraw-Hill, 1966.
15. Becker, R. F., Wilson, J. W., and Gehweiler, J. A.: The Anatomical Basis of Medical Practice. Baltimore, Williams & Wilkins, 1971.
16. Goss, C. M. (Ed.): Gray's Anatomy, 28th Ed., Philadelphia, Lea & Febiger, 1967.
17. Grant, J. C. B., and Basmajian, J. V.: Grant's Method of Anatomy, Baltimore, Williams & Wilkins, 1965.
18. Lockhart, R. D., Hamilton, G. F., and Fyfe, F. W.: Anatomy of the Human Body, Philadelphia, Lippincott, 1965.
19. Romanes, G. S. (Ed.): Cunningham's Textbook of Anatomy, 10th Ed., London, Oxford University Press, 1964.

Chapter 2

JOINTS AND LIGAMENTS

INTRODUCTION

The articular system of the vertebral column is composed of a series of joints and supporting ligaments. With the exception of the special joints situated between the occiput and the atlas and between the atlas and axis, two series of joints unite the individual vertebrae.

Between the vertebral bodies are slightly movable *(amphiarthrodial) joints*, or *symphyses*. A symphysis is a joint consisting of fibrocartilage, usually a disk, held in place by ligaments. A thin lamina of hyaline cartilage separates the disk fibrocartilage from the bone above and below. Such slightly movable joints exist only between the vertebral bodies and between the two pubic bones — that is, the pubic symphysis.

Fibrocartilaginous menisci or small disks generally found in diarthrodial (freely movable) joints should not be considered as symphyses. The "symphysis menti" and the "basioccipital symphysis" are not true symphyses, as fibrocartilage is not involved in these structures.

Freely movable *synovial joints (diarthroses)* of the gliding variety (arthrodial) unite the adjacent vertebral arches. We will call them the *apophyseal joints* (zygapophyseal joints, facet joints, and small joints are synonymous).

All movable joints are enclosed in fibrous capsules lined by a synovial membrane that secretes a synovial fluid into the smooth-lined capsule. These joints may contain fibrocartilaginous menisci or disks separating the ends of opposing bones.

The joint surfaces in a gliding type synovial joint are relatively flat. Movement is permitted by the lax articular capsule and limited by ligaments and osseous processes surrounding the articulation.

Movement between adjacent vertebral bodies is more limited than movement between the articular processes at the apophyseal joints. In the amphiarthrodial joints of the spine, movement is largely dependent upon disk thickness. It follows, then, that movement is freest in the cervical and lumbar regions where the intervertebral disks are the thickest.

While ligaments have no ability to contract like muscles, in life they are somewhat pliant. Yet, they serve as restraints to movement.

ARTICULATIONS BETWEEN THE VERTEBRAL BODIES

The Intervertebral Disks

The fibrocartilaginous *intervertebral disks* are the major connecting bond between adjacent vertebral bodies (Fig. 2–1). The most cranial disk is found between the second and third cervical vertebrae. Remnants of disk tissue are reportedly found in the subdental synchondrosis and in the apical ligament of the dens.[1] We usually think of the most caudal disk as being at the lumbosacral junction, but disks may persist in the adult between the upper sacral segments. Rudimentary disks are often found at the sacrococcygeal junction and between successive coccygeal segments.

The intervertebral disk spaces have varying heights during growth. In the newborn, the disk space is almost equal to the height of the centrum of the vertebra. This 1:1 ratio gradually changes with age; in the adult, the intervertebral disk space is about one-third to one-fourth the height of the vertebral body.

In the cervical region, the intervertebral

disks are taller ventrally than dorsally. They are responsible for the ventral convex cervical curvature (lordosis). While the disks in the thoracic and lumbar regions conform to the cranial and caudal surfaces of the vertebral bodies, this does not apply in the cervical region. The width of cervical intervertebral disks is decreased owing to the presence of the uncinate process adjoining the cranial surface of the third to the seventh cervical vertebrae.

We have established that the thoracic curvature is due to the shape of the vertebral bodies, which are slightly less tall ventrally than dorsally. The intervertebral disks are equal in height ventrally and dorsally; however, they are not of uniform height throughout the thoracic spine. Disks are thinner in the less mobile upper thoracic region.

Intervertebral disks in the lumbar spine are wedge-shaped and are thicker ventrally than dorsally. While these disks contribute to the lumbar curvature, they are aided, in part, in the lower lumbar region by the shape of the vertebral bodies.

The intervertebral disks are described by anatomists as consisting of two parts: the outer laminated portion, the *anulus fibrosus* (old, inaccurate spelling — annulus), and the inner core, or *nucleus pulposus* (Fig. 2–1). Many insist that the hyaline cartilaginous plates on the cranial and caudal surfaces of the vertebral bodies must be considered an integral part of the intervertebral disk.[2, 3]

The cartilaginous plates function with the anulus fibrosus to contain the nucleus pulposus, which is maintained in a state of constant turgor. If the plates remain intact, the nucleus pulposus is prevented from herniating into the vertebral body.

In the fetus, blood vessels supply the disk from the periphery of the anulus fibrosus and from adjacent vertebral bodies. In the latter case the vessels extend through the cartilage plates but do not reach the nucleus pulposus. Shortly after birth these vessels begin to degenerate and they are completely obliterated by age four.[3]

Anulus Fibrosus

The peripheral zone of the intervertebral disk is the fibrocartilaginous *anulus fibrosus* (Figs. 2–1, 2–2). Fibrous tissue predominates in the anulus. Its fibers are arranged in concentric rings; the alternating obliquity of fiber alignment in each ring acts to check motion between the vertebral bodies in various directions.

Superficial fibers of the anulus fibrosus blend into the anterior and posterior longitudinal ligaments. Some of the fibers of the anulus pass over the cartilaginous plates as *Sharpey's fibers* to attach firmly to the bony rim of the body. Deeper fibers insert directly into the hyaline cartilaginous plates.

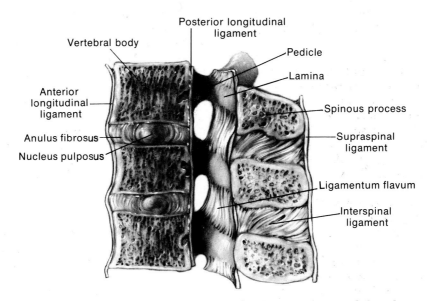

Figure 2–1.   Median sagittal section of three lumbar vertebrae and their ligaments.

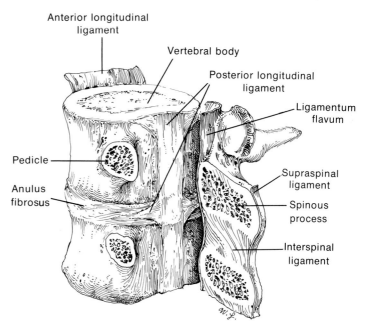

Figure 2-2. Ligaments of the lumbar spine viewed from behind, with the vertebral arch partially removed.

Except in the young person, the nucleus pulposus and the anulus fibrosus blend with each other. A sagittal section through an intervertebral disk shows that the nucleus pulposus is not located centrally in the disk but rather slightly dorsal of the center (Fig. 2–1). The anulus fibrosus is thereby thicker ventrally than dorsally. Strong, thick fibers of the anterior longitudinal ligament strengthen the anulus ventrally. Dorsally the anulus is strengthened by the posterior longitudinal ligament in the midline and to

a lesser extent dorsolaterally (Figs. 2–2, 2–3).

Nucleus Pulposus

The *nucleus pulposus* and anulus fibrosus are derived embryologically from the notochord. In infancy the nucleus pulposus is soft and gelatinous, quite large in relation to the anulus fibrosus, and contains many notochordal cells. These notochordal cells gradually disappear with increasing age,

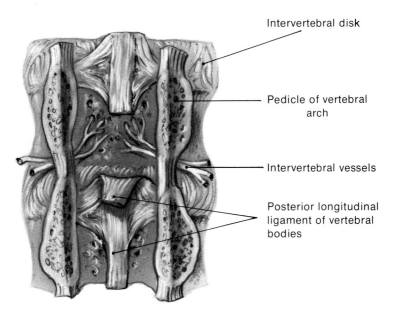

Figure 2-3. Posterior view of the posterior longitudinal ligament. Vertebral arches have been removed.

and surrounding fibrocartilaginous tissues invade their boundaries. The anulus fibrosus grows more rapidly, and the nucleus becomes proportionately smaller.

With aging of the intervertebral disk tissues, a definite decrease in water content occurs. In newborns, the water content of the anulus is 78 per cent and that of the nucleus pulposus is 88 per cent. By the third decade of life, the anulus fibrosus contains 70 per cent water; the nucleus pulposus contains 76 per cent water. For the duration of life, the water content of the anulus remains rather constant at 70 per cent, while the water content of the nucleus pulposus diminishes slowly until it reaches that of the anulus.[2]

Luschka (Uncovertebral) "Joints" or Fissures

A storm of controversy surrounds the joints first described by von Luschka[4] in 1858. Synovial joints were described in that portion of the intervertebral disk situated between the uncinate process and the beveled undersurface of the cervical vertebra above (Figs. 2–4, 2–13). Rathke disputed the concept that true synovial joints were present, and since then the literature has

been filled with arguments. Most authors dispute von Luschka's concept but a few support the original description.[5-14]

Luschka joints have also been termed the *uncovertebral joints; lateral intervertebral half-joints; lateral interbody joints; covertebral joints; lateral intervertebral joints; and uncinate joints.*

Most authorities now agree that Luschka "joints" are actually fissures that do not contain true synovial linings. These fissures are not present at birth. They form in the first decade of life, at about four to seven years of age, and are first seen within the anulus fibrosus near the developing uncinate processes. These clefts enlarge and, eventually, reach the nucleus pulposus. The uncovertebral fissures are felt to represent a functional adaptation by the intervertebral disks to the increased mobility of the cervical vertebrae at the time that the uncinate processes are reaching their full height.

Reactive vertebral body changes (osteophytes) occur in the region of the uncovertebral fissures. These changes are most often seen in the lower cervical vertebrae in association with disk degeneration. They may attain clinical significance if they encroach upon nearby spinal nerves or the vertebral artery (Fig. 2–4).

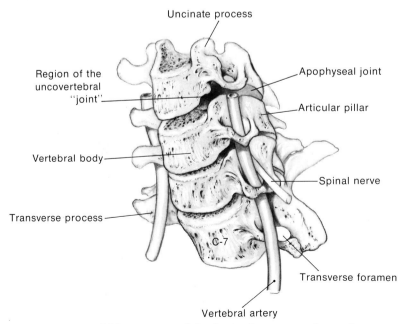

Figure 2–4. Oblique view of the lower four cervical vertebrae.

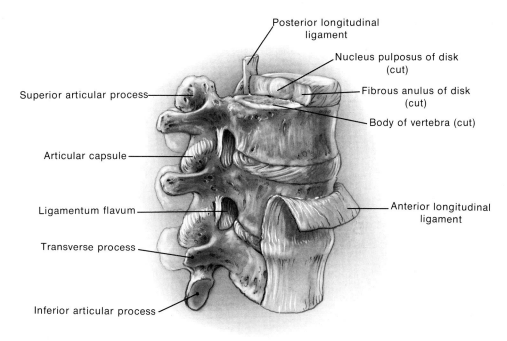

Figure 2–5. Anterior oblique view of the ligaments of the lumbar spine.

Figure 2–6. Anterior view of the anterior longitudinal ligament and the ligamenta flava.

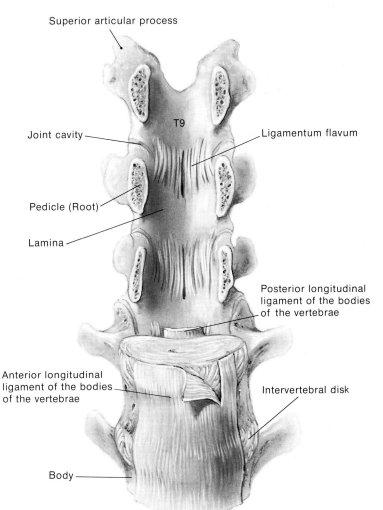

Anterior Longitudinal Ligament

This strong ligamentous band is situated over the ventral and ventrolateral surfaces of the vertebral bodies (Figs. 2–1, 2–5, 2–6). It is narrowest at its attachment to the basilar part of the occipital bone of the skull (Fig. 2–13). From this point, it widens as it descends and terminates on the pelvic surface of the sacrum.

The anterior longitudinal ligament is thicker in the thoracic region than in the cervical or lumbar regions of the vertebral column. It is thickest over the concavity of each vertebral body ventrally, where it is firmly attached, blending with the periosteum.

The anterior longitudinal ligament consists of dense longitudinal, collagenous fibers arranged in layers of several lengths; each layer is interlaced with the others. The deepest fibers, connecting adjacent vertebrae, bind the ligament loosely to the disk and to the rim margins of the vertebral body. Intermediate fibers span two or three vertebrae, while the most superficial fibers extend over four or five vertebrae. At the sides of the vertebral bodies, a few fibers connect adjacent vertebrae and have sometimes been called *lateral ligaments*.

Posterior Longitudinal Ligament

This ligament lies on the dorsal surface of the vertebral bodies within the vertebral canal (Figs. 2–1, 2–3, 2–6). It attaches to the body of the axis, where it is continuous with the tectorial membrane, which covers the dens and attaches to the occipital bone (Fig. 2–11A). Caudally the posterior longitudinal ligament continues onto the ventral wall of the sacral canal.

The posterior longitudinal ligament, unlike the anterior longitudinal ligament, is firmly bound to the intervertebral disks but it is separated from the vertebral bodies by venous plexuses. Like the anterior longitudinal ligament, it consists of fibers of varying lengths. The deepest of these fibers span adjacent vertebrae, while the longest extend over several vertebrae.

In the cervical region, the posterior longitudinal ligament is broad but takes on a different configuration in the remainder of the presacral spine. Remaining narrow over the middle of the vertebral bodies, it widens over the disk spaces (Fig. 2–3). These lateral extensions over the disks are much thinner than the central portion of the ligament. This may account, in part, for the larger number of disk herniations that occur dorsolaterally than occur centrally.

ARTICULATIONS OF THE VERTEBRAL ARCHES

Apophyseal Joints

Between the superior and inferior articular processes of adjacent vertebrae are synovial joints. We will call them the *apophyseal joints* (Fig. 2–4).

Attached not to the margins of the facets but to the outer surfaces of the articular processes of these apophyseal joints is a thin, fibrous articular capsule that has a synovial lining. To allow greater mobility, these articular capsules are looser in the cervical spine than in either the thoracic or lumbar regions.

The articular surfaces of the apophyseal joints are covered by hyaline cartilage. Between these articular surfaces are interposed meniscus-like tabs (Haversian glands or fat pads) of synovium that project inward from the capsule.[3, 15] They are thought to function as shock absorbers that allow for changing pressures within the joint. Since nature abhors a vacuum, these meniscus tabs or disks glide in and out of the joint. If a meniscus becomes incarcerated within an apophyseal joint, the joint locks; that is, motion is severely reduced and the joint becomes painful.

Ligamenta Flava

The *ligamenta flava* are paired ligaments connecting the laminae (Figs. 2–1, 2–5, 2–6, 2–7). Their name refers to their yellowish color, due to their high elastin content. After removal of the bodies of several vertebrae (Fig. 2–6), the right and left ligamenta flava may be seen to greatest advantage. They are heavy, flattened bands that arise from the ventral surface of the lower lamina and attach onto the upper part of the dorsal surface of the next succeeding lamina. In the midline they are separated at intervals by

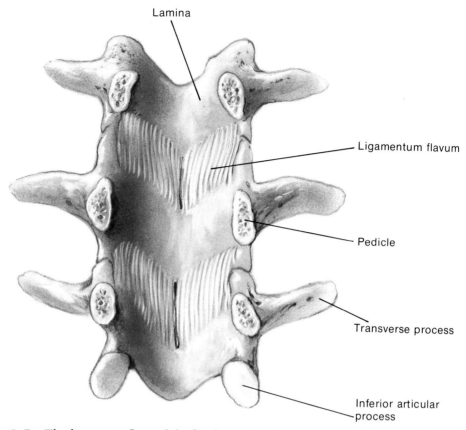

Figure 2-7. The ligamenta flava of the lumbar spine. Anterior aspect. The vertebral bodies have been removed.

the passage of veins from the posterior internal and external vertebral venous plexuses. Laterally the ligamenta flava extend to the articular capsules about the apophyseal joints and blend with them (Figs. 2–5, 2–6).

With the vertebral column in the neutral position these ligaments are under tension. They stretch to allow flexion of the spine with separation of the laminae. When the spine returns to the normal position, they are not folded. In extension, however, the laminae closely approach each other and the ligamenta flava are heaped up into folds.

Supraspinal (Supraspinous) Ligament

This ligament, composed of thin bundles of fibrous tissue, courses over the tips of the spinous processes of the vertebrae. Short fibers of this ligament connect adjacent spinous processes, while longer ones span several vertebrae to connect the spines. They probably do not exist in the lumbar region. Deep fibers blend with those of the interspinal (interspinous) ligament laterally. In the cervical region, the supraspinal ligament becomes continuous with the nuchal ligament.

The *nuchal ligament* (Fig. 2–8), the cervical counterpart of the supraspinal ligament, is a fibroelastic septum separating the dorsal muscles of the neck to each side. Its dorsal border runs between the external occipital protuberance and the seventh cervical spinous process. Deep fibers attach to the posterior tubercle of the atlas and to all of the spinous processes in the cervical region.

In man the nuchal ligament is by no means as heavily elastic in its composition as it is in the necks of grazing animals. These animals have more elastin in their nuchal ligaments. All other ligaments relat-

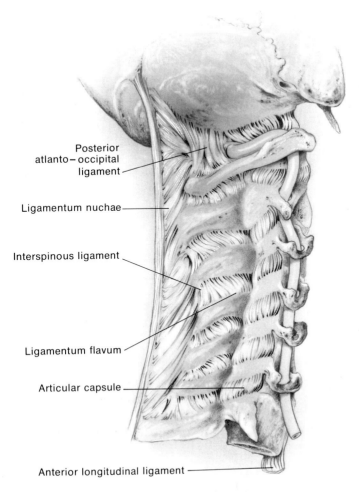

Posterior
atlanto–occipital
ligament

Ligamentum nuchae

Interspinous ligament

Ligamentum flavum

Articular capsule

Anterior longitudinal ligament

Figure 2–8. Posterior oblique view of the ligamentous structures of the cervical vertebral column.

ed to the vertebral column are collagenous in composition (except the ligamenta flava).

At times the nuchal ligament is partly ossified — "ossicula nuchae" (Fig. 2–9 *A*). Such ossifications usually have a smooth outline and should not be mistaken for fractures of the spinous processes. Spinous process fractures usually occur near their bases at the junction with the lamina (Fig. 2–9*B*).

Interspinal (Interspinous) Ligament

This ligament is quite thin and may, in some regions of the vertebral column, actually disappear. The fibers connect adjacent spinous processes. They extend from the root of one spinous process to the apex of the next (Figs. 2–1, 2–8). With advancing age they frequently degenerate — thus iso-

lated tears after trauma are of questionable clinical significance.

Intertransverse Ligaments

Between the transverse processes are interposed fibers that make up the *intertransverse ligaments*. In the cervical region they are sparse, and consist of only a few scattered fibers. They are better developed in the thoracic region, where they are intimately connected with the deep back muscles (Fig. 2–14). In the lumbar region, they are only thin membranous strands.

ATLANTOAXIAL JOINTS

The atlantoaxial articulation is composed of three synovial joints: paired lateral joints and a middle (median) atlantoaxial joint.

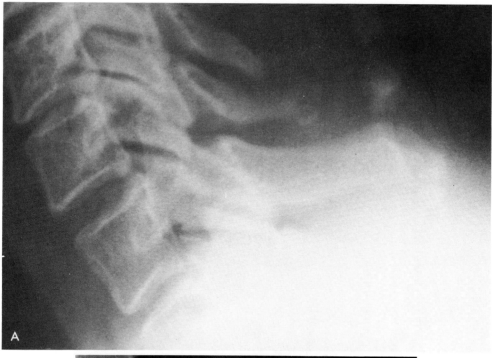

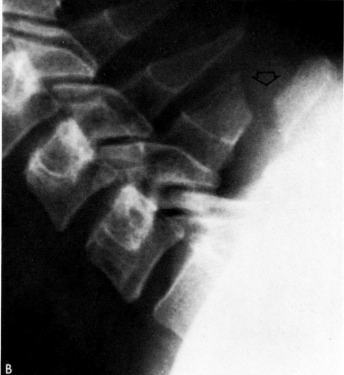

Figure 2-9. A, Ossified nuchal ligament dorsal to the spinous processes of the lower cervical vertebrae. B, Fracture of a spinous process in the lower cervical column (arrow). Note the jagged edges at the fracture site.

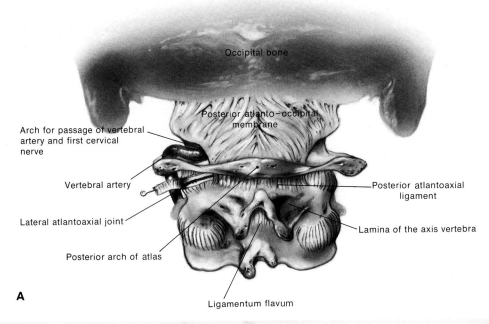

Occipital bone

Posterior atlanto–occipital membrane

Arch for passage of vertebral artery and first cervical nerve

Vertebral artery

Posterior atlantoaxial ligament

Lateral atlantoaxial joint

Lamina of the axis vertebra

Posterior arch of atlas

A

Ligamentum flavum

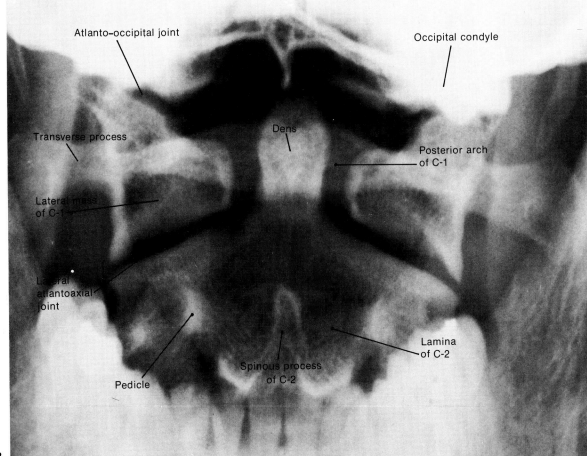

Atlanto–occipital joint

Occipital condyle

Transverse process

Dens

Posterior arch of C-1

Lateral mass of C-1

Lateral atlantoaxial joint

Lamina of C-2

Pedicle

Spinous process of C-2

B

Figure 2–10. *A*, Ligaments of the occipito-atlanto-axial region viewed from behind. *B*, Radiograph of the atlanto-occipital and atlantoaxial joints; anteroposterior view taken through the open mouth. Note the lateral inclination of the atlantoaxial joints.

Lateral Atlantoaxial Joints

These joints are situated between the superior articular surface of the axis and the inferior articular facet of the atlas on each side (Figs. 2–10, 2–13). They are inclined laterally and inferiorly up to about 20° and therefore may not be seen on lateral radiographs. They are best evaluated on the open mouth view (Fig. 2–10 B).

The articular surfaces of these synovial joints are covered by cartilage and surrounded by an articular capsule of fibrous tissue lined by synovium. Although the capsules are loose and thin, they are strengthened posteromedially by the accessory atlantoaxial ligament. This ligament arises from the posterior aspect of the body of the axis near the base of the dens and courses cranially and medially to the inside of the lateral mass of the atlas near the transverse ligament origin (Fig. 2–12A).

Middle (Median) Atlantoaxial Joint

The articulation of the dens with the atlas, the *middle atlantoaxial joint*, is a pivot type joint with two small synovial cavities, each enclosed by a fibrous capsule with a synovial lining (Fig. 2–11 A, B). Between the facets on the posterior surface of the anterior arch of the atlas and that on the anterior surface of the dens is a small synovial cavity. Dorsally there is a larger synovial cavity situated between the dens and the transverse ligament of the atlas.

Ligaments related to the dens are the *tectorial membrane* and the *cruciform ligament* (Figs. 2–11 A, 2–12 A).

Tectorial Membrane

This is a broad band of fibers continuous with the posterior longitudinal ligament on the lower surface of the body of the axis (Fig. 2–11 A). It stretches cranially to attach upon the inner aspect of the base of the occiput and thereby covers over the dens and its other ligaments.

Cruciform (Cruciate) Ligament of the Atlas

Ventral to the tectorial membrane lies the cruciform ligament (Figs. 2–11, 2–12). Its strong, clinically important, transverse part is the *transverse ligament*. The transverse ligament attaches to small tubercles on the medial sides of the lateral masses of the atlas (Figs. 2–11 B, 2–12). It holds the dens against the anterior arch of the atlas. Situated between the transverse ligament and the posterior facet of the dens is a synovial joint.

The *vertical portion* of the cruciform ligament is composed of fibrous bundles coursing downward from the transverse ligament to attach to the body of the axis and coursing upward just inside the foramen magnum to attach to the occipital bone. In Figure 2–12 B, we can see the three ligaments radiating upward and outward from the dens. From the apex of the dens to the basion stretches the *apical ligament* of the dens. It is covered over by the upper extension of the cruciform ligament.

On each side of the apex of the dens are short, stout bands, the *alar (check) ligaments*, coursing cranially and laterally to attach to the medial side of the occipital condyles (Fig. 2–12 B).

ATLANTO-OCCIPITAL JOINTS AND MEMBRANES

The skull and atlas are bound together by synovial joints on each side of the foramen magnum, the atlanto-occipital joints (Fig. 2–12), and by the anterior and posterior atlanto-occipital membrane (Figs. 2–10A, 2–13).

Each *atlanto-occipital joint* is formed by the convex occipital condyle and the reciprocally concave superior articular surface of the atlas. They are enclosed by an articular capsule of fibrous tissue lined by synovium, which is attached to the margins of the articular surfaces. The articular capsule is thin and loose, and is often deficient medially, permitting free communication between the atlanto-occipital joints and the synovial joint between the dens and the transverse ligament of the atlas. These joints are reported to contain menisci also.[3, 15]

The broad, dense, fibrous *anterior atlanto-occipital membrane* (Fig. 2–13) attaches above to the anterior margin of the foramen magnum, and below to the anterior arch of the atlas. Centrally it is thickened

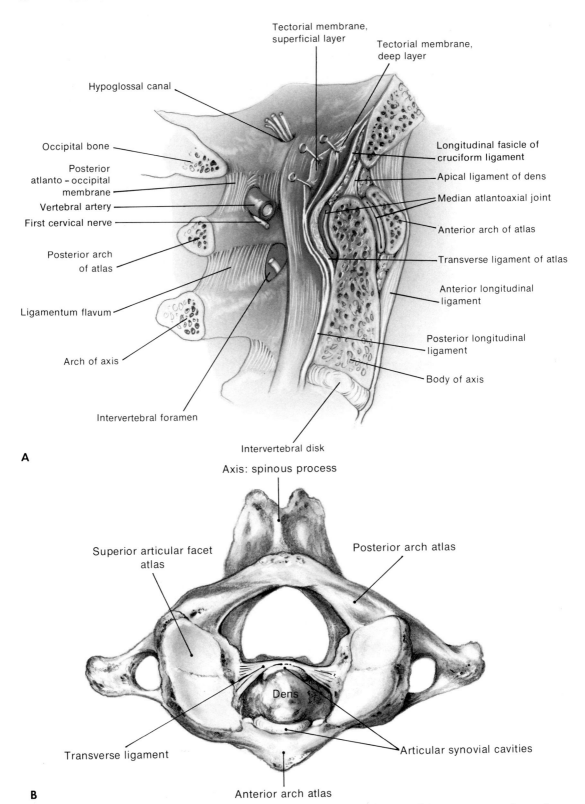

Figure 2–11. *A*, Median sagittal section through the occipital bone and first two cervical vertebrae. *B*, Atlas and axis articulated and viewed from above showing the transverse ligament and synovial joints about the dens.

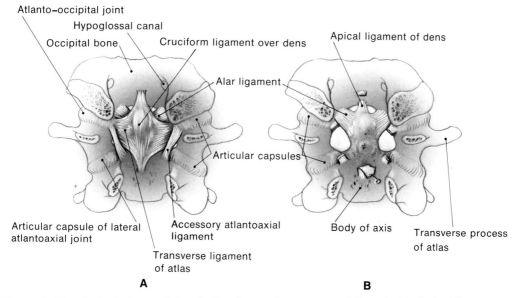

Atlanto–occipital joint

Hypoglossal canal

Occipital bone

Cruciform ligament over dens

Alar ligament

Apical ligament of dens

Articular capsules

Articular capsule of lateral atlantoaxial joint

Accessory atlantoaxial ligament

Body of axis

Transverse process of atlas

Transverse ligament of atlas

A

B

Figure 2–12. Articulations of the skull, atlas, and axis viewed from behind. *A*, After removal of the arches, and of the tectorial membrane and posterior longitudinal ligament. *B*, After removal of the cruciform ligament.

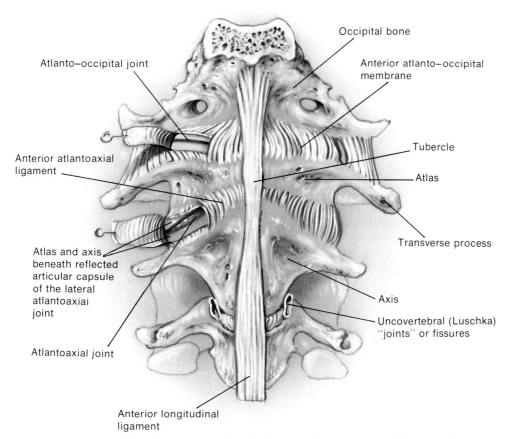

Occipital bone

Atlanto–occipital joint

Anterior atlanto–occipital membrane

Anterior atlantoaxial ligament

Tubercle

Atlas

Transverse process

Atlas and axis beneath reflected articular capsule of the lateral atlantoaxial joint

Axis

Atlantoaxial joint

Uncovertebral (Luschka) "joints" or fissures

Anterior longitudinal ligament

Figure 2–13. The atlanto-occipital and atlantoaxial joints viewed from in front.

by fibers extending upward from the anterior longitudinal ligament. Laterally it blends with the articular capsules of the atlanto-occipital joints.

The *posterior atlanto-occipital membrane* is also broad but thin (Fig. 2–10 A). It is analogous to the ligamenta flava in its relation to the vertebral canal. The posterior atlanto-occipital membrane adheres to the posterior margin of the foramen magnum and below to the posterior arch of the atlas. It blends laterally with the articular capsules, and also arches over the sulcus of the vertebral artery. This membrane is pierced by the vertebral artery and the first cervical spinal nerve.

ARTICULATIONS OF THE RIBS TO THE VERTEBRAL COLUMN

All of the ribs articulate dorsally with the thoracic vertebrae. The typical ribs (two through nine or ten) articulate through their heads with two adjacent vertebrae and their intervening disk. Their articular tubercle also forms a joint with the transverse process of the lower of these vertebrae. The typical plan of articulation varies with respect to the first rib and the last two or three ribs.

Costovertebral Joints

Typical ribs have two *articular facets*, superior and inferior, on their heads that are separated by a crest (Fig. 2–14). Figure 2–14 shows the rib head articulated with the demifacets of the adjacent vertebrae. The rib crest is bound to the intervertebral disk by a short, stout *intra-articular ligament*, dividing the costovertebral joint into two separate synovial joints.

A thin, fibrous *articular capsule* surrounds the costovertebral joint. Ventrally this capsule is thickened by the fan-shaped *radiate ligament* of the head of the rib (Fig. 2–14). The radiate ligament extends medially from the ventral aspect of the rib head to the immediately adjacent vertebral bodies and their intervening disk. Dorsally the capsule merges with the lateral extensions of the posterior longitudinal ligament.

Costotransverse Joints

Figure 2–15 shows a typical articular tubercle of a rib in contact with the facet of the transverse process of the lower vertebra to which the rib head is joined. This small synovial *costotransverse joint* is surround-

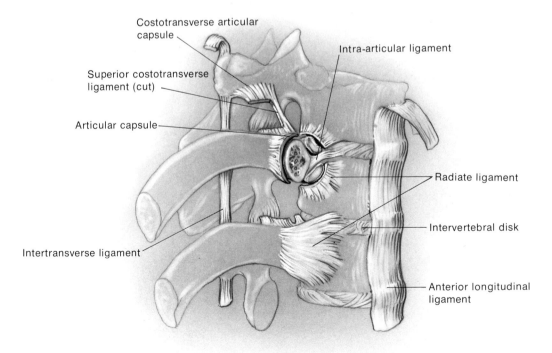

Figure 2–14. Anterior oblique view of the costovertebral articulations.

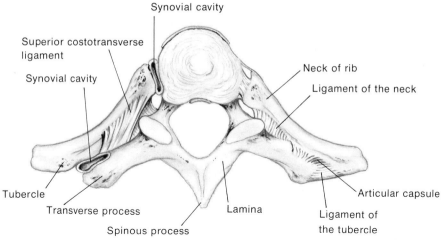

Synovial cavity

Superior costotransverse
ligament

Synovial cavity

Neck of rib

Ligament of the neck

Tubercle

Transverse process

Spinous process

Lamina

Articular capsule

Ligament of
the tubercle

Figure 2–15. The costovertebral and costotransverse articulations; cranial aspect.

ed by a thin articular capsule that is reinforced by the lateral costotransverse ligament dorsolaterally, which joins the tip of the transverse process to the articular tubercle.

Situated between the ventral margin of the transverse process and the dorsal margin of the neck of the rib, short fibers of the costotransverse ligament join rib to transverse process (Fig. 2–14). Each typical rib is also attached to the transverse process above by the *superior costotransverse ligament* (Figs. 2–14, 2–15) extending from the neck of the rib to the lower border of the transverse process.

Since the last two (or occasionally the last three) ribs do not have articular tubercles, they have no costotransverse joints. The heads of the first and the last two or three ribs have only a single facet for articulation with their corresponding vertebra. There are no intra-articular ligaments and thus these costovertebral synovial joints are single.

SACROILIAC JOINT AND ACCESSORY LIGAMENTS

Sacroiliac Joint

The sacrum and hip bone (*os coxa,* innominate bone) are united by the synovial *sacroiliac joint* and several heavy, strong *accessory ligaments* (Figs. 2–16, 2–17).

Between the articular surfaces of the sa-

crum and ilium is a sinuous synovial joint (Fig. 2–17 *A–C*), the sacroiliac joint. These articular surfaces are covered by hyaline cartilage on the sacral side, and by fibrocartilage on the iliac side. The sacroiliac joint has a fibrous capsule and a synovial lining.

The fibrous capsule of the sacroiliac joint is rather thin ventrally but thicker dorsally. The ventral part of the capsule is known as the *ventral (anterior) sacroiliac ligament,* which is a broad band separating the joint space from the pelvic cavity (Fig. 2–16 *A*). This ligament stretches from the sacral ala across the joint to the pelvic surface of the ilium.

Dorsally the fibrous capsule of the sacroiliac joint is stout and strong. Here the *interosseous sacroiliac ligaments* fill the gap between the roughened sacral and iliac tuberosities just behind the articular surfaces of the two bones (Fig. 2–17). Within the substance of this ligament, accessory sacroiliac synovial joints are commonly found.

Accessory sacroiliac joints occur in roughly 35 per cent of patients.[15] They are synovial joints formed either between the posterior superior iliac spine and the sacrum at the level of the second sacral foramen or at the level of the first sacral foramen between the sacral and iliac tuberosities (Fig. 2–18*A*). They often show osteoarthritic changes.

Superficial to the fibers of the interosseous sacroiliac ligament are the *dorsal (posterior) sacroiliac ligaments* (Fig. 2–16 *B*). Their fibers are directed almost verti-

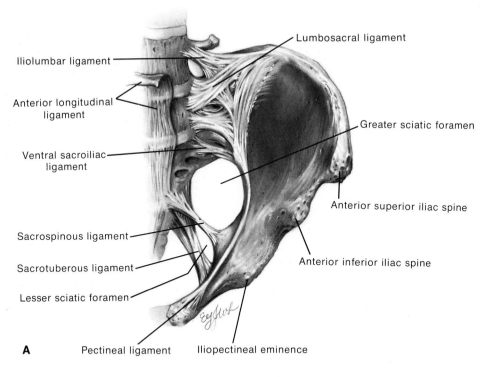

Iliolumbar ligament

Anterior longitudinal ligament

Ventral sacroiliac ligament

Sacrospinous ligament

Sacrotuberous ligament

Lesser sciatic foramen

A

Pectineal ligament

Lumbosacral ligament

Greater sciatic foramen

Anterior superior iliac spine

Anterior inferior iliac spine

Iliopectineal eminence

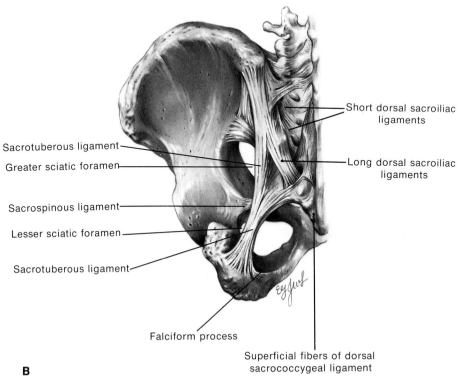

Sacrotuberous ligament

Greater sciatic foramen

Sacrospinous ligament

Lesser sciatic foramen

Sacrotuberous ligament

Falciform process

B

Short dorsal sacroiliac ligaments

Long dorsal sacroiliac ligaments

Superficial fibers of dorsal sacrococcygeal ligament

Figure 2–16. The joints and ligaments of the left side of the pelvis. *A*, Anterior aspect. *B*, Posterior aspect.

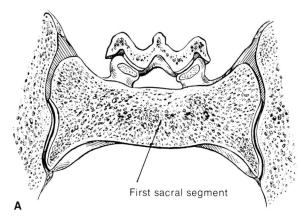

A

First sacral segment

Figure 2–17. Coronal sections through the sacrum and sacroiliac joints. *A*, Anterior sacral segment. *B*, Middle sacral segment. *C*, Posterior sacral segment. (After Gray, H.: Anatomy of the Human Body. Goss, C. M., editor. Philadelphia, Lea & Febiger, 1966.)

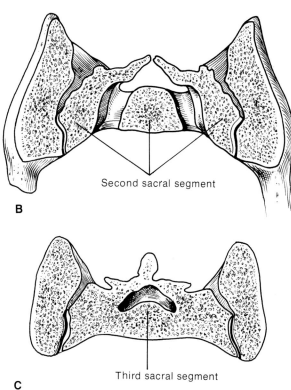

B

Second sacral segment

C

Third sacral segment

cally and connect the posterior superior iliac spine of the ilium to the lateral crest of the third and fourth segments of the sacrum. Here they blend with the *sacrotuberal (sacrotuberous) ligament* (Fig. 2–16 *B*).

Accessory Ligaments

The sacrotuberal (sacrotuberous) ligament has a broad attachment to the posterior superior and posterior inferior iliac spines, the lower three sacral segments, and the coccyx (Fig. 2–16 *B*). Note that it also blends with the fibers of the dorsal sacroiliac ligament. From this upper attachment the fibers converge as they pass downward and laterally toward the ischial tuberosity. Here they diverge to attach to the medial margin of the tuberosity and the lower margin of the ischial ramus. The sickle-shaped extension of these fibers to the ramus of the ischium is called the *falciform process.*

The *sacrospinal (sacrospinous) ligament* has a triangular shape (Fig. 2–16 *B*). Its base is attached to the lateral edge of the lower

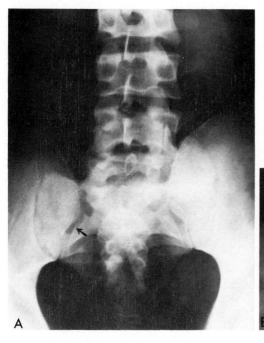
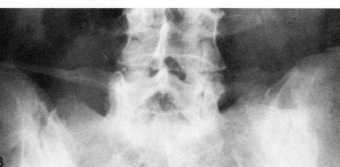

Figure 2–18. A, Accessory sacroiliac joints on the right (arrow) and left. B, Calcified iliolumbar ligament on the right.

sacral and upper coccygeal segments, and its apex is attached to the pelvic surface of the ischial spine.

The *iliolumbar ligament* arises from the transverse process of the fifth lumbar vertebra, and courses laterally to attach anterior to the sacroiliac joint on the inner surface of the ilium (Fig. 2–16 A, B). Some of its fibers blend with the ventral sacroiliac ligament. Calcification in the iliolumbar ligament may be mistaken for an elongated transverse process of the fifth lumbar vertebra (Fig. 2–18B).

REFERENCES

1. Keith, A.: Human Embryology and Morphology, 6th Ed., Baltimore, Williams & Wilkins, 1948.
2. Hollingshead, W. H.: Anatomy for Surgeons, Vol. 3, The Back and Limbs. New York, Harper & Row, 1969.
3. Schmorl, G., and Junghanns, H.: The Human Spine in Health and Disease, 2nd Amer. Ed. Translated and edited by E. F. Besemann. New York, Grune & Stratton, 1971.
4. Luschka, H.: Die Halbgelenke des menschlichen Körpers. Berlin, Reimer, 1858.
5. Boreadis, A. G., and Gershon-Cohen, J.: Luschka joints of the cervical spine. Radiology, 66:181, 1956.
6. Compère, E. L., Tachdjian, M. O., and Kernahan, W. T.: The Luschka joints: their anatomy, physiology and pathology. Orthopedics, 1:159, 1959.
7. Frykholm, R.: Lower cervical vertebrae and intervertebral discs: Surgical anatomy and pathology. Acta. Chir. Scand., 101:345, 1951.
8. Hadley, L. A.: The covertebral articulations and cervical foramen encroachment. J. Bone and Jt. Surg., 39-A:910, 1957.
9. Hall, M. C.: Luschka's Joints. Springfield, Charles C Thomas, 1965.
10. Hirsch, C., Schajowicz, F., and Galante, J.: Structural changes in the cervical spine. Acta Orthoped. Scand. (Suppl.), 109, 1967.
11. Jackson, R.: The Cervical Syndrome, 3rd Ed. Springfield, Charles C Thomas, 1966.
12. Rathke, L.: Zur normalen und pathologischen Anatomie der Halswirbelsäule. Deutsch. Z. Chir., 242:122, 1933.
13. Töndury, G.: Entwicklungsgeschichte und Fehlbildungen der Wirbelsäule. In Die Wirbelsäule in Forschung und Proxis. Bd 7, Stuttgart, Hippokrates, 1958.
14. Töndury, G.: The cervical spine—its development and changes during life. Acta Orthop. Belg., 25:602, 1959.
15. Hadley, L. A.: Anatomico-Roentgenographic Studies of the Spine. Springfield, Charles C Thomas, 1964.

Part II

INJURIES OF THE CERVICAL SPINE

Chapter 3

GENERAL CONCEPTS

"The beginning of wisdom is the definition of terms."

Socrates.

BASIC PRINCIPLES

Introduction

Since biblical times and the Tower of Babel, men have ceased to speak a universal language. This is particularly true in medicine, where the use of medical jargon frequently prevents physicians from communicating accurately. It is not merely an academic exercise to properly describe fractures and dislocations and to recognize variations in the patterns of injury.

In this chapter the descriptive terms relating to fractures and dislocations are reviewed, the methods of reporting these injuries are discussed, and a practical guide to roentgen diagnosis is presented. These basic concepts of cervical spine injury will provide a sound foundation on which to build one's knowledge in the next chapters.

Classification of Fractures

A fracture (L. *fractura,* a break) may be defined as a break, either complete or incomplete, in the continuity of a bone, epiphyseal plate, or cartilaginous joint surface. The same terminology may be applied to all of the five types of bones — long, short, flat, irregular (the vertebrae), and sesamoid.

A *complete fracture* implies that both cortices of the bone have been broken, while an *incomplete fracture* involves only one cortex. Most fractures of the vertebral column are *simple,* or *closed,* fractures; that is,

there is no communication with the exterior of the body (Fig. 3–1). *Compound,* or *open,* fractures communicate with the external environment and are often produced by missile injuries (Fig. 3–2).

Fractures may be caused by either *direct* or *indirect violence.* In direct spinal injury,

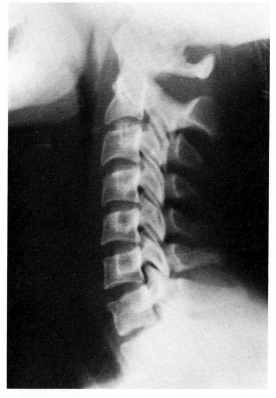

Figure 3–1. Simple (closed) fracture of the superoanterior margin of the C-7 vertebral body. The mechanism of injury in this case was hyperflexion and compression.

91

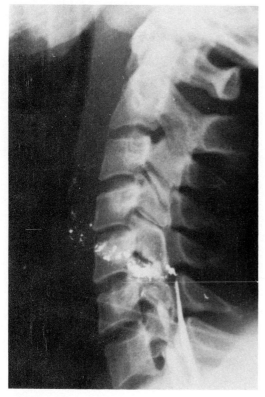

Figure 3-2. Compound (open) fracture of C-5/6 secondary to a gun shot wound. Note the marked retropharyngeal soft tissue swelling.

force is applied directly to the vertebra and the bone fractures at the site of impact. In the cervical spine, the most common fractures resulting from direct injury involve the spinous processes (Fig. 3–3).

In indirect injury, force is applied at a distance from the spine, for example, to the head or trunk in the case of a cervical spine injury. This force is transmitted indirectly to the vertebral column, which is then deformed beyond its normal physiologic range of motion. Excessive movements of the cervical spine are also produced by sudden acceleration or deceleration of the head relative to the trunk, or vice versa, especially in traffic accidents (Fig. 3–4). The excessive movements of the cervical spine to be considered later are as follows: (1) hyperflexion, (2) hyperextension, (3) hyperrotation, and (4) lateral hyperflexion.

Descriptive Terms Relating to Fractures of the Vertebrae

The same terminology that applies to the other bones of the skeleton is used here. In preparing reports relating to vertebral fractures, it is important to mention the level of the injury, the exact anatomic site, its extent and direction, and the relationship of the fracture fragments to each other.[1]

Level of Injury

While the majority of fractures of the vertebral column occur at or near the thoracolumbar junction or in the lower cervical spine, fractures may occur at any level. In Part I of this book, we presented detailed information on the gross anatomy of both typical and atypical vertebrae in each region of the vertebral column. Aided by a knowledge of these anatomic features, one should be able to determine the level of a fracture accurately, even though the entire region is not included on the radiographs.

Site

Fractures of vertebrae may be divided into those that involve the vertebral body and those that involve the vertebral arch. Arch fractures may be further subdivided into those involving the pedicles; laminae; and the spinous, transverse, and articular processes.

Great care should be taken to select the correct anatomic terms. An old Chinese

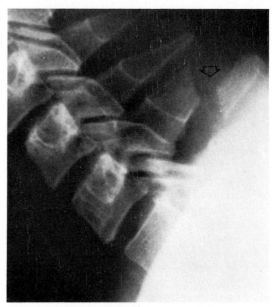

Figure 3-3. Isolated fracture of the spinous process of C-7 (arrow), which resulted from a direct blow to the back of the neck. Note the jagged edges of this fracture. The fragment is distracted and displaced caudally.

Figure 3-4. Indirect violence due to a rear-end automobile accident. The head is moved backward and downward in hyperextension (1). The head is then flexed striking the anterior chest wall (2), and finally the neutral position is assumed (3). This type of trauma may result in soft tissue injury, fracture and/or dislocation of the cervical spine. See Table 3-4, for injuries that may result from this trauma.

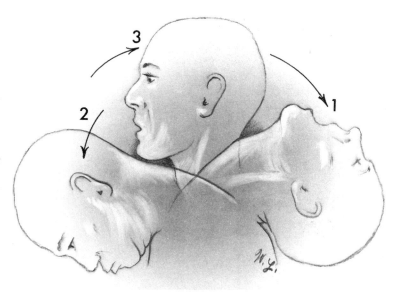

proverb says, *"The beginning of wisdom is to call things by their right names."* Thus in an infant, before the neurocentral synchondrosis has united, fractures of the centrum and the neural arch may be described (Chapter 1, p. 3). The terms centrum and neural arch are not valid, however, when applied to the adult vertebrae.

Vague terms such as the *anterior* and *posterior elements* of a vertebra should be avoided. These terms are occasionally encountered in the literature but are not recognized in medical lexicography at present. Remember, also, that only two vertebrae in the entire vertebral column have *lateral masses,* namely, the atlas and the sacrum.

Extent and Direction

Vertebral fractures, as mentioned earlier, may be complete or incomplete. A *comminuted* fracture has more than two fragments, such as a burst fracture (Fig. 3-5).

In a *transverse* fracture, the cortical break occurs at right angles to the long axis of the bone (Fig. 3-6). *Oblique* fractures, as the name implies, are directed obliquely to the long axis of the vertebra (Fig. 3-7). Rotary forces may produce *spiral* and *vertical* fractures (Fig. 3-8), which usually occur in either the sagittal or the coronal plane.

Relationship of Fracture Fragments

A fracture may be either *displaced* or *undisplaced.* Displaced fractures may be *avulsed, impacted, distracted,* or *rotated.*

The fracture fragment may be shifted anteriorly, posteriorly, laterally, medially, cranially, or caudally. An almost infinite va-

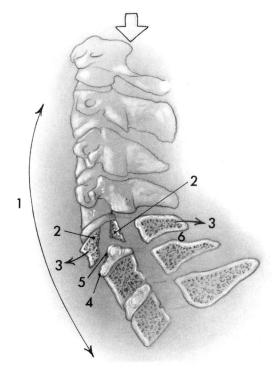

Figure 3-5. A comminuted, or bursting, fracture of the body of C-5. The cervical spine is held rigidly erect (1) while the axial compressive force is applied to the vertex of the head. The C-5 vertebral body is shattered (2) and the bony fragments are displaced (3). The C-5 intervertebral disk is ruptured (4) and has been forced into the vertebral body (5). There is no posterior ligamentous disruption (6).

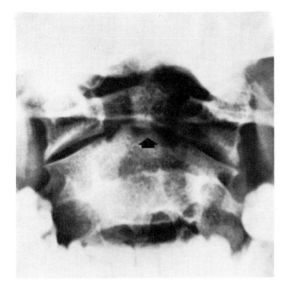

Figure 3–6. Transverse fracture of the base of the dens with left lateral displacement (arrow). The patient was involved in a side car collision and sustained a lateral hyperflexion injury.

Figure 3–7. A supine oblique vertebral arch view showing oblique fractures of the laminae of C-5 and C-6 on the left (arrows). This patient had Type V-A hyperextension fracture-dislocations of C-5 on C-6, and C-6 on C-7. See Chapter 5 for more details.

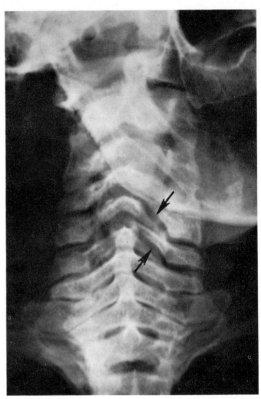

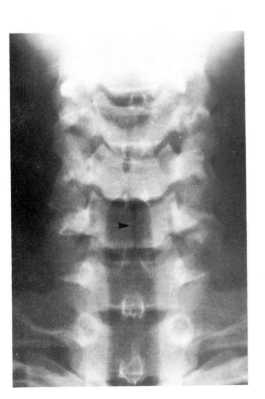

Figure 3–8. A vertical fracture of the body of C-6 in the sagittal plane. The fracture is clearly visualized through the tracheal shadow (arrow head).

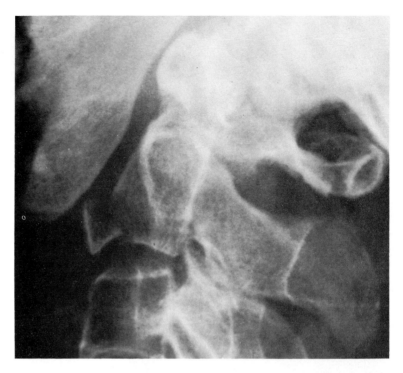

Figure 3-9. Avulsion fracture from the anteroinferior margin of the axis body. The mechanism of injury is disruptive hyperextension. Note the fractures of the posterior arch of the atlas, also caused by hyperextension. The most dorsal fragment is displaced and angled cranially by the pull of the rectus capitus posterior minor muscle.

riety of relations may exist between the fracture fragments.

Many examples of *avulsion fractures* may be seen in the vertebral column. Fragments of bone are pulled off either by violent muscle contraction or, more commonly, by passive resistance of a ligament applied against an oppositely directed force. In Figure 3–9, the anteroinferior border of the body of the axis has been avulsed by a hyperextension injury of the neck. Another type of avulsion fracture is illustrated in Figure 3–10. This is a *clay-shoveler's fracture*, an avulsion of a spinous process. The fractures occurred in a weekend gardener who attempted to throw some thick, sticky North Carolina clay out of a ditch, but the clay adhered to his shovel. The spinous processes were torn off by the sudden pull on the supraspinous ligament of the trapezius and rhomboid muscles. Note that the fracture fragments are *distracted;* that is, they are held apart either by interposed soft tissues or by tendon pull.

Impaction, or compression, fractures are commonly observed in the cervical spine. They result from flexion or extension compressive forces pushing two vertebrae together. In flexion, the intervertebral disk is usually resistant to such forces[2] and the end result is a wedge-shaped vertebral body

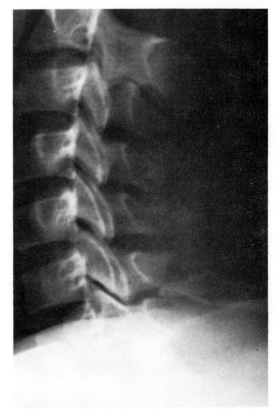

Figure 3–10. Avulsion fractures of the spinous processes of C-6 and C-7.

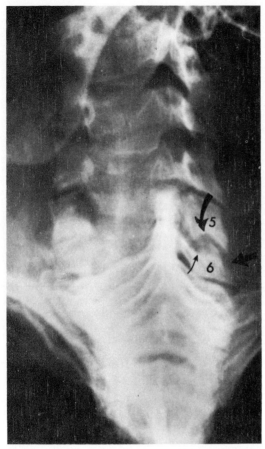

Figure 3–11. An oblique vertebral arch view showing severe compression fractures of the articular pillars of C-5 and C-6 on the left. The mechanism of injury was compressive hyperextension with rotation.

(Fig. 3–1). With an extension compressive injury, one or more articular pillars may be compressed (Fig. 3–11).

Pathologic fractures occur through bone already involved with some disease process, either generalized or local skeletal disease. This bone is, therefore, weaker than normal bone and more susceptible to fracture. Pathologic fractures may be caused by minor injury, major injury, or even normal use. An example of a pathologic fracture of a cervical vertebra is shown in Figure 3–12.

Classification of Joint Injuries

Joint injuries, like fractures, are caused by either direct or indirect violence. In a direct injury, the joint may be contused or, if there is sufficient force, an intra-articular fracture may result.

Indirect violence may cause ligamentous injury of varying degrees of severity. A ligamentous *sprain* results from stretching of ligamentous fibers beyond their normal limits of elasticity, causing tears and hemorrhage. A more severe injury produces a tear or *rupture* of a ligament, which may be partial or complete. Sprain and rupture thus are both ligamentous injuries; they differ only in degree (Fig. 3–13).

Three types of joint instability are recognized:[1] (1) *Occult* joint instability. This can only be recognized on the radiographs when the joint is stressed.[1, 3, 4] (2) *Disloca-*

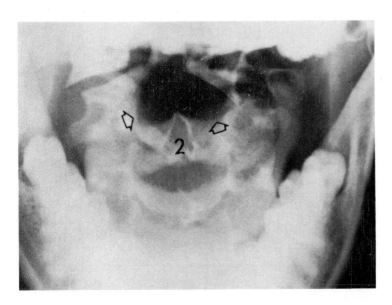

Figure 3–12. Metastatic melanoma to the axis vertebra with fracture (arrows) and rotary dislocation of the atlas on the axis.

tion — a complete disruption of the normal contact between articular surfaces[5] (Fig. 3–14). In the cervical spine, the terms luxation or dislocation may be used if there is disruption of a synovial joint with locking of its articular surfaces. The reader should note that we have used the term "locking" for the abnormal relationship between articular surfaces. We will use "interlocking" for the normal relationship of synovial joint surfaces. (3) *Subluxation*—a partial luxation (dislocation) in which the joint surfaces maintain some degree of contact after injury. Subluxation is a rather vague term when applied to the vertebral column, especially the cervical spine. Consider for a moment the wide range of contact between the opposing articular facets during the normal movement in flexion-extension (Fig. 3–15 *A, B*). What is the difference between the relationships of these joint surfaces in maximum flexion and subluxation? This is difficult to define and, therefore, we will follow the lead of others and avoid the term "subluxation" in this book.

Descriptive Terms Relating to Dislocations

Level of Injury

Traumatic dislocations may occur at any level of the cervical spine (Fig. 3–14); however, they are most common at C-5/C-6 and C-6/C-7 intervertebral joints. Dislocations are often associated with fractures, as we will see shortly.

Extent and Direction

Dislocations may be either *complete* or *self-reducing*. If the articular processes lock, the inferior articular processes will lie in front of the superior articular processes of the vertebra below (Fig. 3–14). These complete dislocations may be unilateral (rotary) or bilateral, and are caused by a disruptive hyperflexion injury. Extension dislocations also occur, as illustrated in Figure 3–16.

Self-reducing hyperflexion dislocations (hyperflexion "sprain" of Braakman and Penning) are produced by the same disruptive hyperflexion mechanism as is a complete dislocation. However, after the force of injury has been dissipated, the articular

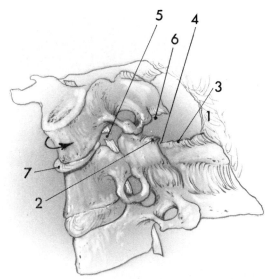

Figure 3–13. Hyperflexion sprain (momentary dislocation) caused by disruptive hyperflexion with concomitant hyperrotation. Rupture of the nuchal ligament at 1, and interspinal ligament (3), apophyseal joint capsule (2), ligamentum flavum (4), and posterior longitudinal ligament (5). There is widening of the apophyseal joint (6) and compression of the intervertebral disk (7).

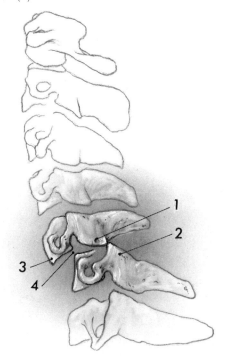

Figure 3–14. Bilateral hyperflexion dislocation (locked facets). The inferior articular processes of C-5 (1) are *locked* in front of the superior articular processes of C-6 (2). The body of C-5 (3) is displaced anteriorly on the C-6 vertebra and the C-5 intervertebral disk is disrupted by the injury (4).

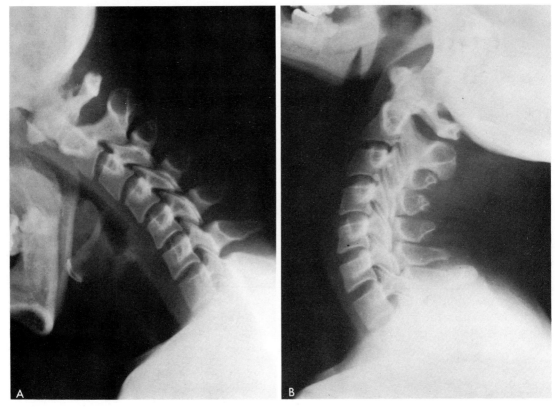

Figure 3–15. Normal lateral views of the cervical spine. *A*, Flexion. *B*, Extension. Examine the wide range of contact between opposing articular facets during the movement in flexion-extension.

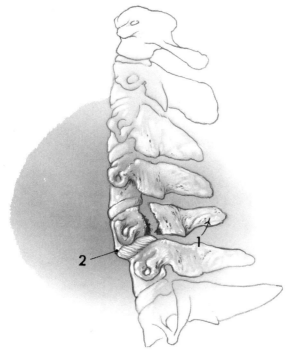

Figure 3–16. Hyperextension fracture-dislocation of C-5 on C-6. The mechanism is compressive hyperextension. The articular pillar and lamina are tilted into a more horizontal plane (1). There is anterolisthesis of the body of C-5 on C-6 (2), and the C-5 intervertebral disk is narrowed. Such cases are frequently misdiagnosed as flexion injuries.

surfaces return to more or less normal contact (Figs. 3–13, 3–17).[63-5]

Relationship of Vertebrae in Dislocation

When reporting dislocations, always *describe the direction taken by the upper vertebra in relation to the one below.* For example, in Figure 3–18, the sixth cervical vertebra is displaced anteriorly on the seventh cervical vertebra.

A PRACTICAL GUIDE TO DIAGNOSIS

Introduction

The roentgen examination of the acutely injured cervical spine is the responsibility of the radiologist and not the surgeon. Before or during the filming of the patient, the

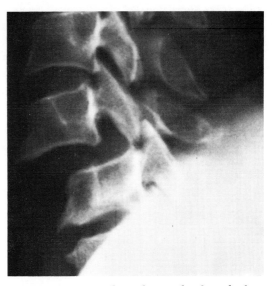

Figure 3–18. Bilateral articular facet locking of C-6 on C-7. Always describe the direction taken by the upper vertebra in relation to the one below.

radiologist should obtain as much clinical information as possible.

Any patient with a suspected cervical spine injury must be managed with extreme care from the moment of trauma to the time that definitive care is instituted. Failure to follow this concept may result in injury to the spinal cord.

Roentgen Examination of the Acutely Injured Patient

What is a "routine" series of radiographs for examining the patient with an acute cervical injury? We are frequently confronted with this question by our colleagues in radiology and surgery. Although there is no definite answer, a practical approach to the problem may be suggested. At the Duke University Medical Center, we have adopted the series shown in Table 3–1.

The most important single projection is

TABLE 3–1. Roentgen Examination of the Acutely Injured Cervical Spine[*]

1. Lateral—cross–table
2. Right and left 30 degree oblique
3. Anteroposterior of the lower cervical spine
4. AP of the atlas-axis
5. Vertebral arch view

[*]All views are made with the patient *supine.* Do not move the head. Protect the spinal cord!

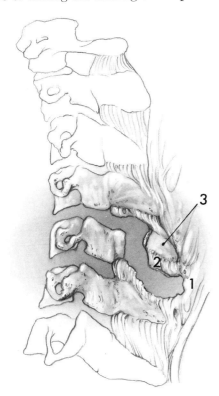

Figure 3–17. Hyperflexion sprain (momentary dislocation) caused by a disruptive hyperflexion injury. Rupture of the supraspinal (supraspinous) and interspinal (interspinous) ligaments is shown at 1 and 2 respectively. Number 3 is an avulsion of the spinous process of C-5. Note the widening of the apophyseal joints at the levels of injury.

the lateral. Two-thirds of significant pathology can be detected on this view (Table 3–2). However, it is usually necessary to obtain additional projections to make a precise morphologic diagnosis.

Often, other clinical problems prevent a complete evaluation of the patient in the emergency room. Thus, a team approach — radiologist, orthopedist, and neurosurgeon in deliberate consultation — is required to decide how far to carry the diagnostic roentgen examination. An ideal radiographic examination may be impossible in certain circumstances. The prudent physician must always put the welfare of the patient first.

It takes only a few minutes to obtain a complete examination of the cervical spine in the acutely traumatized patient. At the Duke University Medical Center we routinely obtain the following projections with the patient *supine*. No special equipment is utilized; indeed, a portable x-ray unit is adequate for filming.

Six projections are obtained:
1. Cross-table lateral view with a grid cassette (Figs. 3–19, 3–20).

TABLE 3–2. Traumatic Lesions of the Cervical Spine—Visibility on Lateral Radiograph

FRACTURE OR DISLOCATION	YES*	NO*
Anterior atlanto-occipital dislocation	+	
"Pure" atlantoaxial dislocations (3 types)	+	
Atlas fractures		
Posterior arch	+	
Horizontal anterior arch	+	
Jefferson fracture	±	+
Lateral mass		+
Transverse process		+
Axis fractures		
Dens		
Anterior fracture-dislocation	+	
Posterior fracture-dislocation	+	
Lateral fracture-dislocation	±	+
Nondisplaced fracture	±	+
Vertebral body		
Anteroinferior margin	+	
Comminuted body	+	
Vertebral arch	+	
Vertebral bodies (lower cervical spine)		
Anterosuperior, anteroinferior margin	+	
Burst	+	
Uncinate process		+
Lateral wedge		+
Vertebral arch (lower cervical spine)		
Articular pillar	±	+
Pedicle		+
Lamina	±	+
Spinous process	+	
Transverse process		+
Hyperflexion sprain	+ erect lat.	
Hyperextension sprain	+	
Locked facets	+	
Hyperflexion fracture-dislocation–teardrop-type	+	
Hyperextension fracture-dislocation—type IV	+	
Hyperextension fracture-dislocation—type V	+	

*± = may be seen
+ = usually visible or not visible

Figure 3-19. Method for obtaining the supine cross-table lateral view of the cervical spine. Note that the grid cassette is held by a sandbag. Arrow indicates central x-ray beam.

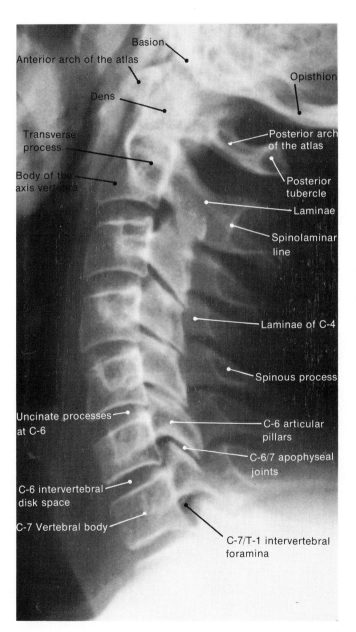

Basion

Anterior arch of the atlas

Opisthion

Dens

Posterior arch of the atlas

Transverse process

Posterior tubercle

Body of the axis vertebra

Laminae

Spinolaminar line

Laminae of C-4

Spinous process

Uncinate processes at C-6

C-6 articular pillars

C-6/7 apophyseal joints

C-6 intervertebral disk space

C-7 Vertebral body

C-7/T-1 intervertebral foramina

Figure 3-20. Normal lateral radiograph obtained with the cross-table projection. Note that the ventral margins of the C-5 and C-6 vertebral bodies are slightly diminished in height relative to those above and below. This is a common variation of the normal.

Figure 3–21. Patient positioning for the supine 30 degree oblique. Because of the angle utilized, the normal anatomic structures are elongated from side to side. Central x-ray beam is indicated by the arrow.

2. Right and left 30 degree oblique views with a nongrid cassette placed flat on the stretcher as close to the neck as possible. The tube is angled from the horizontal, and the central ray enters just behind the larynx (Figs. 3–21, 3–22).
3. Anteroposterior view of the lower cervical spine with 20 degrees of cranial angulation (Figs. 3–23, 3–24).
4. Anteroposterior view of the atlas-axis through the open mouth (Figs. 3–25, 3–26).
5. Anteroposterior vertebral arch view with 25 to 30 degrees of caudal angulation.

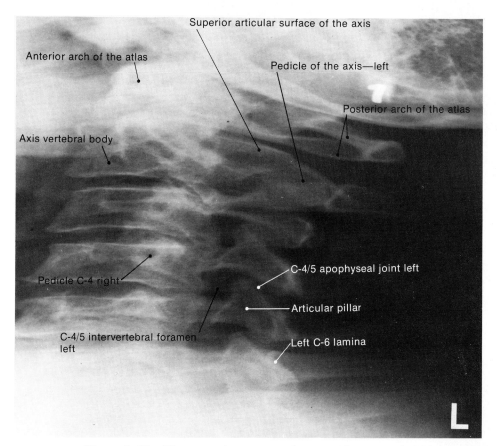

Figure 3–22. The normal supine 30 degree oblique view.

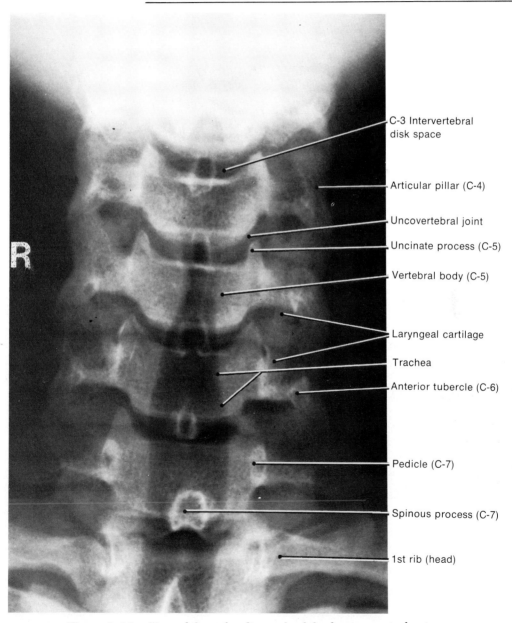

Figure 3–23. Patient positioning for the AP projection of the lower cervical spine. The central ray is angled 20 degrees toward the head (arrow).

20°

R

C-3 Intervertebral disk space

Articular pillar (C-4)

Uncovertebral joint

Uncinate process (C-5)

Vertebral body (C-5)

Laryngeal cartilage

Trachea

Anterior tubercle (C-6)

Pedicle (C-7)

Spinous process (C-7)

1st rib (head)

Figure 3–24. Normal frontal radiograph of the lower cervical spine.

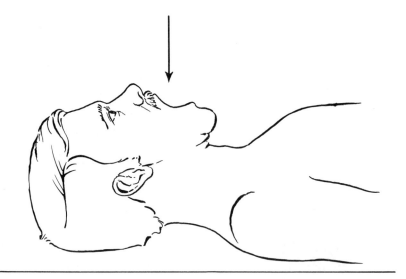

Figure 3–25. Patient positioning for the atlas-axis anteroposterior open mouth projection.

The tube angle can be determined accurately by using the cross-table lateral view. Measure the angles of the lower three apophyseal joints and average these numbers. The central ray is directed at the suprasternal notch (Figs. 3–27, 3–28).

Some among the readers will consider this to be extreme. After all, they will argue, most injuries of the cervical spine are demonstrable on lateral radiographs. It is quite true that about *two-thirds* of cervical spine fractures and dislocations are recognizable on a lateral radiograph (Table 3–2).

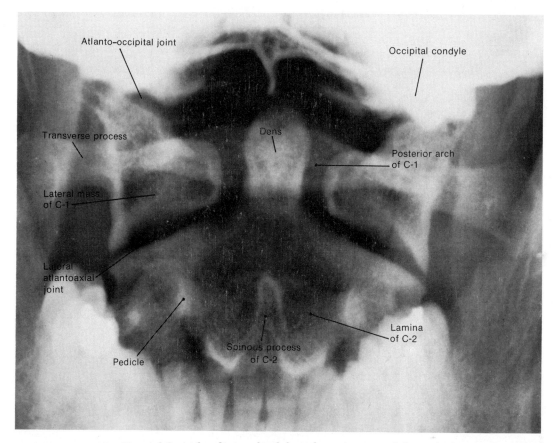

Figure 3–26. Normal frontal radiograph of the atlas-axis viewed through the open mouth.

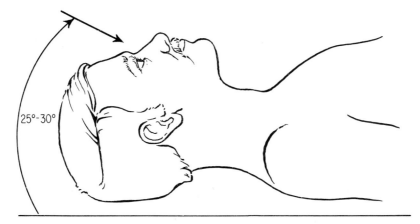

Figure 3–27. Patient positioning for the *supine* anteroposterior vertebral arch projection. The central ray is angled 25 to 30 degrees toward the feet and centered on the suprasternal notch.

However, there are some traumatic conditions of the cervical spine that may look identical on lateral radiographs but require completely different modes of treatment (Fig. 3–29 *A,B*). This is especially true of a type IV hyperextension fracture-dislocation (Chapter 5, p. 218) and of unilateral facet locking (hyperflexion dislocation with rotation). Differentiation of these two lesions requires the use of the other projections.

A computer analysis of 400 patients with recognizable fractures and/or dislocations of the cervical spine showed that 50 per cent of the patients had vertebral arch fractures.[6] Some of these can be diagnosed on one or more of the projections recommended but are usually not apparent on all views.

An Analytic Approach to the Roentgen Diagnosis of Cervical Injuries

We have found that the use of *triangulation* is the most rational approach to diagno-

Figure 3–28. The normal vertebral arch view.

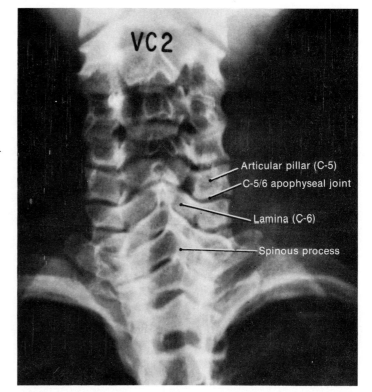

VC2

Articular pillar (C-5)

C-5/6 apophyseal joint

Lamina (C-6)

Spinous process

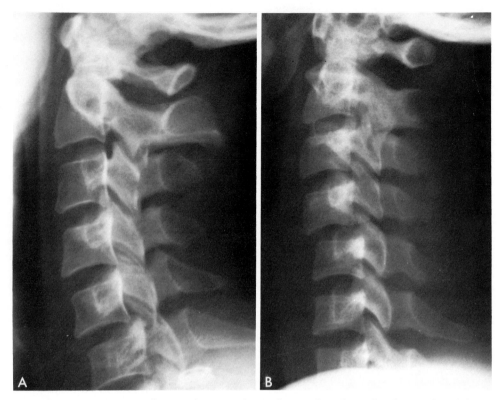

Figure 3–29. Traumatic conditions that may look identical on lateral radiographs of the cervical vertebral column. *A,* Type IV hyperextension fracture-dislocation of C-5 on C-6 with a fractured articular pillar at C-5 on the right. (See Fig. 5–49 for the complete radiographic series). *B,* Unilateral facet locking of C-4 on C-5 (See Fig. 5–50 for the complete radiographic series). In both x-rays, there is anterolisthesis of the injured vertebra on that subjacent, narrowing of the intervertebral disk beneath, and rotation of the vertebrae from the level of injury and above. Never attempt to make an accurate diagnosis on a lateral radiograph alone!

sis. Such an analysis permits the least chance of error in the interpretation of the radiographs (Table 3–3).

Clinical

Look at the patient and try to determine whether there are bruises, cuts, or fractures of the head or thorax. Take a history, if the patient's clinical condition will permit, to determine the mode of injury. Attempt to reconstruct the trauma in order to determine the probable mechanism of injury, whether it be (1) hyperflexion, (2) hyperextension, (3) hyperrotation, (4) lateral hyperflexion, or a combination of these forces. If

TABLE 3–3. An Analytic Approach to the Roentgen Diagnosis of Cervical Spine Injuries

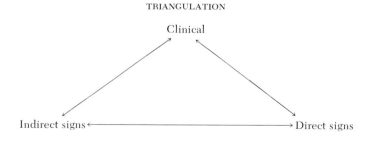

TABLE 3–4. Classification of Injuries Based Upon Mechanism

HYPERFLEXION INJURIES
  Disruptive hyperflexion
    Hyperflexion sprain (momentary dislocation)
    Hyperflexion-dislocation (Locked Facets)
      Bilateral
      Unilateral (with associated rotational force)
    Spinous process fracture
  Compressive hyperflexion
    Wedge-like compression of vertebral body
    Comminuted (teardrop) fracture of vertebral body
    Hyperflexion fracture-dislocation (Type IV)
  Hyperflexion or shearing forces
    Anterior atlanto-occipital dislocation(?)
    "Pure" anterior atlantoaxial dislocation (without associated fracture)
    Anterior fracture-dislocation of the dens

HYPEREXTENSION INJURIES
  Disruptive hyperextension
    Horizontal fracture of the anterior arch of C-1
    Hangman's fracture (traumatic spondylolisthesis of C-2)
    Anteroinferior margin of the body of the axis (C-2)
    Hyperextension sprain (momentary dislocation)
    Spinous process fracture
  Compressive hyperextension
    Posterior arch of the atlas fracture
    Vertebral arch fracture (articular pillar, pedicle, lamina)
    Hyperextension fracture-dislocation (type IV-V)
  Hyperextension or shearing forces
    Posterior fracture-dislocation of the dens
    "Pure" posterior atlantoaxial dislocation (without associated fracture)

HYPERROTATION INJURIES
  Rotary atlantoaxial dislocation
  Anterior and posterior ligament disruption

LATERAL HYPERFLEXION INJURIES
  Fracture of transverse process
  Uncinate process fracture
  Lateral fracture-dislocation of the dens
  Brachial plexus avulsion associated with cervical fractures and/or dislocations
  Lateral wedge-like compression of vertebral body

AXIAL COMPRESSIVE INJURIES
  Isolated fracture of the lateral mass of the atlas
  Bursting fracture of Jefferson (C-1)
  Vertical and oblique fractures of the axis body
  Bursting fracture of a vertebral body

the mechanism of injury can be determined, then specific traumatic lesions may be sought on the radiographs. A classification of cervical spine trauma based on mechanism is shown in Table 3–4. We will elaborate on this shortly.

Indirect Signs

Twelve significant indirect and direct signs of cervical spine trauma have been evaluated over the past several years.[7] The reader must always look for these signs as a clue to underlying trauma. Such a search will be richly rewarding (see Table 3–5).

Direct Signs

Finally, the physician should examine the radiographs of his patient while bearing the most common lesions in mind. These will be described shortly (p. 118).

Classification of Cervical Spine Injuries

"If thou examinest a man having a crushed vertebra in his neck (and) thou findest that one vertebra has fallen into the next one. . . .; his falling head downward has caused that one vertebra crush into the next one; shouldst thou find that he is unconscious of his two arms and his two legs because of it . . . An ailment not to be treated."

Case 33 — *The Edwin Smith Surgical Papyrus. Circa 17th Century* B.C.[8]

The earliest known recorded observations about cervical spine trauma were made fifty centuries ago. The Egyptian surgeons in the Old Kingdom (3000 to 2500 B.C.) utilized a nosologic designation for the injuries that were encountered. They differentiated between the following: (1) penetrating wounds (Case 29), (2) sprain (Case 30), (3) dislocation (Case 31), (4) displaced vertebra (Case 32), and (5) a fatal case of crushed vertebra (Case 33).[8]

In the last case (33), the mechanism of injury is clearly spelled out. A similar classification of cervical spine injuries based upon mechanism (Table 3–4) is still utilized today. The *Edwin Smith Surgical Papyrus* dates from the seventeenth century B.C., and is a manuscript copy of a treatise thought to have originated yet a thousand years before. To this original manuscript, which had been circulating for centuries, had been added a commentary or gloss explaining the meaning of terms apparently no longer clear to the Egyptian surgeons of 1700 B.C. Some examples are given below. Notice how clear the gloss makes the classification. In Case 30, a sprain refers to a "rending of two members." A cervical dislocation (Case 31) is explained as a "separation of one vertebra of his neck from another, the flesh over it being uninjured." The explanation of displacement "in a vertebra in the neck" is a "sinking of a vertebra of his neck (to) the interior of his neck, as a foot settles into cultivated ground. It is a penetration downward."

The document is a truly remarkable one, and the reader is urged to spend a long evening in the company of the ancient surgeon who penned the treatise.

Dr. Breasted speculates that the author of the original treatise may have been the noted architect-physician Imhotep, and that the title of his work was "The Secret Book of the Physician." In this section, we will presume to continue where Imhotep left off.

No single classification of cervical spine injuries has won international acceptance.[5, 9-11] However, one of the most useful classifications, proposed by Whitley and Forsyth[12] and subsequently modified by Braakman and Penning,[5] relates the mechanism of injury to the radiologic findings (Table 3–4).

Vertebrae may be subjected to forces of varying direction and magnitude. We have already mentioned that injuries of the cervical spine may be caused by direct or indirect violence. With direct violence, the force of injury acts directly upon the vertebra. In indirect violence the force may result from injuries to the skull or thorax, causing the cervical spine to move beyond its physiologic range. Similar excessive movements of the cervical spine may result from sudden deceleration or acceleration injuries. The excessive movements of the cervical spine to be considered are as follows: (1) hyperflexion, (2) hyperextension, (3) hyperrotation, and (4) lateral hyperflexion.

We must also consider two additional forces acting along the axis of the cervical spine: (1) compression and (2) disruption. These may be entirely axial in their direction, or may be compounded with other forces of injury to result in compressive hyperflexion, compressive hyperextension, disruptive hyperflexion, and so on.

Definition of Terms

Compression forces (L. *compressio* from *comprimere*, to squeeze together) squeeze parts together, diminishing their volume and increasing their density (Fig. 3–30 *B*). A *disruptive* force (L. *dis* apart; *rumpere* to break apart), on the other hand, rends, ruptures, or bursts apart (Fig. 3–30 *A*).

The terms *flexion* and *extension* refer to bending movements in the sagittal plane, which normally affords the spine its greatest range of mobility. *Hyperflexion* and *hyperextension* denote disruption of ligamentous supports by excessive flexion or extension. *Rotation* (L. *rotatio, rotare* to turn) is a turning about the longitudinal axis. *Shear* injuries result from equal and opposed but displaced forces acting on one level of the

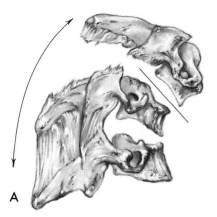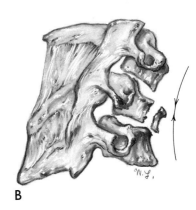

Figure 3–30. A, Disruptive hyperflexion injury with rupture of the posterior ligaments and apophyseal joint capsules. This injury may result in a hyperflexion sprain (momentary dislocation) or locked articular facets. B, Compressive hyperflexion injury with intact ligaments posteriorly. Since the normal intervertebral disks are quite resistant to compression, the compressive force is primarily expended on the vertebral body, resulting in a fracture.

spine. In the cervical spine, horizontal shear forces are thought to produce fractures of the dens. If the head is suddenly displaced forward, the dens may be sheared off by the stronger transverse ligament of

the atlas. The resulting picture is that of forward displacement of the dens (Fig. 3–31 A). When the head is displaced backward on the cervical spine, the anterior arch of the atlas may shear the dens off the body of the

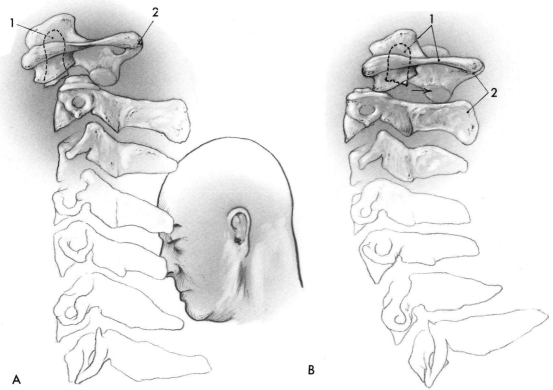

Figure 3–31. Fractures of the dens. A, With anterior atlantoaxial dislocation. #1 = fractured dens. #2 = anterior displacement of the posterior tubercle of the atlas relative to the spinous process of the axis. B, With posterior atlantoaxial dislocation. #1 = atlas and dens are displaced posteriorly. #2 = the most posterior margins of the posterior tubercle of the atlas and the spinous process of the axis may lie in the same vertical plane.

axis and displace the dens backward (Fig. 3–31 *B*).

Flexion Injuries

If the injuring force is directed forward and upward, as with a blow to the occiput from below, a *disruptive hyperflexion* injury results (Table 3–4). At the level of the injury, the spinous processes will be distracted and the posterior ligaments will receive the greatest trauma. Experimentally, Roaf,[2] using thoracolumbar vertebral columns from cadavers, was unable to produce posterior ligamentous tears in flexion without the addition of a concomitant rotary or shear force. Other workers[10] had no trouble producing such tears in their cervical spinal models with pure flexion and compression. In this type of injury, a spinous process may be avulsed.

On the radiographs, disruptive hyper-flexion injury may present in several ways, depending upon the magnitude of the injuring force. When the posterior ligaments are torn locally, a hyperflexion sprain or rupture (momentary dislocation) results.[5] On the erect lateral radiograph of the cervical spine, there is an acute kyphotic hyperangulation at the level of injury, associated with widening of the apophyseal joints and increased separation between two spinous processes (Figs. 3–17, 3–32 *A*). Complete dislocation does not occur. The hyperangulation is characteristically reduced by fully extending the neck. This may not be possible in the erect position if the center of gravity of the head is not situated posterior to the level of injury. Thus reduction may be achieved only by placing the patient supine with the head hanging off the end of the table, as in the hanging head position (Fig. 3–32 *B*).

If a more intense force of injury has been

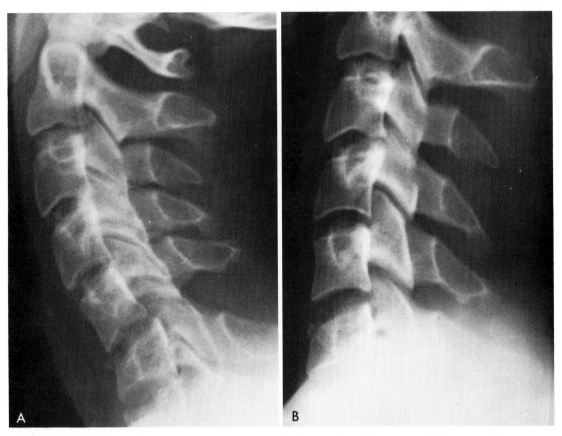

Figure 3–32. Hyperflexion sprain (momentary dislocation) with associated fracture of the supero-anterior margin of the C-6 vertebral body. *A*, Erect lateral view showing the kyphotic hyperangulation at C-5/6. Note the abnormal interspinous distance at C-5/6. Reduction of the hyperangulation could not be obtained in the erect position with attempted extension of the spine. *B*, Hanging head lateral showing reduction of the kyphotic hyperangulation.

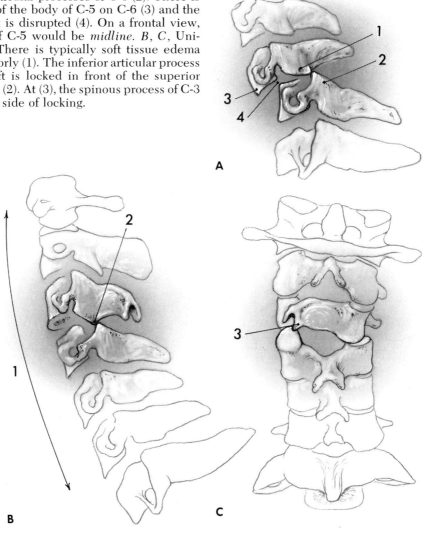

Figure 3–33. Locked articular facets resulting from disruptive hyperflexion forces. *A*, Bilateral locked facets. Note that the inferior articular processes of C-5 (1) are locked in front of the superior articular processes of C-6 (2). There is marked displacement of the body of C-5 on C-6 (3) and the C-5 intervertebral disk is disrupted (4). On a frontal view, the spinous process of C-5 would be *midline. B, C,* Unilateral locked facets. There is typically soft tissue edema and hemorrhage anteriorly (1). The inferior articular process of C-3 on patient's left is locked in front of the superior articular process of C-4 (2). At (3), the spinous process of C-3 is deviated *toward* the side of locking.

applied, the posterior ligaments are torn and the articular surfaces of the apophyseal joints lose all contact and override. After the force is dispelled, the spine springs back toward its normal position and the articular processes lock. If the trauma occurs in hyperflexion without significant rotation, locking of articular processes occurs bilateral-ly — a bilateral hyperflexion dislocation (Fig. 3–33 *A*). Unilateral hyperflexion dislocation results if a rotary component is added to the force (Fig. 3–33 *B,C*).

Compressive hyperflexion injuries are usually caused by a blow to the top of the head. The force is transmitted downward along the cervical vertebral column. This results in varying degrees of compression of the vertebral bodies (Fig. 3–34 A) or even in a hyperflexion fracture-dislocation (Fig. 3–34 B,C). If the force is mainly compressive, the posterior ligamentous structures may remain intact. Since the normal intervertebral disk is usually quite resistant to compression, it is the vertebral body that is disrupted by the compressive force (Fig. 3–1).

The Type IV "teardrop" hyperflexion fracture-dislocation results from hyperflexion compression (Chapter 5, p. 252). The force acting on the spine moves it in an arc (Fig. 3–35 B). At the level of injury, the vertebra is displaced posteriorly, causing disruption of the apophyseal joint capsules

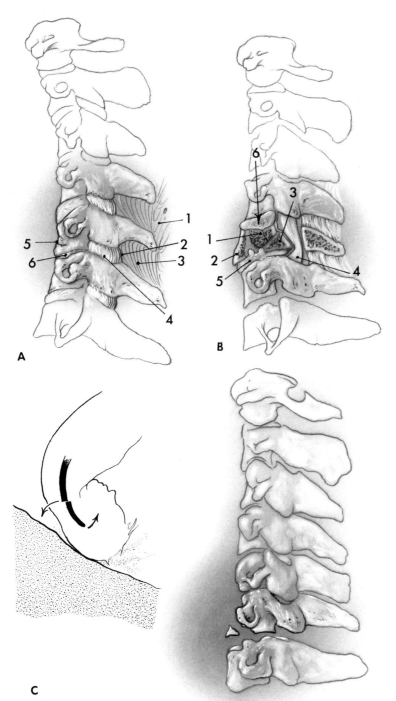

Figure 3–34. A, Wedge compression fracture of C-5 (5). The disk bordering the fracture (6) may be injured. Intact posterior ligaments are shown at 1–4 (1 = nuchal ligament; 2 = ligamentum flavum; 3 = interspinal ligament; 4 = capsule of the apophyseal joint). B, Bursting fracture of C-5 vertebral body. The cervical vertebral body is severely comminuted (1,2,3). The spinal cord (4) may be crushed by the posteroinferior fragment (3). C-5 intervertebral disk is disrupted (5). The direction of the compressive force is shown at 6. C, "Teardrop" hyperflexion fracture-dislocation (Type IV) resulting from a dive into shallow water. For the details of the mechanism of injury see Figure 3–35.

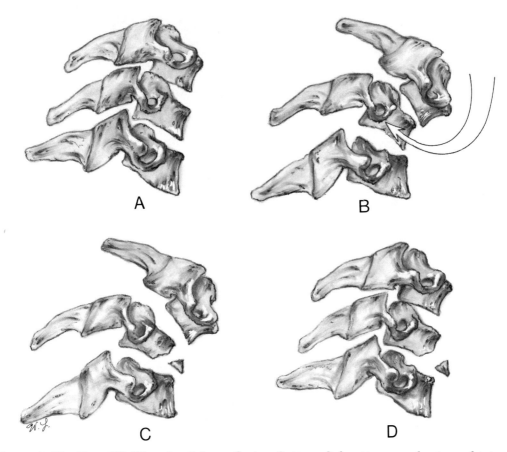

Figure 3–35. Type IV "Teardrop" hyperflexion fracture-dislocation—mechanism of injury. *A*, Normal, prior to injury. *B*, The hyperflexion compressive force moves the cervical spine in an arc. At the level of injury, the vertebra is displaced posteriorly causing disruption of the apophyseal joint capsules and the posterior portion of the intervertebral disk below. Either the anterior or the anteroinferior margin of the involved vertebra is fractured. *C*, The fragment resembles a "teardrop." *D*, After the force passes, the fractured vertebra remains displaced posteriorly on the vertebra below.

and of the posterior portion of the intervertebral disk below. Either the anterior or the anteroinferior margin of the involved vertebral body is fractured (Fig. 3–35 *C*). The fragment, which resembles a "teardrop," is displaced anteriorly. After the force passes, the fractured vertebra remains displaced posteriorly on the vertebra below (Fig. 3–35 *D*). In a few cases, the vertebral arch is fractured by the pull of the posterior ligaments.[14, 15]

Extension Injuries

A distinction may be made between a disruptive and a compressive hyperextension injury. With a blow to the chin, the injuring force is directed backward and upward. If the force is sufficient, the anterior longitudinal ligament and the intervertebral disk may be ruptured. The cervical vertebrae above the ligamentous injury are carried posteriorly with the spinal cord. The cord is pinched between the posteroinferior margin of the vertebral body above and the laminae of the vertebra below[14, 16] (Fig. 3–36). As the force is dissipated, the neck may spring back to its normal position, and subsequent radiographs may appear entirely normal. Since this is primarily a ligamentous injury, it has been termed a hyperextension sprain (rupture).[5]

The hyperextension sprain mechanism helps in understanding what has happened to the emergency room patient with clinical evidence of a severe spinal cord injury and normal radiographs. Subtle changes, such as a tiny avulsion fracture from the anterior

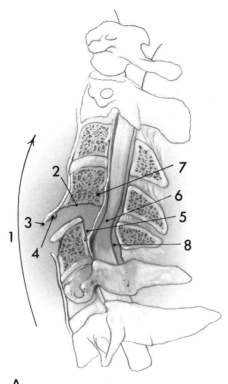

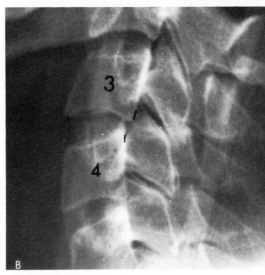

A

Figure 3–36. A, Hyperextension sprain (momentary dislocation) caused by a disruptive hyperextension injury (1). The C-4 intervertebral disk is torn from the caudal endplate of the C-4 body (2); the anterior longitudinal ligament is ruptured (3); an avulsion fracture off the anterosuperior margin of the body of C-5 is seen at (4); the posterior longitudinal ligament is widely separated from the body of C-5 (5); and the spinal cord (6) is pinched between the posteroinferior margin of C-4 (7) and the laminae (8) of C-5. B, Lateral radiograph of patient with an acute central cord syndrome following a severe disruptive hyperextension injury. The C-3 intervertebral disk space is abnormally wide, and there is retrolisthesis of the C-3 vertebra on C-4. Diagnosis: hyperextension sprain.

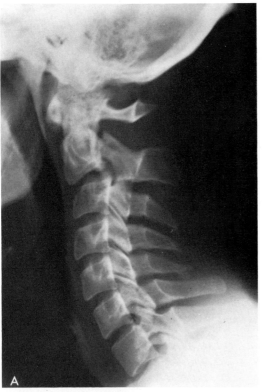

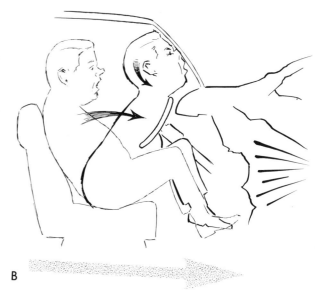

A

B

Figure 3–37. "Classic" hangman's fracture, or traumatic spondylolisthesis of the axis. Note that the vertebral arch of the axis is avulsed from the axis body, and that the axis body is displaced forward on C-3. The C-2 intervertebral disk space has been disrupted and is narrowed. Soft tissue changes are absent. The patient was neurologically normal. B, Mechanism of injury to produce the hangman's fracture.

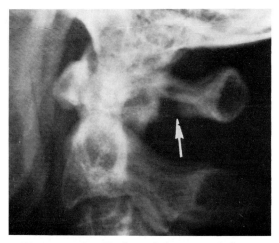

Figure 3–38. Unilateral fracture of the posterior arch of the atlas vertebra (arrow).

margin of a vertebral body or a widened intervertebral disk space (Fig. 3–36 *B*), may offer the only diagnostic clue to the true nature of the patient's injury.

Another quite common type of disruptive hyperextension injury (7 per cent of patients in the Duke series) is the "hangman's fracture" or traumatic spondylolisthesis of the axis (Fig. 3–37).[14, 17-23] Fractures may occur through the pedicles; and, depending upon the magnitude of the force applied, the fragments may be distracted to yield anterior displacement of the body of the axis with respect to the C-3 vertebra below. The remaining portion of the axis remains in place along with the lower cervical spine.

In a compressive hyperextension injury, several types of fracture may occur. In the upper cervical spine, this injury may fracture the posterior arch of the atlas (Fig. 3–38). Lower in the cervical spine, the force of injury is directed posteriorly and downward, crushing the vertebral arch components, especially the articular pillars, spinous process, and laminae (Fig. 3–39).

If the hyperextensive compressive force is of greater magnitude, the head may be forced backward in an arc. Initially the head moves backward, then downward. Assuming that rupture of the anterior longitudinal ligament occurs only late in the course of the trauma if at all, the force of injury is initially expended on the articular processes, then on the spinous processes, laminae, and pedicles (Fig. 3–40 *B*). Once the articular processes have been fractured, the forces still acting through an arc are now free to

displace the vertebral body anteriorly, as it is no longer restrained by an intact vertebral arch. The resulting picture (Fig. 3–40 *C, D;* 3–41) shows anterior displacement of the fractured vertebra on the one below. The lateral view is suggestive of a hyperflexion injury, but the important differentiating diagnostic point is the fracture of one or both articular processes, uncommon occurrences in flexion injuries.[14, 24]

Axial Compressive Injuries

With the cervical spine maintained in the neutral position, an axial compressive force

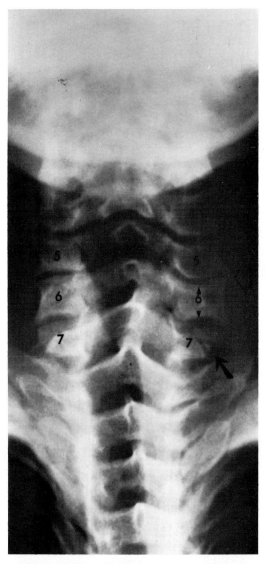

Figure 3–39. Supine vertebral arch view. Fractures of the articular pillars at C-6 and C-7 are present (arrows).

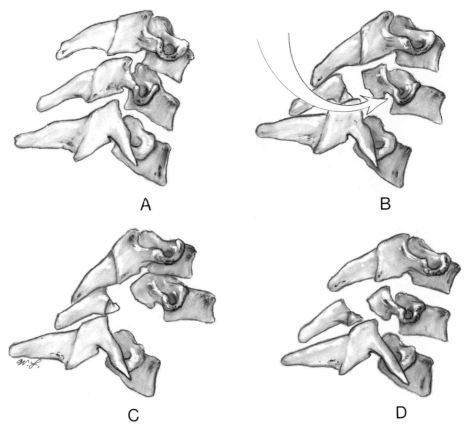

Figure 3–40. Type IV hyperextension fracture-dislocation–mechanism of injury. *A*, Normal. *B*, If the compressive hyperextension force is of sufficient magnitude, the head may be forced backward in an arc. Initially the head moves backward, then downward. Assuming that rupture of the anterior longitudinal ligament occurs only late in the course of the trauma if at all, the force of injury is initially expended on the articular processes, then on the spinous processes, laminae, and pedicles. *C*, Once the articular processes have been fractured, the forces still acting through an arc are now free to displace the vertebral body anteriorly, as it is no longer restrained by the intact vertebral arch. *D*, Post-injury appearance (also see Figure 3–41).

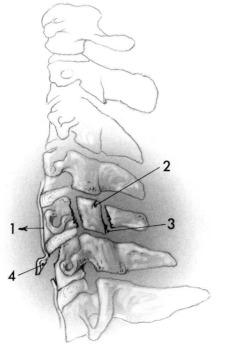

Figure 3–41. Type V-A hyperextension fracture-dislocation. Similar to the Type IV lesion shown in Figure 3–40, however, in this case the vertebral arch is comminuted. Post-injury appearance showing the C-5 vertebral body displaced forward (1); the articular pillar is fractured and rotated into a more horizontal plane (2), and there is a laminal fracture (3); an avulsion fracture of the anterosuperior margin of the C-6 vertebral body is present (4), and the anterior longitudinal ligament is ruptured.

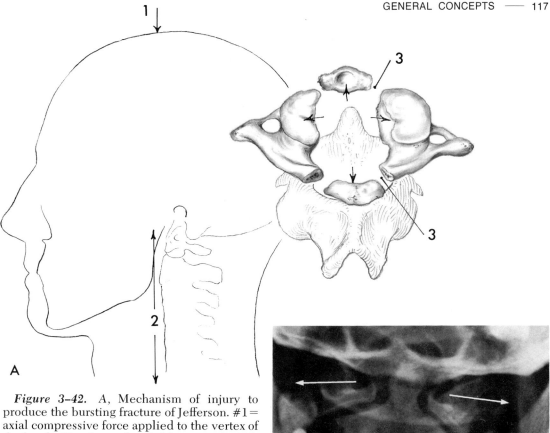

Figure 3–42. A, Mechanism of injury to produce the bursting fracture of Jefferson. #1 = axial compressive force applied to the vertex of the head; #2 = the neck is held erect and rigid; #3 = fractures through the anterior and posterior arch of the atlas. Note the bilateral lateral displacement of the lateral masses of the atlas on the axis. B, Open-mouth view of the atlas-axis showing a Jefferson fracture. Note the bilateral atlantoaxial offset (arrows).

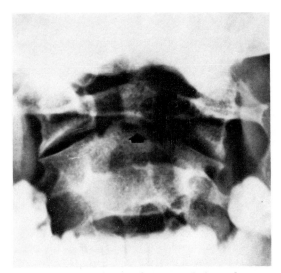

Figure 3–43. Frontal view of the atlas-axis through the open mouth. There is a laterally displaced fracture of the dens to the patient's left side. The mechanism of injury is lateral hyperflexion.

directed caudally through the vertex of the skull may produce a bursting fracture of the atlas. The force of injury is directed to the superior articular facets of the atlas through the occipital condyles. It is opposed by resistance directed upward through the superior articular facets of the axis. Thus the triangular lateral masses of C-1 are forced laterally, resulting in combined fractures of both anterior and posterior arches of the atlas (Fig. 3–42). This type of fracture was described by Jefferson in 1920.[25]

Lateral Flexion Injuries

Lateral flexion injuries result from blows to the lateral aspect of the head or the neck. The resultant lateral flexion forces may produce five possible lesions, including the following: (1) fracture of the dens with lateral displacement (Fig. 3–43); (2) lateral wedge-

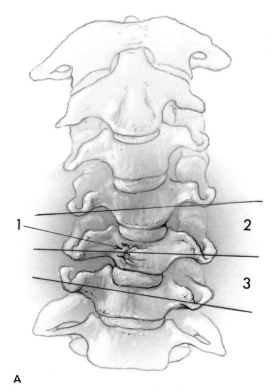 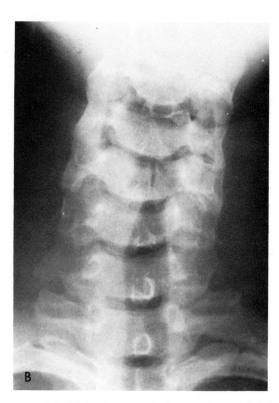

Figure 3–44. *A,* Lateral wedge-compression fracture of C-5 (1). There is slight separation of C-5 from the vertebra above and below (2,3). *B,* Frontal radiograph showing wedging of the C-5 vertebral body on the left. There is also a vertical fracture in the same vertebral body.

compression fracture of a vertebral body (Fig. 3–44); (3) uncinate process fracture (Fig. 3–45); (4) fracture of a transverse process (Fig. 3–46); or (5) brachial plexus avulsions with associated cervical or upper thoracic spine fracture (Fig. 3–47).[26]

Rotary Injuries

Rotational forces may be combined with any other mechanism of cervical spine injury. Experimentally, Roaf[2] showed that the ligaments of the spine are resistant to tear or rupture with a pure flexion or extension mechanism of injury. However, when components of horizontal shear or rotation injury are added, these structures are easily damaged. Thus, with rotation and flexion injuries, the posterior ligaments, apophyseal joint capsules, and the posterior longitudinal ligament may be ruptured, in that order. If the spine is extended and rotated, the anterior longitudinal ligament may be readily torn.

Owing to their normally wide range of rotation, the atlantoaxial joints are not espe-

cially subject to hyperrotational injuries. Locking of the atlas on the axis in rotation is only rarely encountered. The atlas must be rotated beyond 45 degrees on the axis to produce this locking injury.

Signs of Cervical Spine Trauma

There are 12 significant signs of cervical spine trauma. These signs indicate underlying, often occult, trauma. Three major categories will be considered: (1) abnormal soft tissues, (2) abnormal vertebral alignment, and (3) abnormal joint[7] (Table 3–5).

Abnormalities of Soft Tissues

The physician should begin his examination of the cervical spine radiographs with a close perusal of the paravertebral soft tissues. Four signs relate to these tissues.

WIDENED RETROPHARYNGEAL SPACE. The retropharyngeal soft tissue space should be measured from the pharyngeal air column to the anteroinferior aspect

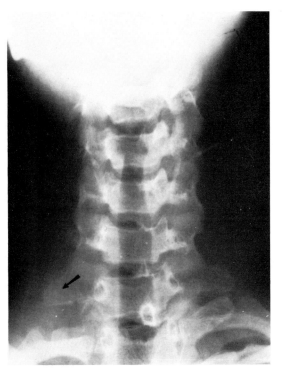

Figure 3–45. Horizontal fracture of the uncinate process of T-1 on the left. Recall that uncinate processes occur from the level of C-3 through T-1!

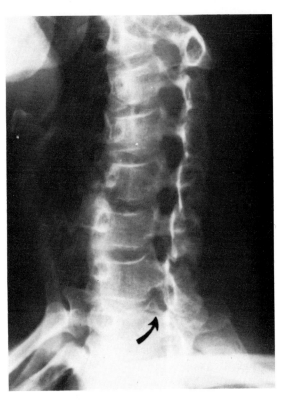

Figure 3–46. Oblique fracture of the transverse process of C-7 on the right. The mechanism of injury is lateral hyperflexion.

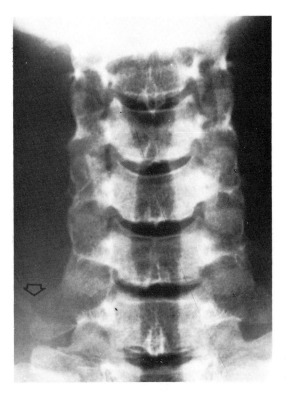

Figure 3–47. Frontal view on a patient with a brachial plexus avulsion and a fracture of the transverse process of C-7 on the right (arrow).

TABLE 3–5. Significant Signs of
Cervical Spine Trauma[7]

ABNORMAL SOFT TISSUES
    Widened retropharyngeal space
    Widened retrotracheal space
    Displacement of prevertebral fat stripe
    Tracheal displacement and laryngeal dislocation

ABNORMAL VERTEBRAL ALIGNMENT
    Loss of lordosis
    Acute kyphotic hyperangulation
    Torticollis
    Widened interspinous space
    Rotation of vertebral bodies

ABNORMAL JOINTS
    Widened middle atlantoaxial joint
    Abnormal intervertebral disk
    Widening of apophyseal joints

of the body of the axis vertebra. A space exceeding 7 mm width in children or adults is abnormal (Fig. 3–48).[27] In Table 3–6 average values are presented. The presence of nasogastric and endotracheal intubation invalidates width measurement of the prevertebral soft tissue space.

WIDENED RETROTRACHEAL SPACE. The retrotracheal soft tissue space is properly measured from the anteroinferior aspect of the body of C- 6 to the posterior tracheal wall. A space greater than 14 mm width in children and 22 mm in adults is considered abnormal, and in the acutely injured cervical spine suggests the presence of edema and/or hemorrhage (Fig. 3–49) (Table 3–6).[27]

DISPLACEMENT OF THE PREVERTEBRAL FAT STRIPE. This thin band of areolar fatty tissue normally parallels the anterior longitudinal ligament to the level of C-6, where it begins to slant anteriorly and inferiorly into the base of the neck. Displacement of this landmark on the lateral radiograph, even in the absence of widening of the prevertebral soft tissues spaces, is a reliable indirect clue to the presence of underlying hemorrhage and/or edema (Figs. 3–49 B, 3–50).

TRACHEAL DEVIATION AND LARYNGEAL DISLOCATION. Following certain hyperextension injuries, the larynx may come to lie immediately adjacent to the anterior aspect of the cervical vertebral bodies as seen on the lateral radiograph. Under these circumstances, the expected band of prevertebral soft tissues will be absent. Lateral deviation of the tracheal air shadow on a true frontal radiograph may indicate displacement resulting from hematoma, or edema formation in the neck following trauma (Fig. 3–51).[10]

Abnormalities of Vertebral Alignment

LOSS OF LORDOSIS. Loss of the normal cervical lordotic curvature is often secondary to spasm of the paraspinal musculature in response to underlying injury (Fig. 3–52). The physician must take great care in evaluating this indirect sign, since straightening or reversal of the cervical lordotic curvature may occasionally be encountered in the normal patient. If the angle of the mandible lies adjacent to the axis vertebral body, the patient's neck is in flexion, which will often reverse the normal lordosis. Unconscious patients also show loss of lordosis due to gravity when the patient is in a supine position.

ACUTE KYPHOTIC HYPERANGULATION. Hyperflexion injuries may disrupt the nuchal and interspinous (interspinal) ligaments and the capsules of the apophyseal joints. As a consequence, there may be kyphotic hyperangulation at one or two levels of the cervical spine (Fig. 3–53). In Figure 3–49 B, another example of acute kyphotic hyperangulation is shown. In both instances rupture of the posterior ligaments has occurred.[5]

TORTICOLLIS. Traumatic torticollis may be the result of unilateral muscle spasm following injury. Although a false diagnosis of cervical subluxation is often made when such an arcuate scoliosis is seen, traumatic changes should always be excluded first. If the injury involves rotation of the head and neck, the possibility of an atlantoaxial rotary fixation should be considered.[29] Specially positioned frontal views of the atlas-axis are required for diagnosis, as shown in Figure 3–54. The example shown is that of a Type II atlantoaxial rotary fixation as defined by Fielding (Chapter 4, p. 144).

WIDENED INTERSPINOUS SPACE. On the lateral radiographs, the presence of widening of the interspace between two adjacent spinous processes should alert the physician to possible rupture of the posterior ligaments at that level (Figs. 3–53 A, 3–57). This finding is usually seen concomitantly with an acute kyphotic hyperangulation of the cervical spine.

Text continued on page 126

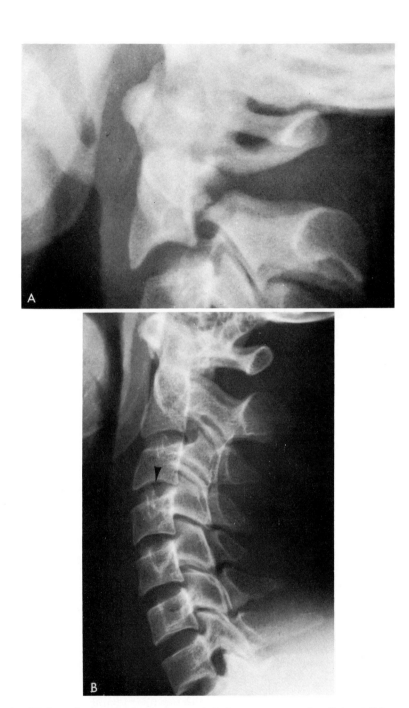

Figure 3–48. Widened retropharyngeal space. *A*, In a patient with a "classic" hangman's fracture. *B*, A patient with a disrupted C-3 intervertebral disk. Note the vacuum sign (arrow), and the very slight widening of the disk space with extension of the spine. Routine plain films and tomograms were normal. The presence of retropharyngeal soft tissue swelling indicated some abnormality, and therefore flexion-extension laterals were done.

TABLE 3–6. Soft Tissue Measurements[27]

	AGE	MEAN WIDTH	RANGE OF NORMAL WIDTH
Retropharyngeal space	<15 yrs >15 yrs	3.5 mm 3.4 mm	2–7 mm 1–7 mm
Retrotracheal space	<15 yrs >15 yrs	7.9 mm 14.0 mm	5–14 mm 5–22 mm

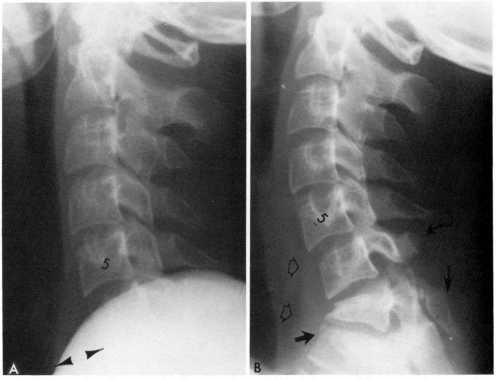

Figure 3–49.   Widened retrotracheal space. *A*, Initial lateral view of the cervical spine. The retrotracheal soft tissue space measured 23 mm, which is abnormal (arrows). *B*, Repeat lateral made while pulling downward on the arms. Note the retrotracheal soft tissue swelling, and displacement of the prevertebral fat stripe (open arrows). There are fractures of the C-7 and T-1 (arrow) vertebral bodies and the spinous process of C-6 (arrows). The acute kyphotic hyperangulation at C-6/7 is due to posterior ligamentous disruption (hyperflexion sprain or rupture).

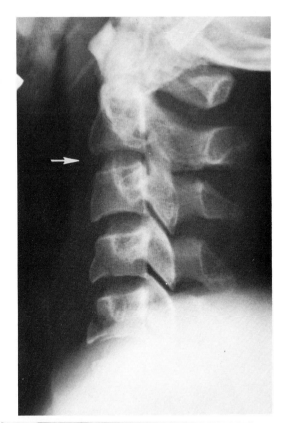

Figure 3–50. Displacement of the prevertebral fat stripe (arrow). There are oblique fractures of the anteroinferior margins of the bodies of C-4 and C-5. Mechanism of injury: hyperextension.

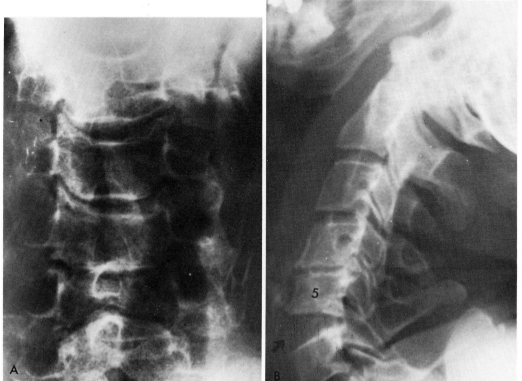

Figure 3–51. Tracheal deviation. *A,* This patient sustained a disruptive hyperextension injury. The frontal view shows tracheal deviation to the left. *B,* Marked widening of the C-5 intervertebral disk space and slight retrolisthesis of C-5 on C-6. Diagnosis: hyperextension sprain. Did you also observe the retropharyngeal soft tissue swelling?

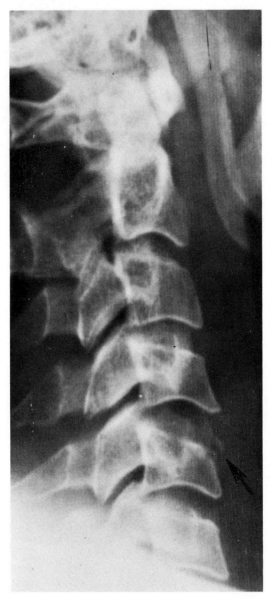

Figure 3–52. Loss of lordosis. This patient had a compressive hyperflexion injury. There is a fracture of the anterosuperior margin of C-5 (arrow). Note the retropharyngeal soft tissue swelling.

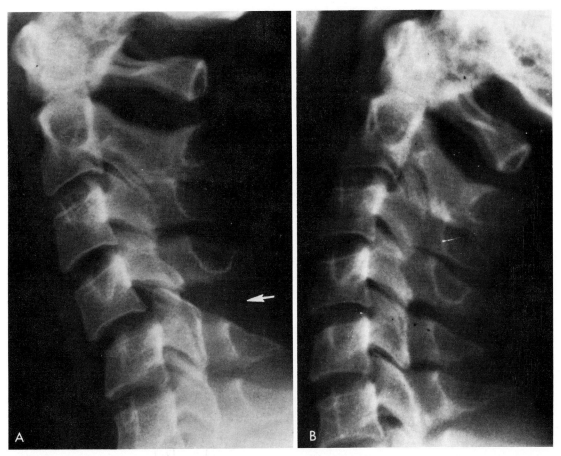

Figure 3–53. Acute kyphotic hyperangulation. *A,* Erect lateral view showing the acute kyphotic hyperangulation at C-4/C-5. There is widening of the interspinous space at C-4/C-5 (arrow), and some decrease in the C-4 intervertebral disk space. No change was seen in attempted extension of the neck. *B,* Supine cross-table lateral view shows reduction of the hyperangulation. Mechanism of injury: disruptive hyperflexion. Diagnosis: hyperflexion sprain.

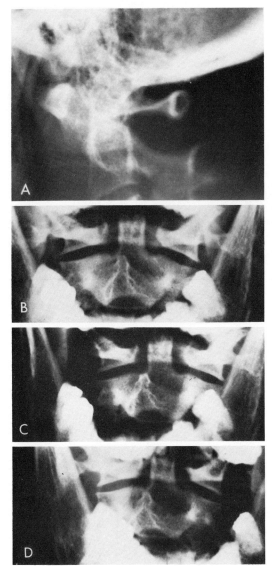

Figure 3–54. Traumatic torticollis. A, Lateral view of the upper cervical spine showing "pure" anterior atlantoaxial dislocation. The predental space measures more than 3 mm. B, Neutral AP view of the atlas-axis showing disparity in the distance between the dens and the lateral masses of the atlas. That distance is slightly greater on the patient's left. The chin and spinous process of the axis are deviated to the right. C, 15 degree rotation to the right. The disparity in the atlas-dens distance persists on this view and with 15 degree rotation to the left (D). Diagnosis: Type II atlantoaxial rotary fixation of Fielding. See Chapter 4 for details of diagnosis.

ROTATION OF VERTEBRAL BODIES. Rotation is manifested on the lateral radiographs as a double contour of the posterior margins of the vertebral body associated with a lack of superimposition of the articular pillars. We have observed this finding in patients with hyperextension fracture dislocations and unilateral facet locking (disruptive hyperflexion dislocation) (Fig. 3–55). Although such rotational changes in alignment may reflect muscle spasm alone, they may also be the first indication of a more serious underlying injury.

Abnormalities of Joints

The third group of signs of cervical trauma involves abnormalities in the cervical articulations.

THE MIDDLE ATLANTOAXIAL JOINT. The middle atlantoaxial joint (predental space) is measured on the lateral radiograph in either of two ways: (a) from the postero-inferior aspect of the anterior arch of the atlas to the adjacent anterior surface of the dens, and (b) from the posterior aspect of the midpoint of the anterior arch of the atlas along the plane of the arch to the anterior surface of the dens. There is no significant difference in the values derived from the two means of measurement. A predental space in excess of 3 mm width in adults and 5 mm width in children is abnormal, and may indicate disruption of the transverse ligament of the atlas (Fig. 3–56). Suppurative pharyngitis, ankylosing spondylitis, rheumatoid arthritis, mongolism, assimilation of the atlas, the presence of an os odontoideum, and mechanical insufficiency of the transverse ligament of the atlas have also been associated with widening of the middle atlantoaxial joint.[5]

WIDENING OR NARROWING OF THE INTERVERTEBRAL DISK. Slight alterations in height and symmetry of the intervertebral disks may be the sole indication of severe traumatic change (Figs. 3–48, 3–51). The disk may "gape" anteriorly or posteriorly with extension and flexion injuries respectively (Fig. 3–55 A). Eccentric or generalized disk space narrowing may follow extrusion of nuclear material from a ruptured intervertebral disk.

WIDENING OF THE APOPHYSEAL JOINTS. Disruptive hyperflexion injuries and some hyperextension injuries may tear the apophyseal joint capsules to widen the apophyseal joint spaces (Fig. 3–57).

As the examples presented well show, signs of cervical spine trauma seldom occur in isolation. Several valuable radiologic

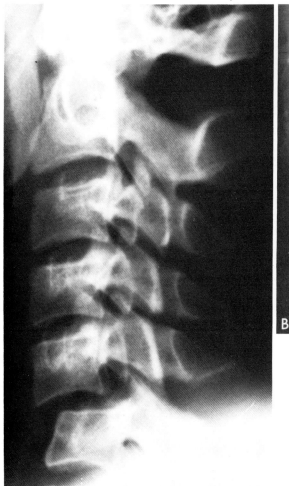

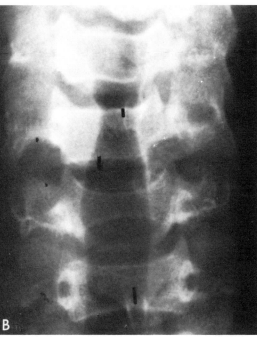

Figure 3–55. Rotation of vertebral bodies. *A*, Lateral view showing the C-5 vertebra displaced forward (anterolisthesis) on C-6, decreased height of the C-5 intervertebral disk space, and rotation of the vertebrae from C-5 cranially. *B*, Frontal view. Black lines have been placed on the spinous processes of C-4, C-5, and C-6. Note the deviation of the C-5 spinous process to the right. Diagnosis: Unilateral facet locking of C-5/C-6 on the right. Compare with Figure 3–33 *B*, *C*.

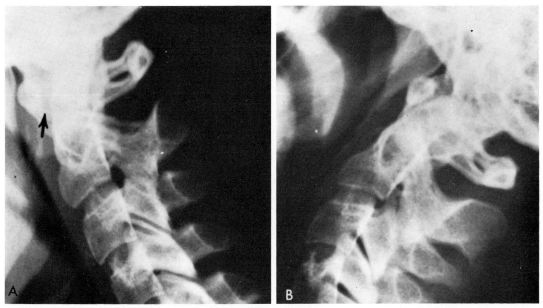

Figure 3–56. Widened middle atlantoaxial joint. *A*, Lateral view in flexion showing widening of the middle atlantoaxial joint (predental space) (arrow). *B*, Extension lateral shows characteristic reduction of the dislocation. In our experience, it is extremely rare to see a traumatic dislocation persist in extension. Mechanism of injury: hyperflexion or shearing forces. Diagnosis: "Pure" anterior atlantoaxial dislocation.

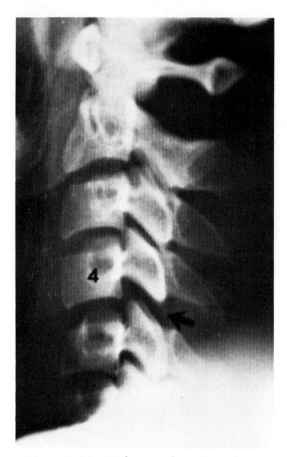

Figure 3–57. Widening of apophyseal joints. Cross-table lateral in a patient with a hyperflexion sprain. Note the widening of the C-4/C-5 apophyseal joints (arrow), and some widening of the interspinous space at C-4/C-5.

clues to significant underlying spinal injury are often visible on one view.

Direct Signs of Cervical Spine Trauma

It will be found helpful when evaluating

TABLE 3–7.   Distribution of Cervical Spine Injuries by Level*

1. C-1—	6%
2. C-2—	27%
3. C-3—	10%
4. C-4—	10%
5. C-5—	18%
6. C-6—	27%
7. C-7—	18%

*Total exceeds 100%, since multiple injuries in the same patient were commonly encountered.

radiographs of the injured cervical spine to keep in mind the data to be presented below concerning the levels and locations of the common fractures, and the most common isolated and combined traumatic lesions. Miller et al. performed a computer analysis of 400 patients with recognized fractures and/or dislocations of the cervical spine. This information will be presented here.[6]

Distribution of Injuries

MULTIPLE LESIONS. Less than one-third of the patients analyzed had only one fracture or dislocation. The average number of injuries per patient was 2.4. One patient in seven had *four or more* cervical injuries. The old radiologic dictum that when one abnormality is found one should search diligently for others is certainly true in cervical trauma patients. Identification of the first fracture or dislocation indicates a need for treatment; however, recognition of the total pattern of injury will determine the mode of therapy to be employed.

LEVELS OF INJURY. The distribution of cervical spine injuries at various levels is shown in Table 3–7. The numbers refer to the percentage of patients with injuries at the levels indicated. The total exceeds 100 per cent, since multiple injuries in the same patient were commonly encountered.

The C-2 and C-6 vertebrae were found to be the most vulnerable to injury. The most common fractures of the axis vertebra were those involving the dens (14 per cent of all patients) and the "hangman's fracture"—traumatic spondylolisthesis—(7 per cent of patients). At the level of C-6, vertebral arch fractures predominated. The articular pillars were the most common site for C-6 vertebral arch fractures. The most protected and therefore least often injured vertebra was the atlas, probably owing to its anatomic position, partially covered by the skull and the heavy neck musculature. Eighty-one of Miller's patients (20 per cent) had injuries at multiple levels. These tended to cluster at adjacent levels, with a significant predilection for the lower cervical spine.

FREQUENCY OF OCCURRENCE. Table 3–8 shows the frequency of injury of each anatomic component in our series. Probably the most startling finding to emerge was the number of vertebral arch fractures; one-half of Miller's patients had such fractures. As a

TABLE 3–8 Distribution of Injury by
Anatomic Structure

LOCATION	PERCENTAGE OF PATIENTS°
Vertebral arch	50%
Vertebral body	30%
Intervertebral disk	29%
Posterior ligaments	16%
Dens	14%
Locked facets	12%
Anterior ligaments	2%

°Because most of the patients had multiple injuries, the total exceeds 100%.

result of this information, the technique of filming acutely injured cervical spines at Duke was drastically changed. This has been mentioned previously (p. 99).

Vertebral body and intervertebral disk injuries each accounted for about 30 per cent of traumatic cervical spine lesions in our series. Injuries to the posterior ligaments, the dens, and locked facets were less common, each occurring in about 13 per cent of the patients studied. Anterior ligament injuries occurred even less frequently, accounting for only 2 per cent of patients in the Duke series.

In the next two chapters, we will study injuries of the cervical spine based on an anatomic classification of lesions.

REFERENCES

1. Salter, R. B.: Textbook of Disorders and Injuries of the Musculoskeletal System. Baltimore, Williams & Wilkins, 1970.
2. Roaf, R.: A study of the mechanics of spinal injuries. J. Bone & Jt. Surg., 42-B:810, 1960.
3. Archer, V. W.: The Osseous System. A Handbook of Roentgen-Diagnosis. Chicago, Yearbook, 1945.
4. Watson-Jones, R.: Fractures and Joint Injuries, 4th Ed. Baltimore, Williams & Wilkins, 1955.
5. Braakman, R., and Penning, L.: Injuries of the Cervical Spine. London, Excerpta Medica, 1971.
6. Miller, M. D., Gehweiler, J. A., Martinez, S., Charlton, O. P., and Daffner, R. H.: Significant new observations on cervical spine trauma. Amer. J. Roentgenol., 130:659, 1978.
7. Clark, W. M., Gehweiler, J. A., and Laib, R.: Significant signs of cervical spine trauma. Skeletal Radiol. 3:201, 1979.
8. Breasted, J. H.: The Edwin Smith Surgical Papyrus. Chicago, University of Chicago Press, 1930.
9. Roaf, R.: International classification of spinal injuries. Paraplegia, 10:78, 1972.
10. Selecki, B. R., and Williams, H. B. L.: Injuries to the Cervical Spine and Cord in Man. Australian Medical Association Monograph, 1970.
11. Holdsworth, F.: Fractures, dislocations and fracture-dislocations of the spine. J. Bone & Jt. Surg., 52-A:1534, 1970.
12. Whitley, J. F., and Forsythe, H. F.: Classification of cervical spine injuries. Amer. J. Roentgenol., 83:633, 1958.
13. Howarth, M. B., and Petrie, J. G.: Injuries of the Spine. Baltimore, Williams & Wilkins, 1964.
14. Gehweiler, J. A., Clark, W. M., Schaaf, R. E., Powers, B., and Miller, M. D.: Cervical spine trauma: the common combined conditions. Radiology, 130:77, 1979.
15. Schneider, R. C., and Kahn, E. A.: Chronic neurologic sequelae of acute trauma to the spine and spinal cord. Part I: The significance of the acute flexion or "teardrop" fracture-dislocation of the cervical spine. J. Bone & Jt. Surg., 38-A:985, 1956.
16. Taylor, A. R., and Blackwood, W.: Paraplegia in hyperextension injuries with normal radiographic appearances. J. Bone & Jt. Surg., 30-B:245, 1948.
17. Von Torklus, D., and Gehle, W.: The Upper Cervical Spine. New York, Grune and Stratton, 1972.
18. Grogono, B. J. S.: Injuries of the atlas and axis. J. Bone & Jt. Surg., 36-B:387, 1954.
19. Wood-Jones, F.: The ideal lesion produced by judicial hanging. Lancet, 1:53, 1913.
20. Schneider, R. C., Livingston, K. E., Cave, A. J. E., and Hamilton, G.: "Hangman's fracture" of the cervical spine. J. Neurosurg., 22:141, 1965.
21. Elliott, J. M., Rogers, L. F., Wissinger, J. P., and Lee, J. F.: The hangman's fracture. Fractures of the neural arch of the axis. Radiology, 104:303, 1972.
22. Brashear, H. R., Venters, G. C., and Preston, E. T.: Fractures of the neural arch of the axis. A report of twenty-nine cases. J. Bone & Jt. Surg., 57-A:879, 1975.
23. Seljeskog, E. L., and Chous, S. N.: Spectrum of the hangman's fracture. J. Neurosurg., 45:3, 1976.
24. Forsyth, H. F.: Extension injuries of the cervical spine. J. Bone & Jt. Surg., 46-A:1792, 1964.
25. Jefferson, G.: Fracture of the atlas vertebra. Report of four cases and a review of those previously recorded. Brit. J. Surg., 7:407, 1920.
26. Schaaf, R. E., Gehweiler, J. A., Miller, M. D., and Powers, B.: Lateral hyperflexion injuries of the cervical spine. Skeletal Radiol., 3:73, 1978.
27. Wholey, M., Bruwer, A. J., and Baker, H. L.: Lateral roentgenograms of neck. Radiology, 71:350, 1958.
28. Whalen, J. P., and Woodruff, C. L.: The cervical prevertebral fat stripe. A new aid in evaluation of the cervical prevertebral soft tissue space. Amer. J. Roentgenol., 109:445, 1970.
29. Fielding, J. W., and Hawkins, R. J.: Atlanto-axial rotary fixation. Fixed rotatory subluxation of the atlanto-axial joint. J. Bone & Jt. Surg., 59-A:37, 1977.

Chapter 4

INJURIES OF THE OCCIPITO-ATLANTO-AXIAL REGION

"If thou examinest a man having a displacement in a vertebra of his neck, whose face is fixed, whose neck cannot turn for him, ... An ailment which I will treat."

The Edwin Smith Surgical Papyrus.
Circa 17th Century B.C.[1]

INTRODUCTION

The occipito-atlanto-axial region is unique — morphologically, developmentally, and functionally. Therefore, injuries to the region must be considered separately from those of the lower cervical spine.

During the movements of flexion, extension, lateral flexion (abduction), and rotation the occipito-atlanto-axial joints function as a single unit. The atlas serves as a washer or bearing between the occipital condyles and the axis vertebra.

As we have learned earlier, the only direct connections between the occiput and the axis are the tectorial membrane (the cranial extension of the posterior longitudinal ligament), the cruciate ligament, the apical dental ligament, and the paired alar ligaments (Fig. 4–1, 4–2 A,B).

The occipital condyles articulate with the superior articular facets of the atlas to form the atlanto-occipital joints. These joints permit motion in two planes — flexion-extension and lateral flexion. Rotation of the skull upon the atlas is blocked by the oblique alignment of the occipital condyles upon the medially tilted facets of the atlas.

The average range of flexion-extension in the atlanto-occipital joints is 13 to 15 degrees.[2, 3] Flexion is limited by contact between the dens and the basion, while extension is limited by bony contact between the basiocciput and the posterior arch of the atlas, as well as by the tectorial membrane. Lateral flexion of the atlanto-occipital joints is controlled by the alar ligaments. Experimentally, Werne[2] showed that removal of the tectorial membrane and division of the alar ligaments produced instability of the atlanto-occipital joints, thereby permitting luxation (dislocation) to occur.

The atlas articulates with the axis through three joints — one middle atlantoaxial and two lateral atlantoaxial joints. By far the most important ligamentous connection of the atlas is the stout transverse ligament, which makes up the horizontal part of the cruciate (cruciform) ligament. The transverse ligament holds the dens in close contact with the anterior arch of the atlas during all movements in the upper cervical spine. Thus, in adults the predental space never normally exceeds 2.5 to 3.0 mm. In children increased laxity of the ligament permits greater movement of the dens relative to the anterior arch of the atlas; however, the predental space normally never exceeds 5 mm. Disruption of the transverse ligament permits atlantoaxial luxation to occur.

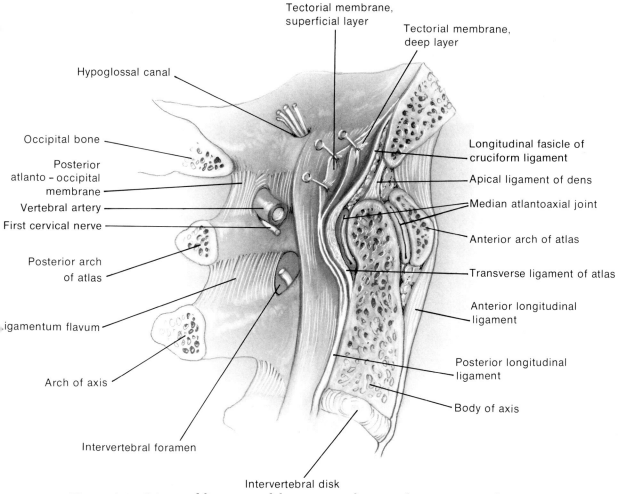

Figure 4–1. Joints and ligaments of the occipito-atlanto-axial region — sagittal section.

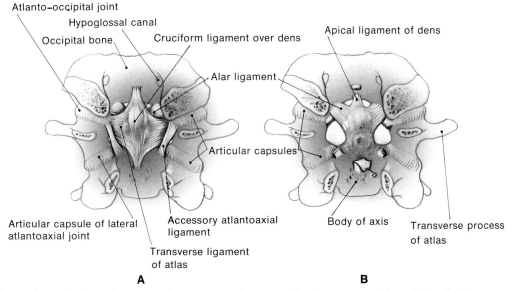

A   **B**

Figure 4–2. *A*, Articulations at the occipito-atlanto-axial region, viewed from behind. The posterior arch of the atlas and the laminae of the axis have been removed along with the tectorial membrane and the posterior longitudinal ligament. *B*, After removal of the cruciform ligament.

Movement at the atlantoaxial joints is limited to flexion, extension, rotation, and lateral shifting (abduction) of the atlas on the axis. The tectorial membrane allows approximately 10 degrees of flexion-extension. The average range of rotation is 47 degrees. This movement is checked by the alar ligaments.[2]

With slight rotation of the skull and atlas (which move as a unit in rotation) upon the axis, the contralateral alar ligament tenses. As rotation continues, the contralateral alar ligament is wrapped around the dens. Ultimately the ipsilateral alar ligament also becomes taut. With rotation of the skull-atlas unit and tightening of the alar ligaments, some lateral flexion of the atlanto-occipital joints occurs.

Keep your eyes straight ahead and slowly turn your head to one side until it approaches 90 degrees. Half of this rotation occurs at the atlanto-axial joints, the remainder in the lower cervical spine. After about 20 to 30 degrees of rotation of the skull-atlas, rotation of the axis and lower cervical vertebrae occurs from above downward and in decreasing amounts.[5] This rotation in the lower cervical spine also produces some ipsilateral lateral flexion in the same direction as the rotation. The vertebral spinous processes are therefore deviated away from the side of rotation and lateral flexion.

Lateral shifting (abduction) of the atlas on the axis requires a combination of movements — lateral bending and rotation.[5, 6] This may occur because of vertical approximation of the atlas and axis in the rotated position, allowing some laxity of the capsular ligaments about the lateral atlantoaxial joints. Atlas shift on the axis may occur to a lesser degree without atlantoaxial rotation.[3] Since this movement is a physiologic one, it should not be mistaken for a "subluxation" of the atlantoaxial joints.

Before we examine the traumatic conditions occurring at the occipito-atlanto-axial region, the reader should be aware of some interesting facts. In our series of 400 patients with fractures and dislocations of the cervical spine (1) 35 per cent involved the occipito-atlanto-axial region, (2) the vast majority of the lesions could be diagnosed on lateral views of the cervical spine, (3) most of the trauma resulted from hyperextension injuries, and (4) the axis vertebra was injured four times more commonly than was the atlas vertebra.

ANTERIOR ATLANTO-OCCIPITAL DISLOCATION

Traumatic atlanto-occipital dislocation is rare and usually fatal. There are, however, six case reports of patients who survived this injury.[7-12] Until the paper of Powers et al.,[12] the criteria for roentgen diagnosis of anterior atlanto-occipital dislocation have been unclear.

In the Duke series of 400 patients, 1 per cent (four patients) had atlanto-occipital dislocation. Two of our four patients survived the injury without significant neurologic deficit (Fig. 4–3).

Atlanto-occipital dislocation is most commonly caused by traffic accidents and falls. The mechanism of injury is conjectural. In the few autopsied cases available, death was apparently due to transection of the medulla oblongata.[13] In the surviving cases, a wide spectrum of neurologic findings[7-12] may result.

The roentgen diagnosis of anterior atlanto-occipital dislocation was not clearly defined until the work of Powers et al.[12] They determined that a ratio $\overline{BC}/\overline{OA}$ was required to evaluate accurately the normal and pathologic relationships between the atlas and basiocciput. The validity of the ratio was proved mathematically, statistically, and through clinical application in a host of normal adults and children and confirmed in all available cases of atlanto-occipital dislocation.

In Figure 4–4, the normal atlanto-occipital anatomy is shown. The landmarks for determining the Powers ratio, $\overline{BC}/\overline{OA}$ are superimposed. B is the *basion*, the midline anterior margin of the foramen magnum. To find the basion, find the point where the inner and outer tables of the basiocciput join. C is the midpoint of the *arch-canal line* of the *atlas*, the junction line of the posterior arch of the atlas and the posterior tubercle. O is the *opisthion*, the midline posterior margin of the foramen magnum. To find the opisthion on the lateral radiograph, trace the inner table of the occipital bone forward and downward to the point where it joins the outer table. A is the *midpoint* of the *posterior surface* of the *anterior*

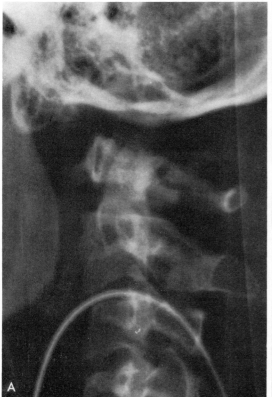

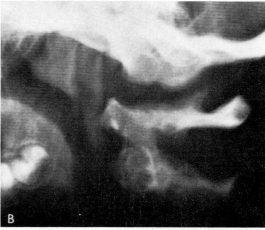

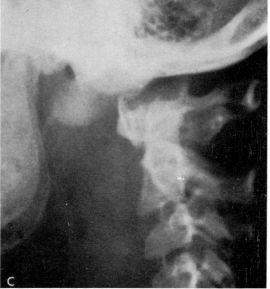

Figure 4–3. Traumatic anterior atlanto-occipital dislocation. *A*, Lateral radiograph of a patient involved in a car-motorcycle accident. This patient did not survive the trauma; however, he was alive at the time this radiograph was made. The *Powers ratio* ($\overline{BC}/\overline{OA}$) is greater than 1. *B*, A five year old boy was struck with an automobile and his head was reportedly ground into the road surface. He survived the incident with minor neurologic deficit. The *Powers ratio* exceeds 1. *C*, A nine year old girl was struck by an automobile. She was dead on arrival in the emergency room. The ratio $\overline{BC}/\overline{OA}$ is greater than 1.

arch of the *atlas*. In some cases it may be difficult to clearly see the basion and opisthion. Stereoscopic views and tomography may be needed for accuracy in diagnosis.

If the ratio $\overline{BC}/\overline{OA}$ is *less than 1*, no anterior atlanto-occipital dislocation exists. If the ratio is *greater than 1*, the skull is dislocated anteriorly on the atlas. This ratio is valid for all age groups. Target-film distance need not be considered, since this is a ratio.

The Powers ratio numbers are valid even in the presence of an upper cervical spine fracture, or anterior atlantoaxial dislocations.

The Powers ratio applies only in cases of *anterior* atlanto-occipital dislocation. Only one case of a *posterior* atlanto-occipital dislocation has been reported.[84] The ratio $\overline{BC}/\overline{OA}$ does not apply.

ATLANTOAXIAL DISLOCATIONS

Classification and Incidence

Atlantoaxial dislocations are classified into three types: (1) atlantoaxial fracture-dislocations, which are complicated by fracture of the dens (11 per cent of all patients

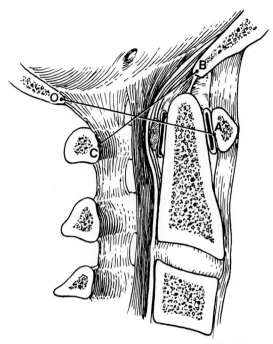

Figure 4-4. The Powers ratio $\overline{BC}/\overline{OA}$ for determining *anterior* atlanto-occipital dislocation. B = basion; C = arch-canal line (midpoint); O = opisthion; A = midpoint of the posterior surface of the anterior arch of the atlas.

in the Duke series of 400 patients); (2) traumatic (pure) atlantoaxial dislocation without associated fracture (2.5 per cent); and (3) nontraumatic atlantoaxial dislocation (Table 4–1).

The atlantoaxial fracture-dislocations are considered on p. 160.

Traumatic (Pure) Atlantoaxial Dislocations

Three types of traumatic (pure) atlantoaxial dislocations are recognized: (1) anterior, (2) posterior, and (3) rotary. In the last two types, the transverse ligament of the atlas is probably intact, while in cases with anterior atlantoaxial dislocation it is postulated that the transverse ligament is ruptured.[14, 15]

Anterior Atlantoaxial Dislocation

In the Duke series, this traumatic dislocation was found in 2.5 per cent of all patients. It is thought to be rare because the transverse ligament of the atlas is probably stronger than the dens itself, although some

recent work by Fielding et al. questions this concept.[14, 15] A displacement of 3 mm or more of the atlas on the axis is evidence of disruption of the transverse ligament of the atlas[15] (Figs. 4–5, 4–6, 4–7).

The most common cause of traumatic anterior atlantoaxial dislocation is a severe head injury. The patients complain of upper neck pain and limitation of motion. Those patients without pain have neurologic symptoms. Patients with the most severe neurologic symptoms show the greatest displacement of the atlas on the axis.

The roentgen diagnosis of traumatic (pure)· anterior atlantoaxial dislocation is made on lateral radiographs of the cervical spine. In some instances, the neutral view may reveal widening of the middle atlantoaxial joint (predental space). In other cases, gentle flexion of the neck is necessary to demonstrate the abnormality (Figs. 4–6, 4–7).

Measured along the midplane of the atlas, the distance from the posterior margin of the anterior arch of the atlas to the anterior surface of the dens, the *predental space*, should not normally exceed 3 mm in adults nor 5 mm in children.[16, 17]

Always evaluate the *retrodental space*, the sagittal diameter of the vertebral canal of the atlas, in all cases of anterior atlantoaxial dislocation. The retrodental space is measured along the midplane of the atlas from the posterior surface of the dens to the arch-canal line (the curvilinear junction line

TABLE 4–1. A Classification of Atlantoaxial Dislocations

TYPE	PERCENT OF PATIENTS (*Duke Series*)
Atlantoaxial fracture-dislocations (associated with dens fracture)	11
Anterior	7
Posterior	3
Lateral	1
Traumatic (pure) atlantoaxial dislocation	
Anterior	2.5
Posterior	0
Rotary	0
Nontraumatic atlantoaxial dislocation	Unknown

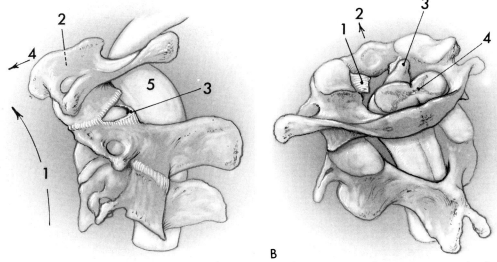

Figure 4–5. "Pure" anterior atlantoaxial dislocation (luxation). *A*, The upper cervical column is flexed (1). Displacement of the atlas (2) anteriorly (4) on the axis. Rupture of the atlantoaxial joint capsules (3). The spinal cord (5) may be traumatized by the posterior arch of the atlas. *B*, Schematic view from above and behind. The transverse ligament (1) is torn, and the atlas dislocated anteriorly on the axis vertebra (2). The spinal cord (4) may be compressed between the dens (3) and the posterior arch of the atlas vertebra.

of the posterior arch of the atlas and the posterior tubercle). If the diameter has been reduced to less than 18 mm in the adult, there are usually neurologic signs and symptoms.[18]

Posterior Atlantoaxial Dislocation

Traumatic (pure) posterior atlantoaxial dislocation is exceedingly rare. In the literature, there are only three case reports in

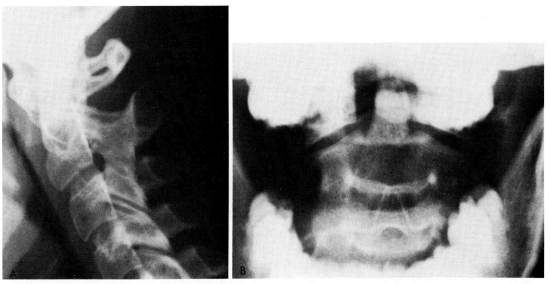

Figure 4–6. "Pure" anterior atlantoaxial dislocation. This 19 year old was hit in the occipital region with an ax. *A*, Flexion lateral roentgenograph showing an abnormal middle atlantoaxial joint (predental space) which measures 4 mm. *B*, Frontal view of the atlas-axis through the open mouth showing normal relationships of the atlas and axis.

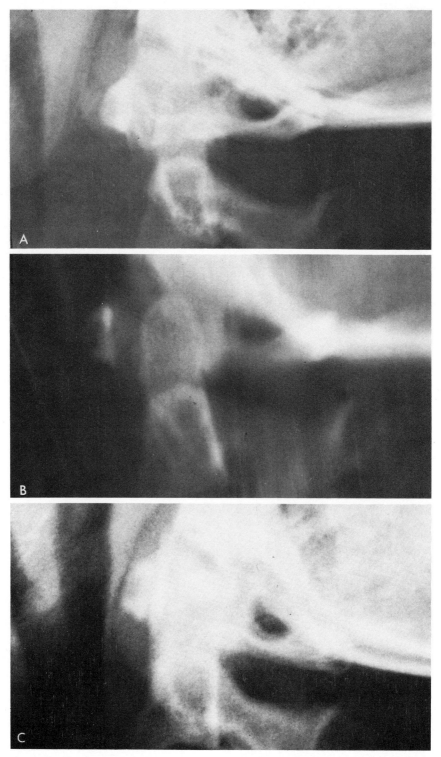

Figure 4–7. "Pure" atlantoaxial dislocation. *A*, Neutral lateral view showing abnormal widening of the middle atlantoaxial joint (predental space) to 6 mm. *B*, Lateral midline tomogram. *C*, Extension lateral showing typical reduction of the dislocation.

which the patient survived. Our artist's concept of one such case is shown in Figure 4–8. These unusual dislocations are believed to result from a disruptive hyperextension injury. All of the ligamentous bonds between the atlas and axis are torn. Interestingly, none of the reported cases showed any significant neurologic deficit. In each case reduction was achieved by skeletal traction.[19-21]

A lateral radiograph of the cervical spine shows the anterior arch of the atlas behind the intact dens. An abnormal basiondens distance may be observed.

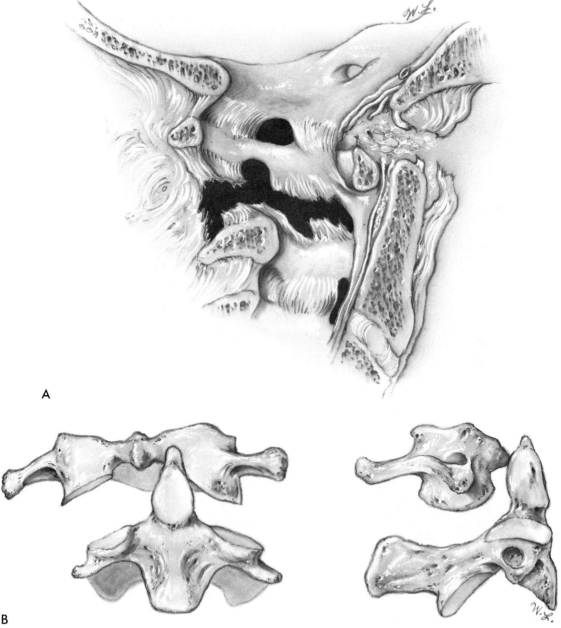

A

B

Figure 4–8. "Pure" posterior atlantoaxial dislocation. *A*, Sagittal section to show the anterior arch of the atlas situated behind the intact dens. Note the probable ligamentous disruption (schematic). *B*, Frontal and lateral drawings based upon the case reported by Haralson and Boyd.[19]

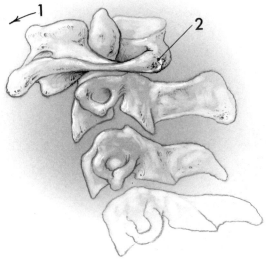

Figure 4–9. "Pure" rotary atlantoaxial dislocation. The atlas is rotated and locked on the axis. There is anterior displacement of the atlas on the axis (1). The posterior tubercle of the atlas can be seen rotated from the midline (2).

Rotary Atlantoaxial Dislocation

Traumatic (pure) atlantoaxial rotary dislocations are rare.[6, 22, 23] The atlas must be rotated on the axis more than 45 degrees to allow locking of the lateral mass(es) of the atlas over the superior articular surface(s) of the axis vertebra to occur (Fig. 4–9).[6]

This condition should not be confused with atlantoaxial rotary fixation (see p. 144).

The roentgen diagnosis depends upon noting the rotation of the atlas more than 45 degrees.[6] The atlas may be tilted and may overlap the superior articular surface of the axis. Stereoscopic and tomographic views may be invaluable in defining the full extent of the dislocation.

We have not observed such a case in our series with injury to the cervical spine. However, a patient with metastatic melanoma and minor trauma showed these changes (Fig. 4–10).

When evaluating patients with traumatic (pure) atlantoaxial dislocation, the physician must keep in mind the possibility of some preexisting condition, which may only be revealed after a neck or head injury. Pure traumatic atlantoaxial dislocations are rare; nontraumatic causes of atlantoaxial dislocations are more common.

Nontraumatic Atlantoaxial Dislocations

Conditions associated with nontraumatic atlantoaxial dislocation include the following: (1) os odontoideum; (2) aplasia of the dens; (3) occipitalization of the atlas; (4) Down's syndrome (trisomy-21, mongolism); (5) rheumatoid arthritis or ankylosing spondylitis; and (6) inflammatory processes in the craniovertebral region.

Os Odontoideum

The *os odontoideum (separate dens)* is generally considered to be a congenital malformation;[40, 64-66] however, there are strong arguments to support the opinion

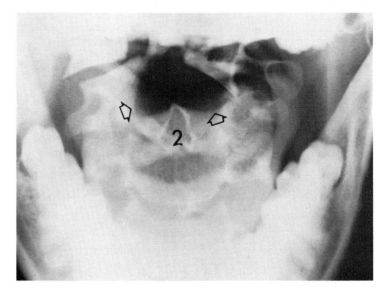

Figure 4–10. Frontal view of the atlas-axis through the open mouth. Note the area of destruction in the body of the axis vertebra (arrows). The atlas is rotated and locked on the axis. In addition there is unilateral right atlantoaxial offset. This patient had melanoma metastatic to multiple bones of the skeleton, including the axis.

that it may be *acquired* as a result of an old fracture of the dens,[53, 67, 68] infection,[40] or rheumatoid arthritis.[69]

Radiographs show a round to oval independent bone situated cranial to the axis atop a hypoplastic dens (Fig. 4–11). Two distinct types of os odontoideum are described:[40] (1) *orthotopic* (G. *orthos* correct, normal + *topos* place): the os lies near the tip of the bony cupola at the upper anterior aspect of the body of the dens, which is hypoplastic; and (2) *dystopic* (G. prefix *dys* bad or difficult + *topos* = malplaced or out of place): The os lies near the basion and may be separate or fused.[40, 70]

How can we explain an os odontoideum developmentally? In Chapter 1 (Developmental Anatomy, p. 54), we described in some detail the development of the dens. With those facts clearly in mind, it would be ridiculous to state that an os odontoideum or separate dens is the result of failure of fusion between the centrum of the atlas and the centrum of the axis, since their junction site lies deep in the body of the axis (Fig. 1–35).[40, 71] Wollin[65] theorizes that a band of mesenchymal tissue persisting in the primitive dens fails to chondrify or ossify, resulting in a divided dens. Von Torklus and Gehle[40] argue that the os odontoideum is a manifestation of occipital vertebra and that the os corresponds to faulty development of the terminal ossicle of the dens.

Os odontoideum is frequently confused in the world literature with *absence of the dens,* which is an extremely rare congenital anomaly. Most published cases of congenital absence of the dens prove, in fact, to be examples of os odontoideum. Although tomography is required in some cases to demonstrate the presence of the os odontoideum, in others it is clearly seen above the hypoplastic dens on conventional views. We agree with Minderhoud et al.[64] that without tomographic proof that an os odontoideum does not exist, cases of "absence of the dens" should be considered to represent os odontoideum.

The term *atlantoaxial instability* has been coined to describe the constantly altered relation of the atlas to the axis in patients with os odontoideum.[64] Depending upon the movement of the skull and cervical spine, the patient may have anterior, lateral, or posterior atlantoaxial luxation. Note should always be made of the size of the vertebral canal at the level of the atlas and axis. This distance is determined by measuring the space between the os odontoideum and the arch-canal line of the atlas. The normal vertebral canal should measure 22.7 mm (mean value) at the level of the atlas and 10.2 mm at the axis.[5] The vertebral canal may be compromised at the C-1 and C-2 levels in patients with an os odontoideum.[64] There is some correlation of symptoms with this finding, although there does not seem to be any constant correlation between the patient's symptomatology and the degree of atlantoaxial instability.

Patients with os odontoideum have variable symptoms: posttraumatic neck pain and torticollis; transient paresis after trauma; myelopathy, slowly progressive or permanent; and findings suggesting a higher level lesion, for example, bulbar symptoms, without cervical myelopathy or nerve root compression.[64, 72]

Aplasia of the Dens

This condition is extremely rare. Note that the defect in the body of the axis conforms almost exactly with the locus of the synchondrosis between the dens and the axis body (Fig. 4–12). In the case illustrated in Figure 4–12 A, the oval bony mass above the axis, separated by a gap, may be an os odontoideum.

Occipitalization of the Atlas

Occipitalization of the atlas is due to failure of segmentation between the last occipital (hypoglossal or anteproatlantal) segment and the first cervical (proatlantal) segment. Degenhardt[73] regards it as a craniad or progressive variant and not a malformation, but others disagree.[40]

Occipitalization of the atlas is rare, occurring in about 0.75 per cent of the population.

The roentgen diagnosis of occipitalization of the atlas depends upon demonstrating some degree of bony union between the atlas and the occipital bone, rather than simply lack of movement at the atlanto-occipital joint. The most frequent finding is a fusion of the basion with the anterior arch of the atlas.[74-77]

Occasionally the entire atlas is fused to the occipital bone (Fig. 4–13, 4–14) and the

Text continued on page 144.

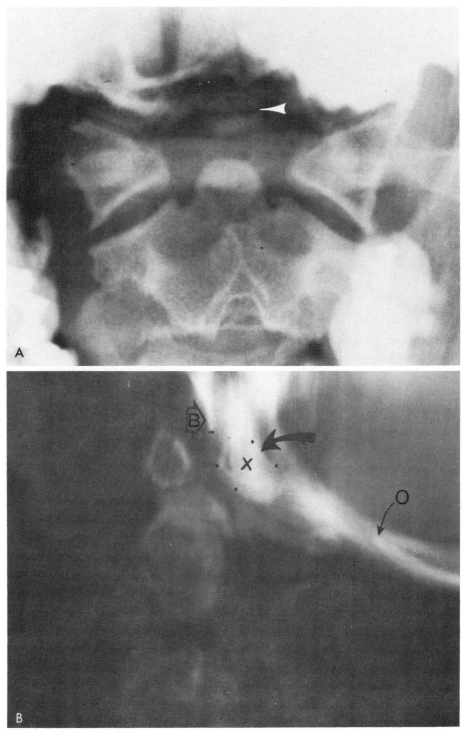

Figure 4–11. Os odontoideum. *A*, Frontal view showing the hypoplastic dens and the os odontoideum (arrow). *B*, Lateral view. Os odontoideum (X), basion (B), opisthion (O).

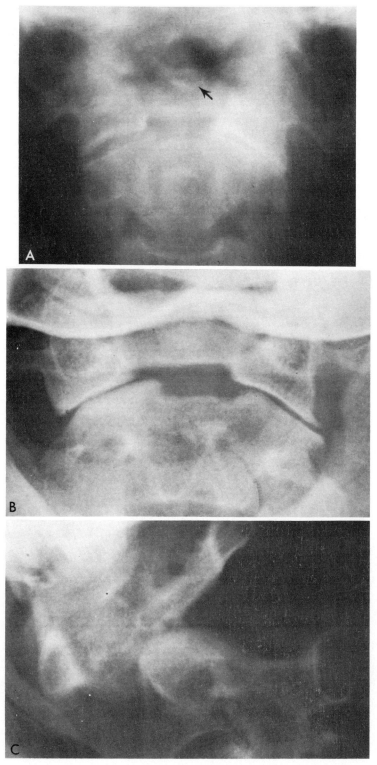

Figure 4–12. Aplasia of the dens — two cases. *A*, Case one. Frontal tomogram showing the bony defect in the body of the axis vertebra, and an os odontoideum (arrow). *B*, *C*, Case two. Frontal and lateral views, respectively, to show the dens aplasia and anterior atlantoaxial dislocation.

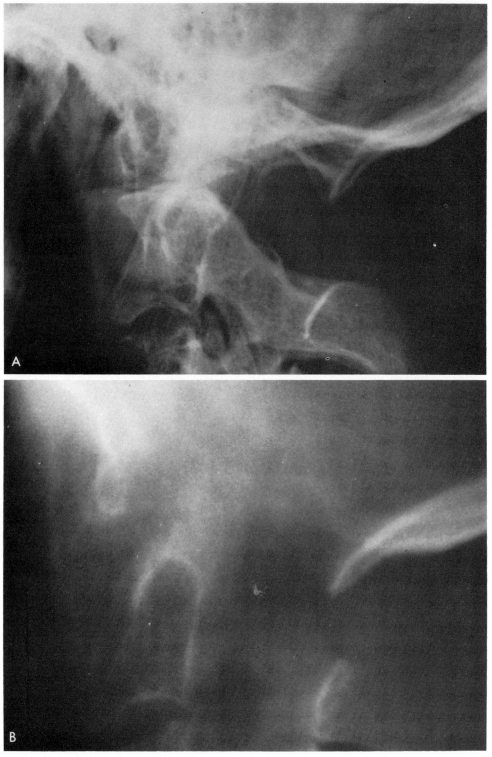

Figure 4–13. Occipitalization of the atlas. *A*, Lateral radiograph showing abnormal middle atlanto-axial joint (predental space), which measured 7 mm. *B*, Lateral midline tomogram showing fusion of the atlas to the occipital bone.

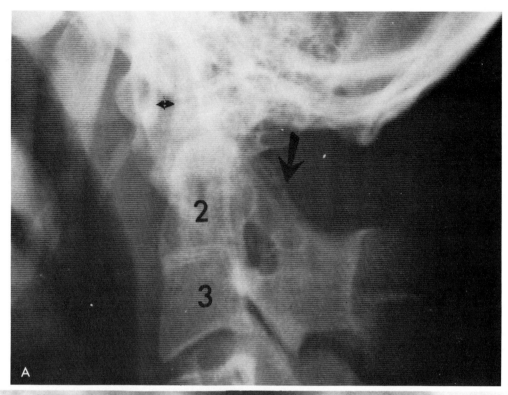

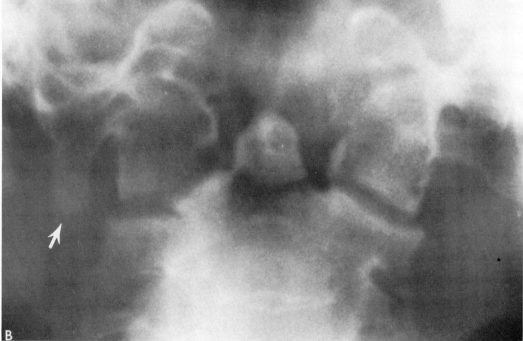

Figure 4–14. Occipitalization of the atlas. *A,* Lateral radiograph showing fusion of the atlas to the occiput, widening of the middle atlantoaxial joint (predental space) to 4 mm, block vertebra at C-2/C-3 involving bodies and vertebral arches, and a fracture of the pedicle of C-2 (large arrow). *B,* Frontal tomogram showing fusion of the atlas to the occiput. Note that there is a large paraoccipital process on the right (arrow). There is also asymmetry of the atlantoaxial joints.

foramen magnum may be encroached upon and distorted by the lateral masses of the atlas.[77, 78] Other findings include the following: (1) partial or complete fusion of the atlanto-occipital joints;[74, 77, 79] (2) fusion of the posterior arch of the atlas to the margins of the foramen magnum (this is often associated with a thickened dural band at the level of the assimilation pressing upon the medulla oblongata);[40] (3) absence of the transverse process and the presence of a paracondyloid process[74, 75, 80] (Fig. 4–14 B); (4) rachischisis of the atlas; (5) os odontoideum;[81] and (6) block vertebra, particularly involving the second and third cervical vertebrae[75, 78] (Fig. 4–14 A). Indeed, C-2/C-3 block vertebrae are so often associated with occipitalization of the atlas that a special effort should be made to look for it when a block vertebra is noted at that level.[70]

Platybasia and basilar impression are uncommon with occipitalization of the atlas and, when present, are usually unimportant clinically.[70, 73]

Generally, patients with occipitalization of the atlas are asymptomatic and have no associated anomalies of the meninges or central nervous system. About one-third of the cases will have symptoms due to a dural band at the level of the foramen magnum compressing the medulla oblongata. This is best demonstrated by gas myelography. Other patients show an abnormally wide predental space of 3 mm or more, or a decrease in the *effective foramen magnum* to less than 19 mm. McRae[70] defines the effective foramen magnum as the shortest distance between the dens to the opisthion or to the posterior arch of the atlas, presumably to the *arch-canal line*. Measurements are made on lateral radiographs taken at a six foot target-film distance.

Inflammatory Conditions in the Craniovertebral Region

Inflammatory processes in the craniovertebral region, for example, pharyngitis, pharyngeal abscess, coryza, otitis media, mastoiditis, cervical adenitis, parotitis, and alveolar abscess may be associated with atlantoaxial dislocation (Grisel's syndrome).[25, 26] Dislocation of the atlas may be noted 8 to 10 days after the onset of symptoms. Numerous hypotheses have been ad-

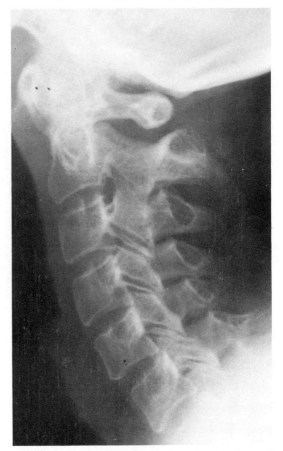

Figure 4–15. Rheumatoid arthritis. Lateral view of the cervical vertebral column showing abnormal widening of the middle atlantoaxial joint (predental space) to 5 mm.

vanced to explain the dislocation. Hydrops of the middle atlantoaxial joint,[27] hyperemia or periostitis resulting in decalcification of the atlas and loosening of the insertions of the transverse ligament of the atlas,[28] or a combination of muscle spasm and laxity of the transverse ligament may be the mechanism of atlantoaxial dislocation.[4] Patients with rheumatoid arthritis may exhibit atlantoaxial dislocation (luxation) during the course of their disease (Fig. 4–15).

ATLANTOAXIAL ROTARY FIXATION

The term atlantoaxial rotary fixation was coined in 1977 by Fielding and Hawkins.[31] They preferred that designation, since fixation of the atlas on the axis may occur with relatively normal atlantoaxial positions, with "subluxation," or with dislocation.

Earlier in 1968, Wortzman and Dewar termed persistent rotation of the atlas-axis as rotary fixation of the atlantoaxial joint.[32]

As mentioned earlier, the primary stabilizer of the atlas-axis complex is the transverse ligament of the atlas. The transverse ligament holds the dens tightly against the anterior arch of the atlas, preventing excessive shift of the atlas on the axis. The alar ligaments also serve to prevent shift of atlas on axis and excessive rotation. Coutts[33] noted that in the presence of an intact transverse ligament of the atlas, the atlantoaxial articulation pivots on the dens and dislocation occurs bilaterally when 65 degrees of rotation have been attained. The vertebral canal at the level of the atlas is at this time decreased to 7 millimeters — sufficient to produce spinal cord injury. If the transverse ligament is deficient, allowing 5 millimeters of forward displacement of the atlas on the axis vertebra, then unilateral dislocation may occur when only 45 degrees of rotation have been attained. In this instance, the vertebral canal at the level of the atlas is narrowed to 12 millimeters.

Atlantoaxial rotary fixation is not common. Fielding's series consisted of 17 patients, and we have had three cases that clearly fit into Fielding's criteria.

Fielding and Hawkins classify atlantoaxial rotary fixation into four types (Fig. 4–16):

TYPE I. Rotary fixation without anterior displacement of the atlas. This was the most common type, in which fixed rotation was within the normal range of atlantoaxial rotation. The transverse ligament of the atlas was intact (Fig. 4–16 A).

TYPE II. Rotary fixation with anterior displacement of the atlas of 3 to 5 mm. This, the second most common type of fixation, was associated with deficiency of the transverse ligament of the atlas and anterior displacement of one lateral mass of the atlas. The opposite, intact atlantoaxial joint acted as a pivot of rotation (Fig. 4–16 B). The amount of fixed rotation exceeded the normal maximum rotation.

TYPE III. Rotary fixation with anterior displacement of the atlas of more than 5 mm. This type is associated with deficiency of both the transverse ligament of the atlas and the secondary, or alar, ligaments. Both lateral masses of the atlas were displaced forward on the axis, one more than the other (Fig. 4–16 C).

TYPE IV. Rotary fixation with posterior displacement of the atlas. Deficiency of the dens is required to allow posterior shifting of the atlas on the axis (Fig. 4–16 D).

Clinically, atlantoaxial rotary fixation may

Figure 4–16. Atlantoaxial rotary fixation. (a) Type I—rotary fixation without anterior displacement of the atlas. The dens acts as the pivot. (b) Type II—rotary fixation with anterior displacement of the atlas of 3 to 5 mm. One lateral mass of the atlas acts as the pivot. (c) Rotary fixation with anterior displacement of the atlas of more than 5 mm. (d) Rotary fixation with posterior displacement of the atlas. (From Fielding, J. W., Hawkins, R. J.: Atlanto-axial rotary fixation (Fixed rotary subluxation of the atlanto-axial joint). J. Bone & Jt. Surg. 59–A:37, 1977.)

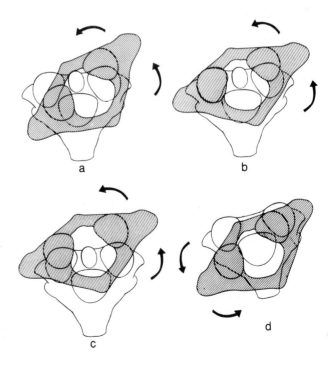

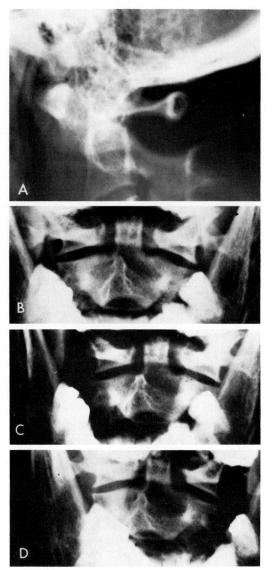

Figure 4–17. Atlantoaxial rotary fixation. *A*, Lateral view showing anterior atlantoaxial dislocation. *B*, Neutral AP view showing disparity in distance between the dens and the lateral masses of the atlas. The patient's chin and the spinous process of the axis are to the right of midline. *C*, 15 degrees of rotation to the right. The disparity in the atlas-dens distance persists on this view and with 15 degrees of rotation to the left (*D*). The spinous process of the axis remains to the right of midline. Diagnosis: Type II atlantoaxial rotary fixation of Fielding-Hawkins.

be caused by a variety of conditions; included among these are that it may be (1) spontaneous, (2) associated with upper respiratory infections, (3) caused by trauma (Fig. 4–17), (4) caused by surgical procedures, including

orthodontic appliance installation, repair of a cleft palate and removal of a body cast in a patient with neurofibromatosis.[31] The diagnosis of atlantoaxial rotary fixation may be delayed after onset of torticollis and diminished range of neck motion. The typical clinical picture is that of persistent torticollis, with its onset after trivial trauma or an upper respiratory infection.

These patients typically assume the "cock robin" position of the head and neck, that is the head is tilted to one side, rotated to the opposite side, and slightly flexed. Neurologic deficits are not common, and are usually limited to weakness of the limbs and radiculopathy.

The radiographic diagnosis of atlantoaxial rotary fixation is based upon demonstrating lack of normal motion between the atlas and the axis during attempted rotation. Fielding prefers cineradiography in the lateral position as the most useful procedure for diagnosis. In the normal patient, the atlas can be readily seen to move independently of the axis. We have done this and it is a most rewarding procedure. However, we also like to obtain the open-mouth views of the atlas-axis described by Wortzman and Dewar, shown in Figure 4–17. Views of the atlas-axis are obtained in neutral position and with the head turned 15 degrees right and left. In patients with fixation, there is a disparity in the distance between the dens and the lateral masses of the atlas. This asymmetric relationship persists in all views. Fielding and Hawkins also point out other features on frontal radiographs: (1) one lateral mass is rotated anteriorly and it appears wider and nearer to the dens in the midline (medial offset), while the opposite lateral mass appears narrower and farther away from the dens in the midline (lateral offset) (Fig. 4–17 *B*); (2) the lateral atlantoaxial joint on the side where the atlas is rotated backward may be partially obscured by overlapping of the structures; and (3) the spinous process of the axis is tilted in one direction and rotated in the other, and the chin and spinous process remain on the same side of the midline (Fig. 4–17).

On lateral radiographs it is imperative to look for atlantoaxial dislocation.

The etiology of the fixation is unknown, although there are numerous theories. Wittek suggested that a hydrops of the synovial joints caused stretching of the ligaments.[27]

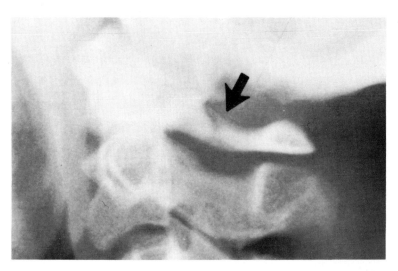

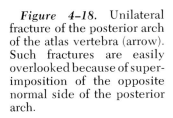

Figure 4–18. Unilateral fracture of the posterior arch of the atlas vertebra (arrow). Such fractures are easily overlooked because of superimposition of the opposite normal side of the posterior arch.

Coutts suggested that the synovial fringes blocked reduction when inflamed or adherent.[33] Hyperemic decalcification with subsequent ligamentous loosening has been suggested.[28] Grisel suggested that severe muscle contracture could follow an upper respiratory infection.[34] Hess et al. thought that a combination of factors, including muscle spasm, prevented reduction.[29] Fielding and Hawkins felt that reduction is prohibited in the early stages by distended synovial and capsular tissues and associated muscle spasm.[31]

FRACTURES OF THE ATLAS VERTEBRA

In 1970, Sherk and Nicholson[35] reported that 191 cases of atlas fractures had appeared in the literature. They found that fractures of the atlas constitute 2 to 13 per cent of fractures of the cervical spine. In the Duke series, atlas fractures accounted for 6 per cent of cervical fractures and dislocations.[36] In Sherk's experience, fractures of the posterior arch made up two-thirds of the cases, with Jefferson fractures accounting for most of the remainder. These findings are in contrast to the experience of Gehweiler *et al.* who found an almost equal incidence of bursting fractures of Jefferson, horizontal fractures of the anterior arch, and posterior arch fractures. Lateral mass and transverse process fractures are rare, and no examples of transverse process fracture could be found in the Duke cases (Table 4–2).

The unique morphology of the atlas was discussed earlier, in Chapter 1. The atlas lies deep within the neck, well protected by several layers of muscle and bone — the occiput above, the axis below, and the mandible and mastoid processes in front and behind. This location makes injury by direct violence unlikely, except in projectile injuries. Therefore, most injuries of the atlas are the result of indirect violence, caused by a blunt injury to the head by a soft or semi-compressible object.

The symptoms and physical findings in patients with atlas fractures are nonspecific. The patient may complain of stiffness of the neck, headache, sub-occipital pain, occipital neuralgia or anesthesia, and dysphagia. Dysphagia occurs secondary to retropharyngeal soft tissue swelling from hemorrhage and edema.[36]

TABLE 4–2. A Classification of Fractures of the Atlas Vertebra[36]

TYPE	PERCENT OF PATIENTS (*Duke Series*)
Fractures of the posterior arch	2
Unilateral	
Bilateral	
Horizontal fracture of the anterior arch	2
The bursting fracture of Jefferson	2
Lateral mass fracture — isolated	0
Transverse process fracture	0

Classification and Incidence

In order of occurrence, atlas fractures may be divided into five types: (1) fractures of the posterior arch (2 per cent of patients in the Duke series); (2) horizontal fracture of the anterior arch (2 per cent); (3) the bursting fracture of Jefferson (2 per cent); (4) lateral mass; and (5) transverse process fractures (Table 4–2).

Fractures of the Posterior Arch of the Atlas

Two per cent of patients in the Duke series had fractures of the posterior arch of the atlas. A combination of axial compression and hyperextension forces is thought to account for these fractures.[37, 38] The posterior arch is crushed between the heavy spi-

nous process of the axis vertebra and the basiocciput. The arch fractures through the weakest point of the atlas ring, the sulcus of the vertebral artery.

Posterior arch fractures may be unilateral or bilateral. Unilateral fractures are often difficult to diagnose on a true lateral radiograph owing to the superimposition of the opposite normal side (Figs. 4–18, 4–19). If there are bilateral arch fractures, the dorsal fragment may be displaced cranially owing to the pull of the rectus capitis posterior minor muscle (Fig. 4–20).

In our series of cases, five had isolated posterior arch fractures. Two patients had associated fractures — a traumatic spondylolisthesis (hangman fracture) of the axis vertebra, in one case, with avulsion of the anteroinferior margin of the axis body. These fractures are also the result of hyperextension forces. The other patient had

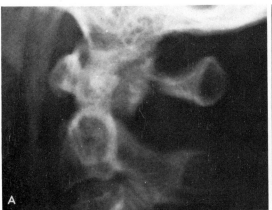
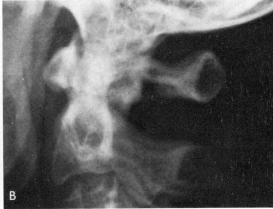

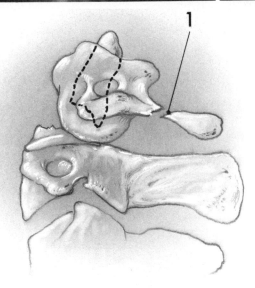

Figure 4–19. Fractures of the posterior arch of the atlas. *A,* True lateral radiograph to show how easily a unilateral posterior arch fracture may be overlooked when superimposed upon the opposite normal side. *B,* Off-centered lateral radiograph showing the unilateral posterior arch fracture. *C,* Schematic drawing showing a posterior fracture-dislocation of the dens and a fracture of the posterior arch of the atlas through the sulcus of the vertebral artery (1).

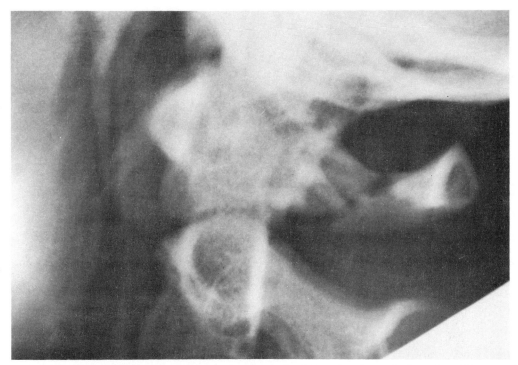

Figure 4–20. Bilateral fractures of the posterior arch of the atlas through the sulci of the vertebral arteries. Note that the most dorsal fragment of the posterior arch is tilted cranially owing to the pull of the rectus capitus posterior minor muscle.

compression fractures of lower cervical vertebral bodies. Figure 4–21 shows a recent case with fractures of the axis body and atlas posterior arch.

Fractures of the posterior arch of the atlas must be differentiated from congenital clefts. Two to four per cent of patients have clefts of the posterior arch of the atlas.

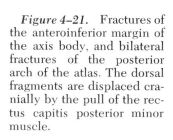

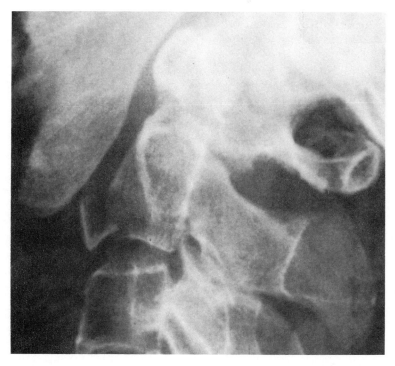

Figure 4–21. Fractures of the anteroinferior margin of the axis body, and bilateral fractures of the posterior arch of the atlas. The dorsal fragments are displaced cranially by the pull of the rectus capitis posterior minor muscle.

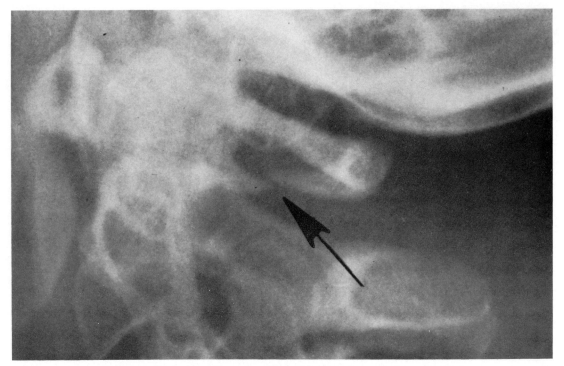

Figure 4–22. Congenital cleft of the atlas through the sulcus of the vertebral artery. Note the smooth borders, which are corticated (arrow).

Ninety-seven per cent of these occur dorsally near the midline (rachischisis), whereas 3 per cent occur laterally through the sulcus of the vertebral artery (Fig. 4–22). Characteristically, the edges of a cleft are smooth with a cortical bony margin, while fractures have jagged edges or may be comminuted.

At times patients with total or partial aplasia of the posterior arch of the atlas are suspected to have atlas fractures. Superimposition of the right and left sides of the posterior arch of the atlas produces Mach bands that may simulate fracture (Figure 4–23 A). Other problems in the diagnosis of posterior arch fractures may be caused by *manifestations of occipital vertebra,* such as a *proatlas* (Fig. 4–23 B), and a partial *ponticulus* or *posticus* (Kimmerle anomaly shown in Fig. 4–23 C).

Horizontal Fracture of the Anterior Arch of the Atlas

In the Duke series of 400 patients, 2 per cent had fractures of the anterior arch of the atlas of the horizontal type. We had no examples of isolated vertical fracture of the anterior arch.

Horizontal fractures of the anterior arch of the atlas are usually associated with other hyperextension fractures of the cervical spine, especially dens fracture (Figure 4–24 A). Two mechanisms of injury have been suggested, but not experimentally proved: (1) The inferior margin of the anterior arch may be shorn off by the dens as the neck is hyperextended. Simultaneous fractures of the dens were present in three of our seven patients (Fig. 4–24 A); (2) The anterior tubercle of the atlas may be avulsed by forces applied by the anterior longitudinal ligament and the defensive contraction of the longus colli muscles (Fig. 4–25). The latter mechanism seems the more likely.[36, 39]

There are only 11 cases reported in the literature of horizontal fracture of the anterior arch of the atlas;[36, 39-42] seven are from the Duke series. Of the 11 cases, four were isolated (Fig. 4–26), four had extension-type fractures of the dens, two had extension-type avulsions of the anteroinferior margin of the axis body, and one had associated hyperextension fractures of the lower cervical vertebral arches.

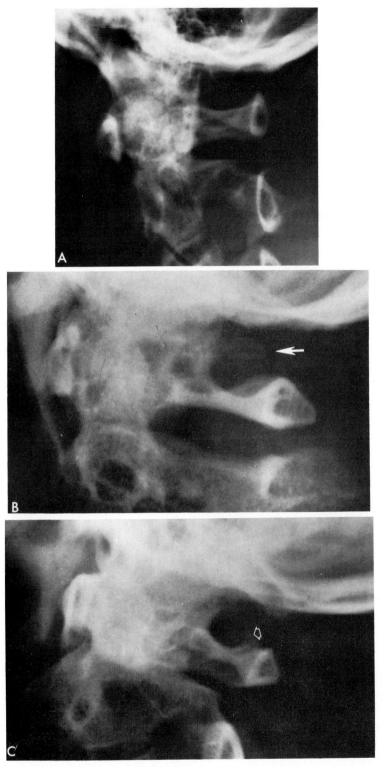

Figure 4–23. Conditions that may be confused with fractures of the posterior arch of the atlas. *A,* Mach band. *B,* A smooth oval-shaped ossicle above the level of the sulcus of the vertebral artery is termed a "proatlas." It is a manifestation of occipital vertebra as is the partial ponticulus posticus (Kimmerle anomaly) shown in *C.*

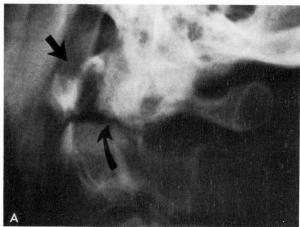

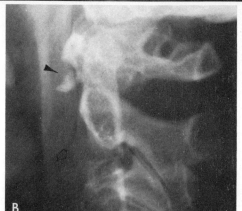

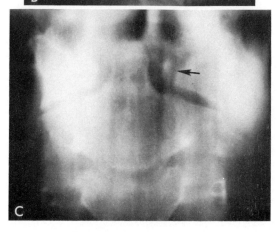

Figure 4–24. Horizontal fractures of the anterior arch of the atlas and associated injuries. *A,* This patient was struck by a car and suffered abrasions of the forehead and scalp lacerations. This lateral radiograph shows a horizontal fracture of the anterior arch of the atlas (arrow) and a dens fracture (curved arrow). The dens is displaced posteriorly and there is posterior atlantoaxial dislocation. *B, C,* After jumping from an airplane, this patient's parachute failed to open and she fell 1000 feet into a soybean field. Her mandible was bruised when it struck her knee. She also sustained bilateral os calcis and thoracolumbar vertebral column fractures. The lateral radiograph (*B*) shows a horizontal fracture of the anterior arch of the atlas (arrow), which is distracted and rotated, and an avulsion fracture of the anteroinferior margin of the axis body (open arrow). There is also retropharyngeal soft tissue swelling. The frontal tomogram (*C*) shows a fracture of the lateral mass of the atlas on the left side.

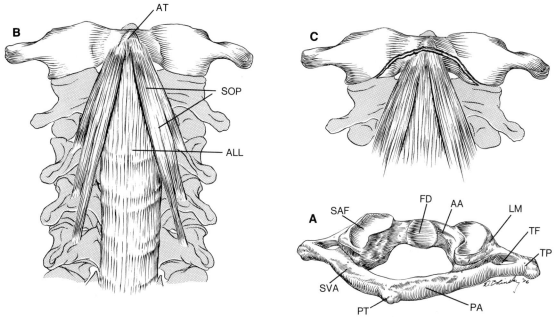

Figure 4-25. *A,* The first cervical vertebra (atlas) from behind. FD: facet for the dens; AA: anterior arch; LM: lateral mass; TF: transverse foramen; TP: transverse process; PA: posterior arch; PT: posterior tubercle; SVA: sulcus of the vertebral artery; SAF: superior articular facet. *B,* Anterior view of the upper cervical spine showing the ligamentous and tendinous insertions on the anterior tubercle of the anterior arch of the atlas. AT: anterior tubercle; SOP: superior oblique portion of the longus colli muscle; ALL: anterior longitudinal ligament. *C,* Schematic drawing illustrating the horizontal fracture of the anterior arch of the atlas.

Horizontal fractures of the anterior arch of the atlas may be overlooked on lateral radiographs because of superimposition of structures. Always look for the significant soft tissue signs (Chapter 3) as a clue to the diagnosis (Figs. 4–24, 4–26). The anterior arch as it appears on the lateral view is normally a distinct semilunar-shaped mass with a cortical rim. Horizontal fractures cause separation of the rim and result in jagged edges. The inferior fragment is distracted and may be rotated (Figs. 4–24, 4–26).

There are only a few conditions that must be distinguished from a fracture, including overlapping structures producing the Mach effect, and manifestations of occipital vertebra, such as the third condyle, occipital basilar processes and accessory ossicles (Fig. 4–27).

The Bursting Fracture of Jefferson

Combined fractures of the anterior and posterior arches of the atlas accounted for 2 per cent of the patients in our series. The mechanism of injury is shown in Figure 4–28. In this injury, an axial compressive force is applied to the vertex of the skull with the head held erect and the neck erect and rigid. As the axial force is transmitted to the spine, the atlas is compressed between the occipital condyles of the skull and the superior articular surfaces of the axis vertebra. Owing to the obliquity of these articular surfaces, the wedge-shaped lateral masses of the atlas are forced laterally. If the force is great enough, both the anterior and the posterior arches fracture and the lateral masses are displaced laterally, appearing laterally offset (usually both sides) on the axis (Fig. 4–29).

Lateral mass displacement of greater than 6.9 mm relative to the axis indicates probable tearing of the transverse ligament of the atlas.[15] Occasionally, only marked unilateral atlantoaxial offset may be seen, with subsequent tomography clearly showing the arch fractures (Fig. 4–30). Avulsion fracture of the lateral mass may also be observed. It is important for the reader to realize that the fractures of the anterior and posterior arches of the atlas in the Jefferson fracture may not be seen in the lateral radiograph. This is

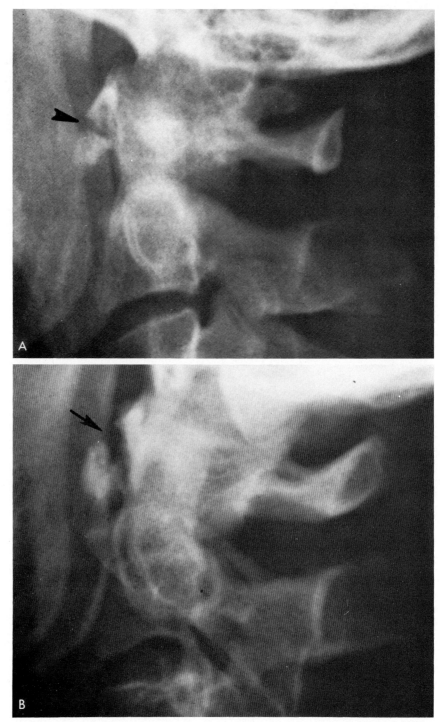

Figure 4–26. *Isolated* horizontal fractures of the anterior arch of the atlas. *A,* The patient also sustained a fracture of the mandible. There is retropharyngeal soft tissue swelling. *B,* The patient was involved in an automobile accident. He had a traumatic enucleation of the left eye. Note the retropharyngeal soft tissue swelling.

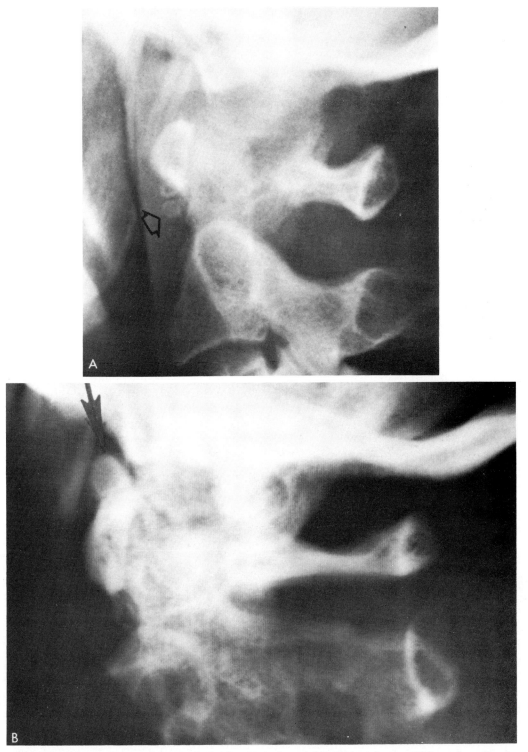

Figure 4-27. Accessory ossicles about the anterior arch of the atlas. *A,* Below the atlas (open arrow). *B,* Above the anterior arch of the atlas (arrow).

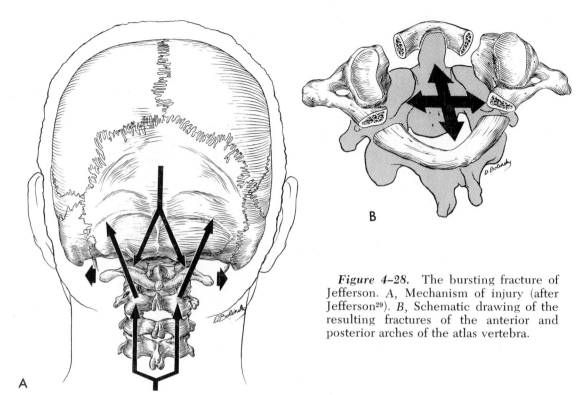

Figure 4-28. The bursting fracture of Jefferson. *A*, Mechanism of injury (after Jefferson[29]). *B*, Schematic drawing of the resulting fractures of the anterior and posterior arches of the atlas vertebra.

because arch fractures usually occur near the junction of the arches with the lateral masses of the atlas. In order to see the fractures on the lateral radiograph, the x-ray beam must pass tangentially through the vertical fracture line (Fig. 4–31). The best view to visualize the Jefferson fracture is the open-mouth view of the atlas-axis.

Only two conditions must be considered in the differential diagnosis of the bursting fracture of Jefferson: (1) bilateral pseudo-offset due to a disparity in growth of the atlas and axis in children[43] (Fig. 4–32), and (2) bilateral atlantoaxial offset due to congenital clefts of the atlas arches (Fig. 4–33).

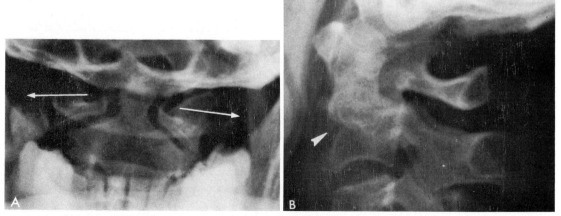

Figure 4-29. Bursting fracture of Jefferson. *A*, Frontal view through the open-mouth showing bilateral atlantoaxial offset; the lateral margins of the lateral masses of the atlas do not align properly with the lateral margins of the axis vertebral body. *B*, Lateral radiograph fails to show the anterior and posterior arch fractures as is often the case. There is a fracture of the dens (arrow), which is anteriorly displaced.

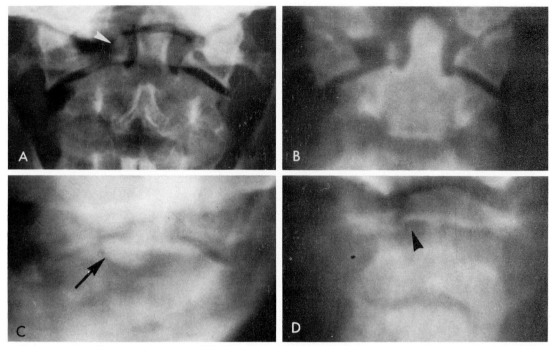

Figure 4–30. Bursting fracture of Jefferson. *A*, Frontal view showing unilateral right atlantoaxial offset. There is an avulsion fracture of the medial aspect of the right lateral mass of the atlas. *B*, Tomogram confirms the plain film findings. *C*, Tomograms showing the anterior arch fracture (arrow) and posterior arch fracture (*D*) (*arrow*) on the right side.

Simultaneous *clefts of the anterior and posterior arches of the atlas* are extremely rare.[40, 43] These congenital defects (Fig. 4–33) are often referred to as anterior and posterior spina bifida. However, since the atlas does not have a spinous process, the term *rachischisis* (G. *rachis* spine + *schisis* cleft) is preferred.

The anterior cleft may be suspected on lateral radiographs if the cortex of the anterior arch cannot be seen in its entirety about the periphery of the arch (Fig. 4–33 *C*). Clefts in the posterior arch are more common than anterior arch clefts. These posterior clefts are easily diagnosed in lateral views by the absence of the *arch-canal line* (Fig. 4–33 *C*). The dorsal aspect of the arch has a paddle-shaped appearance.

Simultaneous anterior and posterior arch clefts may occasionally be accompanied by lateral spread of the lateral masses of the atlas.[43]

Isolated Fractures of the Lateral Masses

Isolated lateral mass fractures are rare. These fractures probably result from asym-

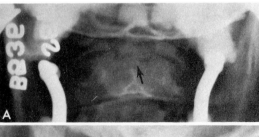

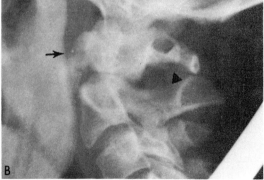

Figure 4–31. Multiple fractures of the atlas and axis. *A*, Frontal view showing a "low-type" transverse fracture of the dens, and bilateral atlantoaxial offset. *B*, Lateral view shows fractures of the anterior and posterior arches of the atlas and posterior atlantoaxial luxation. Diagnosis: bursting fracture of Jefferson, and fracture of the dens with posterior atlantoaxial luxation.

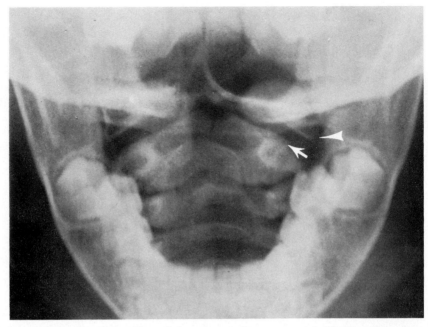

Figure 4–32. Bilateral pseudo-offset of the atlas on the axis in a child. The white arrowhead points to the right lower margin of the lateral mass of the atlas. The white arrow indicates the upper lateral margin of the axis body. These margins should be in the same sagittal plane; however, in this child disparity in growth is causing these changes.

metric axial compressive forces.[38] We have no examples of isolated fracture of a lateral mass of the atlas. However, we have seen four cases with lateral mass fractures associated with other fractures of the cervical spine — three were associated with Jefferson fractures (Fig. 4–30) and one with a dens fracture.

The roentgen diagnosis may be difficult unless both lateral masses of the atlas are clearly visualized. This may be possible only with tomography. Compression of the lateral mass may be present and there may also be an avulsion of the tubercle of the transverse ligament.

The differential diagnosis of an avulsion of the attachment of the transverse ligament is shown in Figures 4–34, 4–35. This is merely a prominent tubercle made even more prominent by a Mach band. Note that the finding is bilaterally symmetrical.

Fracture of the Transverse Process

A few cases of transverse process fractures are described by Abel.[44] The mechanism of injury is probably lateral hyperflexion. The best view for demonstrating the fracture is the basal projection of the skull.

FRACTURES AND DISLOCATIONS OF THE AXIS VERTEBRA

Fractures and dislocations of the axis vertebra were found in 27 per cent of patients in the Duke series.[45] The most common fracture of the axis is the dens fracture (13 per cent of all patients). There were equal numbers of hangman's fractures (traumatic spondylolisthesis) and a group of less common fractures; each group made up about 7 per cent of the total patients.[46]

The axis vertebra is an "atypical" cervical vertebra. The gross morphology has been described in Chapter 1.

Classification and Incidence

In Table 4–3, an anatomic classification of axis fractures and dislocations is presented. Four major types are recognized:[46] (1) dens, (2) vertebral body, (3) vertebral arch, and (4) locked articular facets. The latter are discussed in Chapter 5, p. 239.

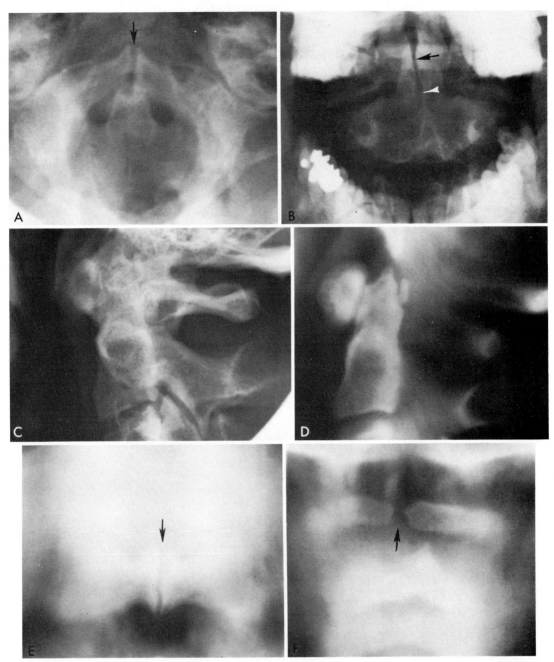

Figure 4-33. Simultaneous clefts of the anterior and posterior arches of the atlas. *A,* Basal view of the skull showing the anterior arch cleft (arrow). *B,* Frontal view through the open mouth. Note the cleft at the arrow. There is slight atlantoaxial offset. *C,* Lateral view of the upper cervical column. An anterior cleft may be suspected if the cortex of the anterior arch cannot be seen in its entirety about the periphery of the arch. *D,* Lateral tomogram showing the abnormal cortical appearance of the anterior arch of the atlas at site of the cleft. Dens is dysplastic. *E,* Frontal tomograms showing the irregular cleft through the anterior arch of the atlas in the midline. *F,* The rachischisis of the posterior arch is noted just to the right of the midline.

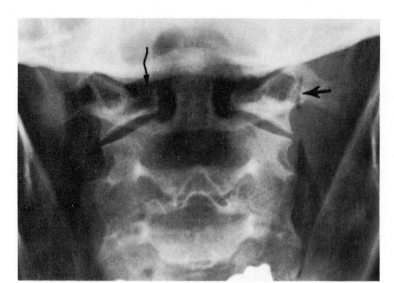

Figure 4–34. Frontal view of the atlas-axis through the open mouth. On the right the prominent tubercle of the lateral mass of the atlas (curved arrow) simulates a fracture. On the left an air shadow crosses the base of the transverse process (arrow) simulating a fracture. Fractures of the transverse process of the atlas are best demonstrated on basal views of the skull.

Fractures of the Dens

Miller et al. reported that fractures of the dens were found in 13 per cent of 400 patients in the Duke series.[45] The classification and incidence of the four types of dens fractures are shown in Table 4–3.

Dens fractures are most commonly

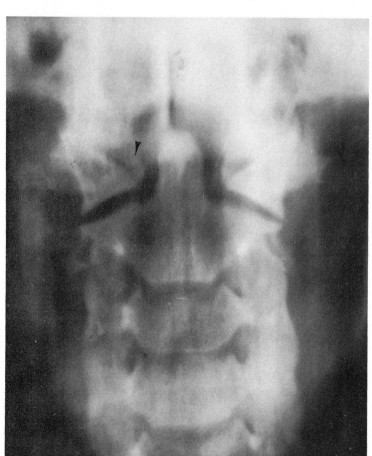

Figure 4–35. Prominent tubercle for attachment of the transverse ligament of the atlas (arrow).

TABLE 4–3. A Classification of Fractures and Dislocations of the Axis

TYPE	PERCENT OF PATIENTS (Duke Series)
Dens	13
Anterior fracture-dislocation	7
Posterior fracture-dislocation	3
Laterally displaced	1
Nondisplaced	2
Vertebral body	5
Anteroinferior margin	2
Other	3
with unilateral arch fracture	2
with bilateral arch fracture	1
Vertebral arch	
Unilateral	1
Bilateral pedicle (hangman's)	7
"Atypical" bilateral	< 1
Vertebral arch appendages	
Spinous process	< 1
Transverse process	0
Inferior articular process	0
Locked articular facets (C-2/C-3)	< 1
Unilateral	
Bilateral	

caused by traffic accidents and falls. The mechanism of injury determines the direction of displacement of the dens. Anterior fracture-dislocations of the dens may result from sudden flexion, during which the dens is sheared off by the strong transverse ligament of the atlas[47] (Fig. 4–36). Posterior fracture-dislocations may result from hyperextension forces, during which the anterior arch of the atlas shears off the dens (Fig. 4–37). Laterally displaced dens fractures are thought to result from lateral hyperflexion trauma.[48]

Dens fractures may be further subclassified into those occurring at *high* and at *low levels* of the dens.[49, 50] A high dens fracture occurs at or above the level of the lateral atlantoaxial joints (Fig. 4–38), while the low type extends into the body of the axis (Fig. 4–39). The latter group exhibit better osseous healing.

Patients with dens fractures may have no neurologic signs or symptoms, or only mild cord symptoms. They may only seek clinical evaluation days or even weeks after injury, complaining of upper neck stiffness, dysphagia, and torticollis.

In patients with neurologic signs and

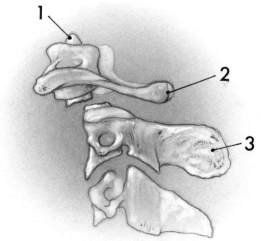

Figure 4–36. Anterior fracture-dislocation of the dens. The apex of the dens is seen at 1; there is displacement of the posterior tubercle (2) of the atlas relative to the spinous process of the axis (3).

symptoms (and these are a minority of the cases), the primary damage is to the anterior spinal artery, the spinal cord, and the first and second cervical spinal nerves. Surprisingly, the posterior spinal cord escapes relatively unscathed.[6] Two points are worthy of mention relative to the lack of neurologic findings even if the dens is displaced more than 10 mm. The dimensions of the vertebral canal are greater than those of the spinal

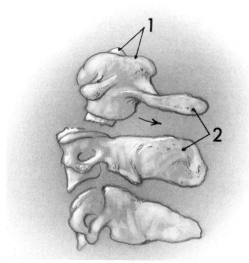

Figure 4–37. Posterior fracture-dislocation of the dens. The atlas and dens (1) are displaced posteriorly; the most posterior margins of the posterior tubercle of the atlas and the spinous process of the axis (2) may lie in the same vertical plane.

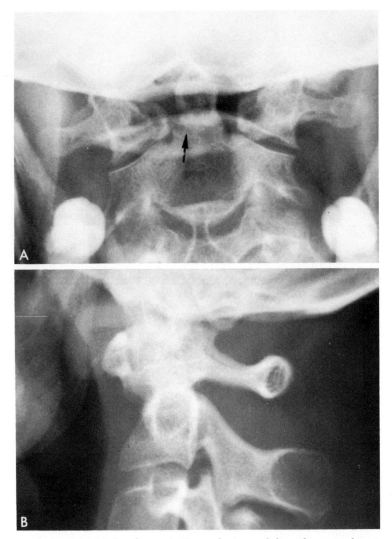

Figure 4–38. High fracture of the dens. *A,* Frontal view of the atlas-axis showing the transverse fracture through the "waist" of the dens above the level of the lateral atlantoaxial joints (arrow). *B,* Lateral view showing the kyphotic angulation of the dens fracture. Note the absence of soft tissue swelling.

cord. The sagittal diameter of the vertebral canal of the atlas is about 22 mm (mean diameter); the spinal cord at the same level is about 10 mm (mean).[5, 6] At the moment of displacement of the dens, the anterior or posterior arch of the atlas moves cranially, bending the cord into an S-shape rather than crushing it.

Fractures of the dens may be subtle, and easily overlooked on lateral views of the skull or cervical spine (Fig. 4–40). Always approach every case of head injury with a high index of suspicion for upper neck fractures. Stereoscopic lateral views of the skull

are excellent for evaluating the upper cervical column. Look carefully for indirect signs of trauma, that is, widening of the retropharyngeal soft tissues and displacement of the prevertebral fat stripe (Fig. 4–41). If there is a strong clinical suspicion of fracture, even though the plain films are normal, we would recommend tomography.[51, 52] The patient who enters the emergency room holding his head on his neck between his hands is an excellent candidate for a fracture in the upper cervical spine. All too often, patients with dens fractures have normal lateral radiographs of the cervical spine.

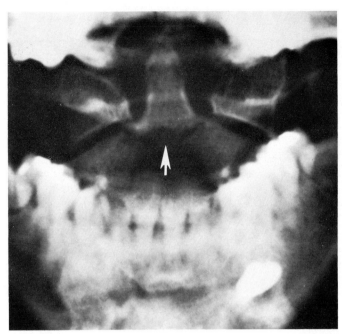

Figure 4–39. *Low* fracture of the dens.

Therefore, we again urge you to obtain at least six projections of the cervical vertebral column (see Chapter 3).

The roentgen diagnosis of a fracture of the dens is determined by the anatomic relationship of the dens to the body of the axis. The posterior surface of the dens should form a straight line with the posterior surface of the axis body (Fig. 4–42A). In the frontal view, the normal morphology of the dens should be carefully checked; note its apex, waist, and base. Is the cortex interrupted? Is it properly aligned, as in the normal radiograph shown in Figure 4–42B? The degree of displacement of a fractured dens is quite variable (Figs. 4–41, 4–43). If there is no displacement or angulation of the dens, the diagnosis is difficult.

Recall the normal anatomy of the dens in children (Chapter 1). The normal subdental synchondrosis has often been mistaken for a dens fracture. (We have done it; so we know.) The terminal ossicle too has caused many a radiologist some sleepless nights (Fig. 4–44). In children under seven years of age, trauma to the cervical spine may produce a separation through the subdental synchondrosis. This condition has been termed *epiphysiolysis dentis.*[6] Remnants of this subdental synchondrosis may persist

into adult life (Fig. 4–45), representing a weakened area in the axis, and a site of fracture. Epiphysiolysis dentis may lead to complete disappearance of the dens, resulting in the erroneous diagnosis of congenital dens aplasia.[53]

Fractures of the dens may be overdiagnosed if great care is not exercised. A myriad of overlapping shadows occur in this region that may simulate a fracture (Fig. 4–46), for example, the tongue, posterior arch of the atlas, upper border of the laminae of the axis, teeth, and the remnant of the subdental synchondrosis. The Mach bands produced provide the greatest source of error.[54]

Other problems in differential diagnosis are the os odontoideum, which has been discussed earlier in Chapter 4 (p. 138). The os odontoideum is an independent bone situated atop a hypoplastic dens (Fig. 4–47). The os is typically round to oval in shape. It may be clearly demonstrable only on tomograms. There are two types of os odontoideum: (1) *orthotopic,* which lies close to the hypoplastic dens, and (2) *dystopic* — the os lies near the basion. This latter type should not present any problem in differential diagnosis owing to the shape of the bone, the wide gap between the os and the hypo-

Text continued on page 171.

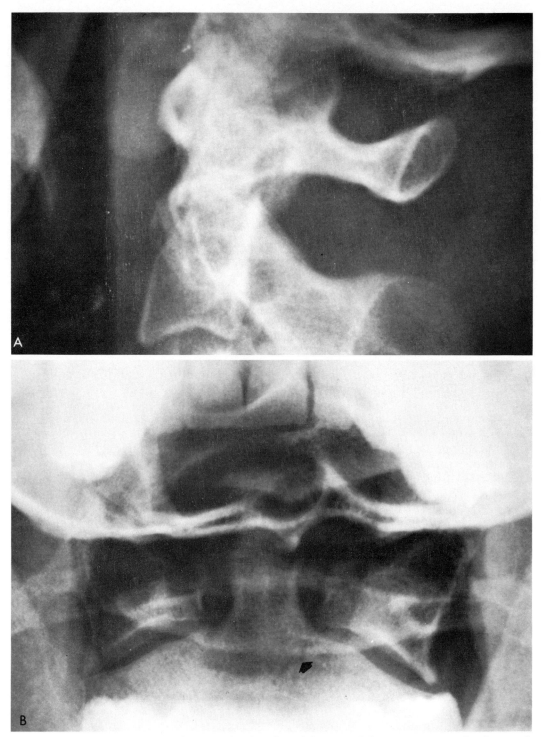

Figure 4–40. Fracture of the dens, *undisplaced.* A, Closeup of the upper cervical column taken from a lateral skull x-ray. There is a subtle low fracture of the dens without associated retropharyngeal soft tissue swelling. *B*, Frontal view. The fracture (arrow) is still difficult to see.

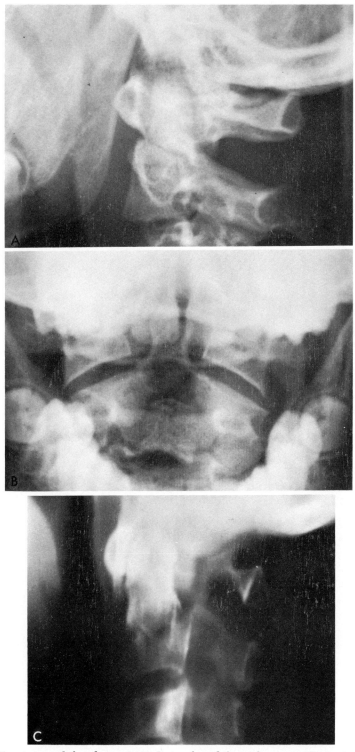

Figure 4–41. Fractures of the dens. *A, B,* Lateral and frontal views of a patient with a *posterior* fracture-dislocation of the dens. *C,* Lateral tomogram in another patient with a low *anterior* fracture-dislocation of the dens.

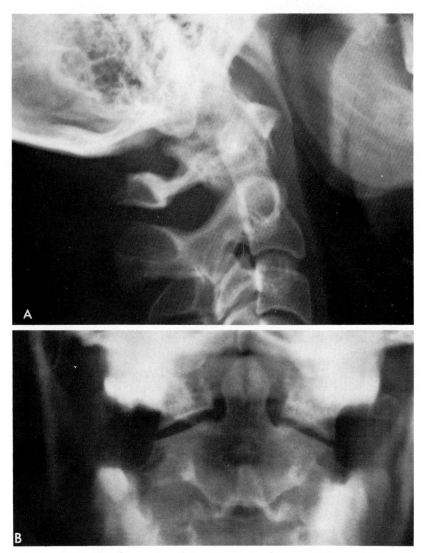

Figure 4–42. *Normal* radiographs of the atlas-axis. *A*, Lateral view. *B*, Frontal view.

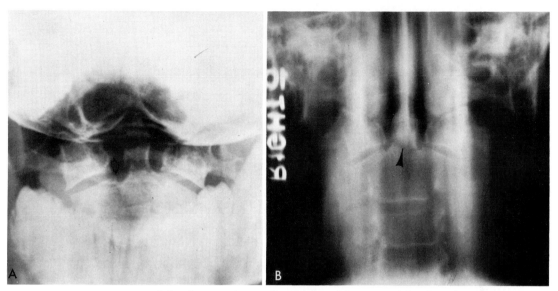

Figure 4-43. Fractures of the dens. *A,* Laterally displaced fracture of the dens (arrow). *B,* Frontal tomogram showing a nondisplaced fracture of the dens (arrow).

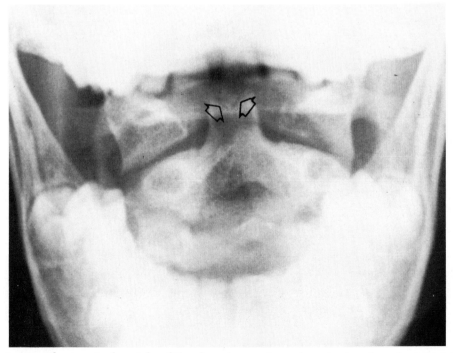

Figure 4-44. The terminal ossicle of the dens (arrows) may be mistaken for a fractured dens. It is found in 26 per cent of children. The terminal ossicle (of Bergman) is usually not visualized before two years of age, although it has been reported at birth. Normally the terminal ossicle fuses with the dens at or before age twelve.

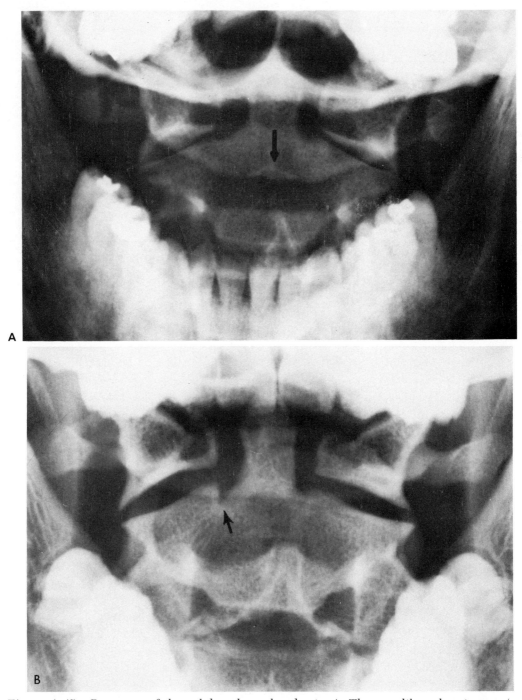

Figure 4–45. Remnants of the subdental synchondrosis. *A*, The tent-like sclerotic area (arrow) deep in the axis vertebral body is a common finding on radiographs. *B*, The exaggerated cleft at the base of the dens on the right (arrow) is often mistaken for a fracture, especially in patients with a history of trauma. Tomograms of this patient were normal.

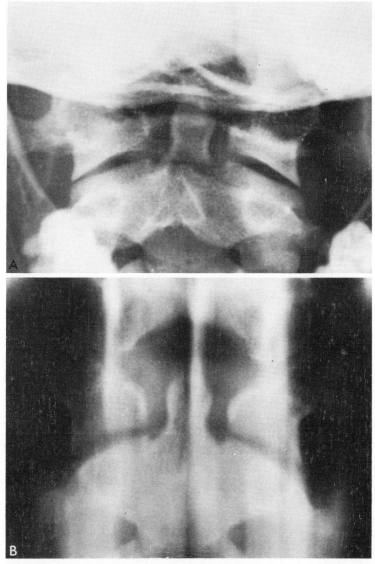

Figure 4–46. Mach band simulating a fractured dens. *A,* Open mouth view of the atlas-axis. The Mach band is produced by the posterior arch of the atlas, and the upper surface of the laminae of the axis. *B,* Tomogram showing the normal dens.

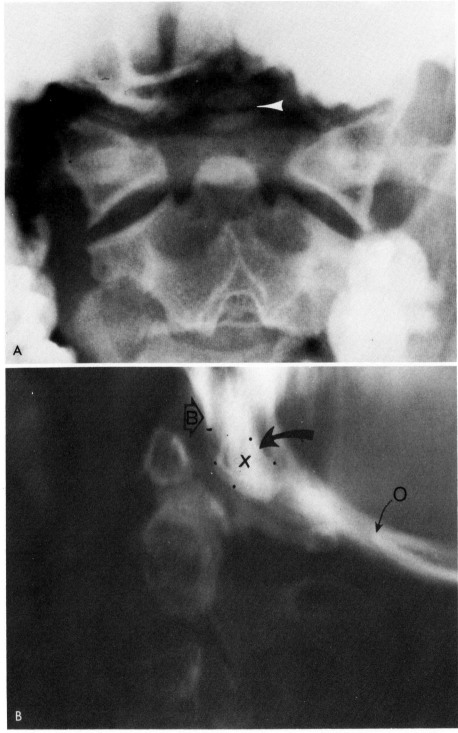

Figure 4–47. Os odontoideum. *A,* Frontal view showing the hypoplastic dens and the os odontoideum (arrow). *B,* Lateral view. Os odontoideum (X), basion (B), opisthion (O).

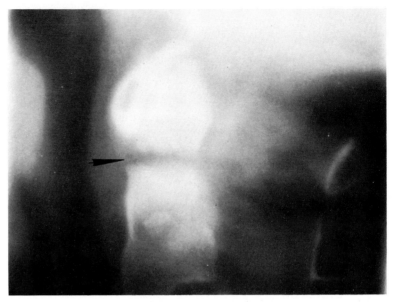

Figure 4-48. Old ununited fracture of the dens. Note the sclerotic margins about the fracture site (arrow) in this midline sagittal tomogram. The dens retains its normal shape, and in no way resembles an os odontoideum (see Figure 4-47).

plastic dens, and the distinct cortical bone surrounding both the os and the small cupola-shaped hypoplastic dens.

It is the orthotopic-type of os odontoideum that presents the greatest challenge to diagnosis. Recent fractures of the dens are usually easy to distinguish, since the fragments should fit together nicely and there should not be any marginal cortical bone at the fracture site. An old, ununited fracture of the dens can be distinguished from an os odontoideum, since it will usually retain the normal configuration of the dens (Fig. 4-48).

Dens dysplasia and asymmetry of the atlantoaxial joints may be mistaken for fractures (Fig. 4-49).

Fractures of the Axis Vertebral Body

Anteroinferior Margin

Two per cent of our patients had fractures of the anteroinferior margin of the axis body. Falls and vehicular accidents caused the majority of these injuries. All of the patients complained of upper cervical pain. None had neurologic deficit referable to the fracture. Two of the nine patients were paraplegic as the result of locked articular facets in the lower cervical spine.

The mechanism of injury in these cases is most often disruptive hyperextension (Fig.4-50). In two cases, the mechanism

may have been compressive hyperflexion (Fig. 4-51).

Fractures of the anteroinferior margin of the axis body are best demonstrated on the lateral radiograph of the cervical spine or skull. There are usually indirect signs of upper cervical trauma, for example, retropharyngeal soft tissue swelling and/or displacement of the prevertebral fat stripe. The fracture line passes obliquely through the anteroinferior margin of the axis body. The avulsed fragment is quite variable in size. It is triangular in shape and may be distracted anteriorly or displaced and rotated (Figs. 4-50 to 4-52). The C-2 intervertebral disk space will show evidence of injury on the initial or followup radiographs.

There may be associated fractures, for example, "hangman's fracture," or horizontal fracture of the anterior or posterior arch of the atlas (Figs. 4-52, 4-53).

Other Axis Body Fractures

WITH UNILATERAL ARCH FRACTURE. In our series of 400 patients, 2 per cent had this variety of fracture.[46] None of the patients had any other associated cervical spine injuries.

Based upon clinical findings and history, we determined that this unique group of fractures was probably produced by a combination of forces: lateral hyperflexion, rotation, and compression.

Figure 4-54 shows an example of the sim-

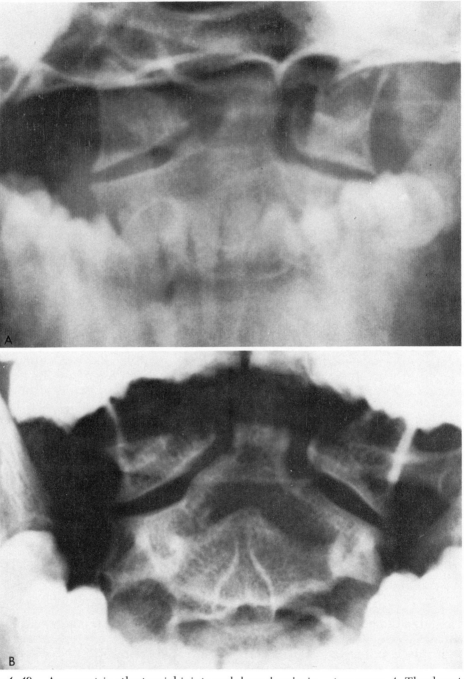

Figure 4–49. Asymmetric atlantoaxial joints and dens dysplasia — two cases. *A*, The dens is "scoli-otic" to the left and the normal sulcus at its base is filled with a hummock of bone. The lateral masses of the atlas vertebra are asymmetric as are the lateral atlantoaxial joints. *B*, Another example showing the same features as *A*.

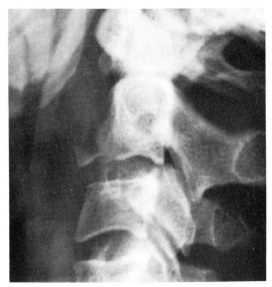

Figure 4–50. Fracture of the anteroinferior margin of the axis vertebral body. Note the retropharyngeal soft tissue swelling.

plest of these fractures. In the oblique and frontal views (Fig. 4–54 A, B), the oblique fracture is seen coursing downward from the superior articular surface medial to the inferior vertebral notch and into the caudal end-plate of the axis. Thus the fracture has passed through the deep hollow located on

either side of the midline on the anterior surface of the axis body. This fracture divides the axis body into two unequal parts: a seemingly undisplaced large fragment to which the dens is attached, and a smaller lateral fragment. The latter is usually displaced laterally and inferiorly on the frontal views (Fig. 4–54 B). Lateral views (Fig. 4–54 C, D) reveal that the fragments are distracted, and that the larger fragment is displaced forward (anterolisthesis) on C-3. The smaller lateral fragment has a very characteristic triangular shape, and it is always displaced backward into the vertebral canal. Note that the C-2 intervertebral disk space is diminished in height, indicating an injury. The radiographic picture is not unlike the Type IV hyperflexion fracture-dislocation described in Chapter 5 (p. 252). Because of the unique morphology of the axis body, these oblique body fractures, when viewed on the lateral radiograph, may appear anterior or posterior in position. The closer the fracture occurs to the midline, the more anterior it will appear on the lateral radiograph (Fig. 4–54 C, D).

The more complex axis body fractures are comminuted. One part of the fracture appears similar to the simplest variety described above. The other fracture lines course obliquely through the vertebral body (Figs. 4–55, 4–56). In both the simple and

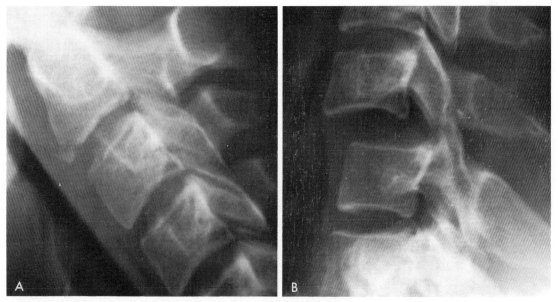

Figure 4–51. Fracture of the anteroinferior margin of the axis vertebral body (A), and associated bilateral locked facets at C-6/7 (B).

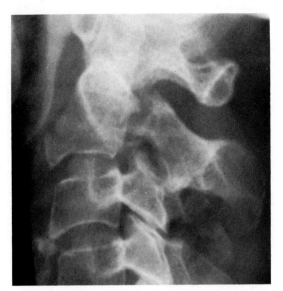

Figure 4–52. Avulsion fracture of the antero-inferior margin of the axis vertebra, and traumatic spondylolisthesis (hangman's fracture). There is also a fractured spinous process of C-3.

comminuted types, the fractures extend horizontally into the pedicle and/or lamina on one side (Figs. 4–54 to 4–56).

WITH BILATERAL ARCH FRACTURES. Patients with bilateral arch fractures of the axis vertebra accounted for 1 per cent of the Duke series. These patients were similar to those with unilateral arch fractures described above, except for the presence of bilateral arch fractures (Fig. 4–57).

Fractures of the Axis Vertebral Arch

Unilateral Arch Fractures

Unilateral arch (pedicle or lamina) fractures accounted for about 1 per cent of all patients in the Duke series. They result from falls and traffic accidents. Clinically the patients complain of upper neck pain; they are neurologically intact.[46]

Compressive hyperextension and rotation is the probable mechanism of injury in these cases.

The roentgen diagnosis is not as easy as one might imagine. Since these are unilateral fractures, they are difficult to evaluate on true lateral radiographs because of the superimposition of the opposite normal side. Stereoscopic views and tomography may be necessary for diagnosis. Look for indirect signs of upper cervical spine trauma.

In some cases, they may resemble classic "hangman's fractures", but evaluation on frontal and oblique views will show that they are unilateral in location (Fig. 4–58).

Bilateral Arch Fractures (the classic "Hangman's fracture")

In a 1954 paper, Grogono described and illustrated a case with avulsion of the vertebral arch of the axis and displacement of the C-2 body forward on C-3.[55] He noted the similarity of his cases to those in an earlier paper by Wood-Jones entitled "The ideal

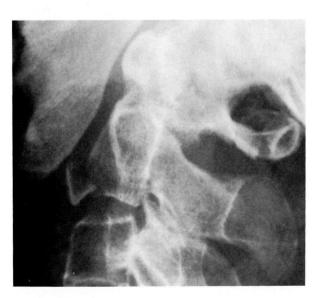

Figure 4–53. Avulsion fracture of the anteroinferior margin of the axis vertebra, and bilateral fractures of the posterior arch of the atlas.

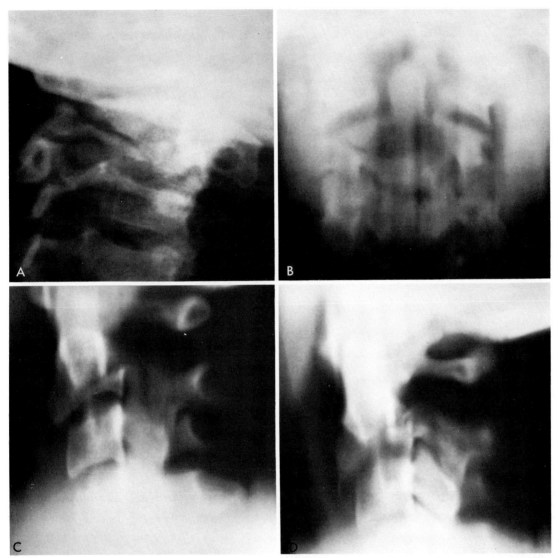

Figure 4-54. Axis vertebral body fracture with unilateral pedicle fracture. *A,* Oblique view showing an oblique fracture passing from the superior articular surface medial to the inferior vertebral notch and into the caudal end-plate of the axis. *B,* Frontal tomogram shows the oblique linear fracture of the right side of the axis body. Note that the smaller lateral fragment is displaced laterally. *C, D,* Lateral tomograms. The larger anterior fragment is displaced forward on C-3, and the C-2 intervertebral disk space is narrowed. The smaller fragment is triangular in shape. The body fracture extends into the right pedicle.

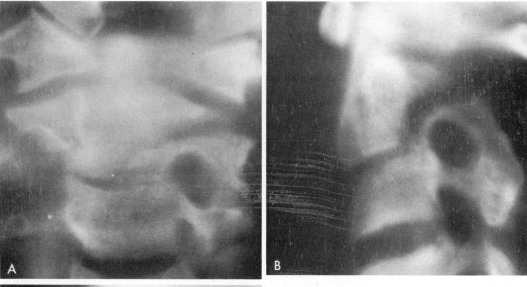

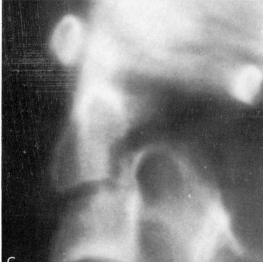

Figure 4–55. Axis body fracture with uni-lateral pedicle fracture. *A,* Frontal tomogram. The axis body is comminuted; there is an oblique linear fracture on the left, and another vertical fracture on the right. *B, C,* Lateral tomograms. The larger fragment is displaced forward on C-3, and the C-2 intervertebral disk space is narrowed. The smaller triangular posteroinferior fragment is clearly seen extending into the pedicle.

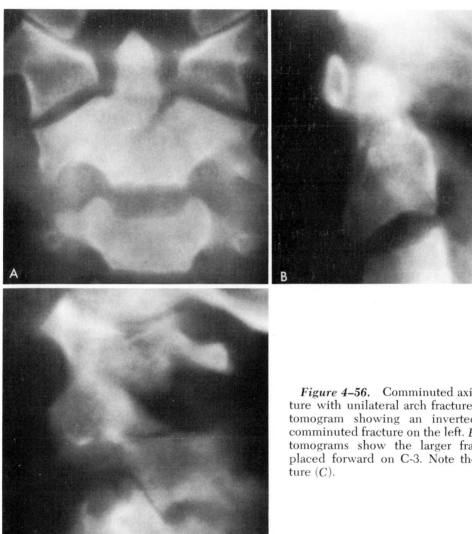

Figure 4–56. Comminuted axis body fracture with unilateral arch fracture. *A*, Frontal tomogram showing an inverted Y-shaped comminuted fracture on the left. *B*, *C*, Lateral tomograms show the larger fragment displaced forward on C-3. Note the arch fracture (*C*).

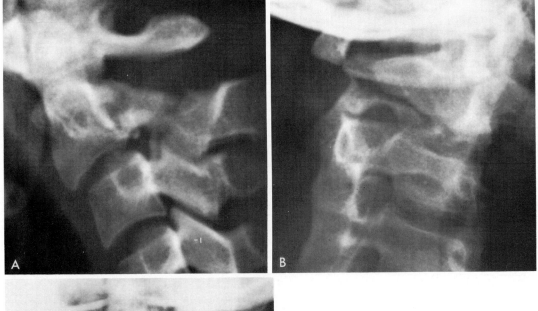

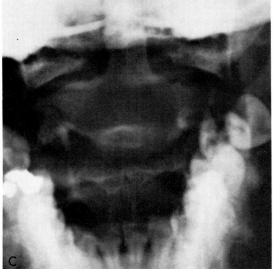

Figure 4-57. Axis vertebral body fracture with bilateral arch fractures. *A*, Lateral view showing the vertebral arch fractured at different levels. There is a small triangular-shaped fragment off the posteroinferior margin of the axis body. *B*, Oblique view. Note the similarity to the fracture in Figure 4–54*A*. *C*, Frontal view shows the linear oblique fracture on the right lateral aspect of the axis vertebral body.

lesion produced by judicial hanging."[56] The characteristic lesion was thought to result from the violent submental jerk of the head backward at the moment the person was hanged, so as to snap the arch of the axis.

Schneider et al., in a 1965 paper, reported eight cases of "hangman's fracture" of the axis vertebra in patients who had suffered hyperextension trauma.[57] They too noted the remarkable resemblance of their patients' radiographs to the drawings in Wood-Jones' report. Nearly identical lesions have been reported by others.[58-62] In general, most of the papers agree that the most common cause of "hangman's fracture" is acute hyperextension of the skull on the upper cervical spine. A few cases may result from flexion trauma.[60]

Neurologic sequelae are rare in the literature and in our own series of 32 cases. Schneider thought the "hangman's fracture" to be rare, but we have found that it was present in 7 per cent of all patients in the Duke series.[58] In order to qualify as a "hangman's fracture" (traumatic spondylolisthesis), the case had to comply with the description of Schneider.

The essential feature is bilateral avulsion of the arch of the axis through the pedicles with or without dislocation of the C-2 body on C-3. The C-2 intervertebral disk or the C-3 vertebral body may be involved.

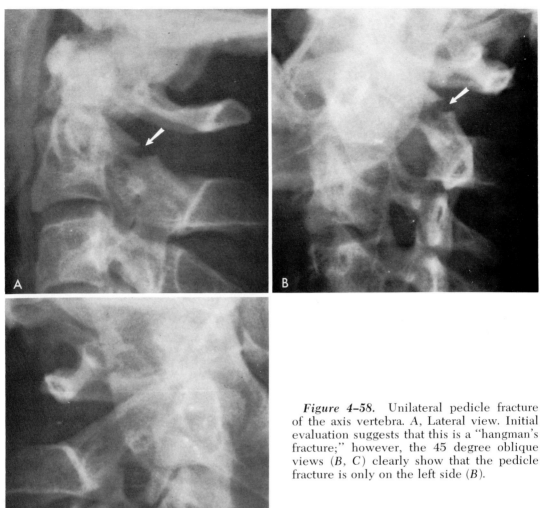

Figure 4-58. Unilateral pedicle fracture of the axis vertebra. A, Lateral view. Initial evaluation suggests that this is a "hangman's fracture;" however, the 45 degree oblique views (*B*, *C*) clearly show that the pedicle fracture is only on the left side (*B*).

Characteristically, the dens and transverse ligament of the atlas are intact. All of the cases show the pedicle fractures to be close to the axis body.[57, 58]

The bilateral fractures of the pedicles may be vertical, oblique, and in rare cases horizontal in direction.[40] The vertebral arch of the axis is avulsed and remains attached to the vertebral arch of C-3. The body and dens of the axis remain articulated to the atlas. The C-2 intervertebral disk space is diminished in vertical height, and the axis body is dislocated forward on the C-3 verte-bra, resulting in widening of the sagittal diameter of the vertebral canal (Figs. 4–59 to 4–61). Oblique views confirm the fractures of the pedicles. Anterior displacement of the axis body causes distortion of the C-2–C-3 intervertebral foramina bilaterally.

The only condition simulating a "hangman's fracture" is a congenital spondylolisthesis of the axis vertebra (Figs. 4–62, 4–63). The senior author has two such cases. Bony defects occur through the pars interarticularis bilaterally. The edges of the bony defects are well corticated, as opposed to the

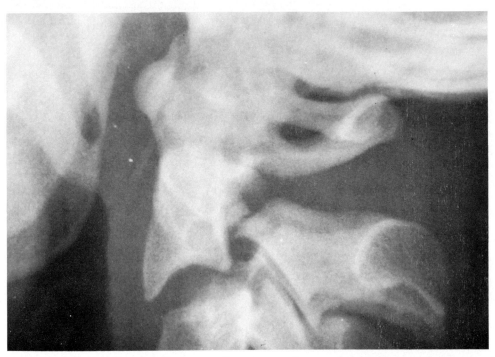

Figure 4–59. Classic "hangman's fracture" or traumatic spondylolisthesis of the axis vertebra. There are bilateral fractures through the pedicles of C-2, slight anterolisthesis of C-2 on C-3, and some narrowing of the C-2 intervertebral disk space. Note the retropharyngeal soft tissue swelling.

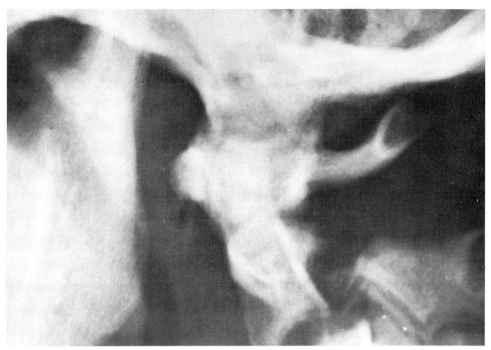

Figure 4-60. Hangman's fracture (traumatic spondylolisthesis).

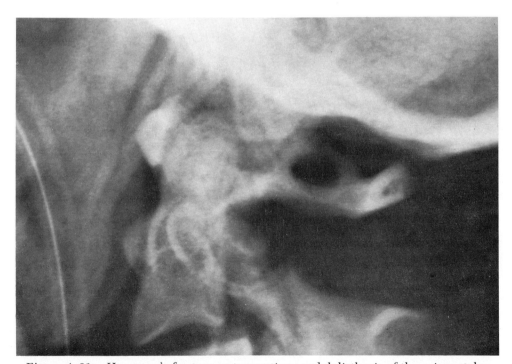

Figure 4-61. Hangman's fracture or traumatic spondylolisthesis of the axis vertebra.

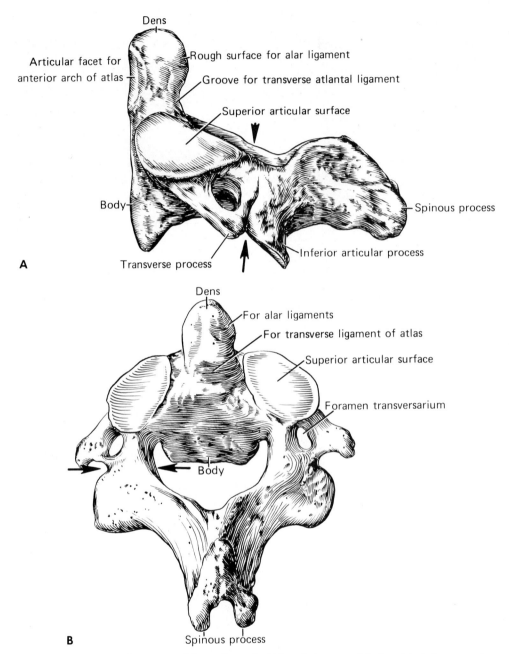

Figure 4–62. Axis vertebra viewed from the side (A) and above and behind (B) showing the region of the pars interarticularis (arrows). Compare with Figure 4–63. The pars interarticularis is that region of the lamina between the superior articular surface and the rest of the lamina (arrows).

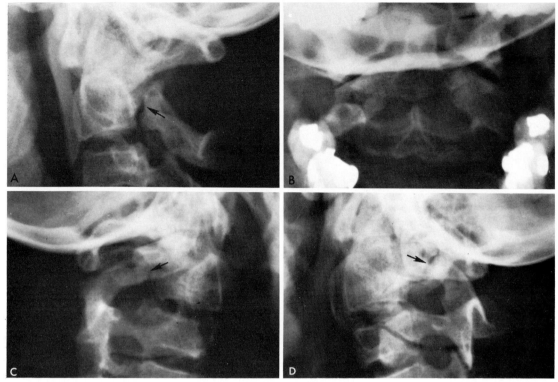

Figure 4–63. Spondylolisthesis of the axis vertebra. *A*, Lateral view showing the pars interarticularis defects bilaterally (arrow). Note the well-corticated bony margins of the bony defects. *B*, Frontal view. *C*, *D*, 45 degree obliques also showing the bony defects (arrows). Compare with Figure 4–62.

jagged edges of fractures. The C-2 vertebral body is displaced anteriorly on C-3, and the C-2 intervertebral disk is preserved.[63]

"Atypical" Bilateral Arch Fractures

Less than 1 per cent of patients exhibited this type of fracture. All of our patients complained of upper cervical spine pain but were neurologically intact. The probable mechanism of injury in this group is compressive hyperextension.[46]

While similar in roentgen appearance to the classic "hangman's fracture," these cases do differ in several aspects. On one side there is a pedicle fracture located anteriorly near the axis vertebral body; on the opposite side, a laminal fracture is present that lies close to the spinolaminar line (Fig. 4–64). Other cases showed bilateral fractures in the laminae anterior to the spinolaminar line (Fig. 4–65). None of the patients had a C-2 intervertebral disk injury, or anterolisthesis of the axis body on C-3.

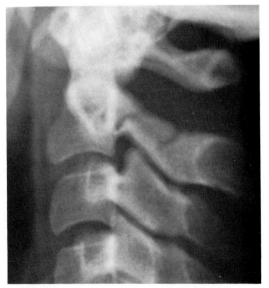

Figure 4–64. "Atypical" bilateral arch fractures. On the lateral view an anterior pedicle and a more posterior laminal fracture are seen. Neither fracture is sharply radiolucent, since there is overlapping of normal bone on the side opposite the fractures.

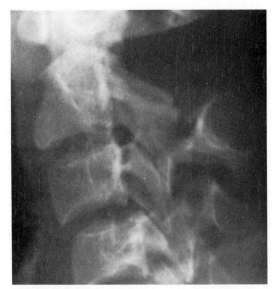

Figure 4–65. "Atypical" bilateral arch fractures. Lateral view showing bilaterally symmetrical laminar fractures close to the spinolaminar line of the axis vertebra. There is also a vertebral arch fracture at C-3.

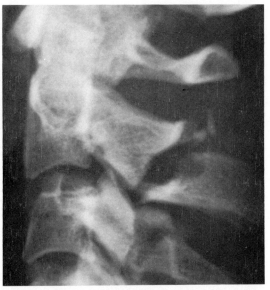

Figure 4–66. Spinous process fracture of the axis vertebra. On the lateral view there is a comminuted fracture of the spinous process that obliterates the spinolaminar line. Note the vertebral arch fracture at C-3.

Spinous Process

Fractures of the spinous process of the axis vertebra account for less than 1 per cent of patients in the Duke series. Spinous process fractures elsewhere in the cervical spine occurred more frequently and were present in 13 per cent of our patients.[45]

These fractures were caused by a direct blow and hyperextension trauma. They

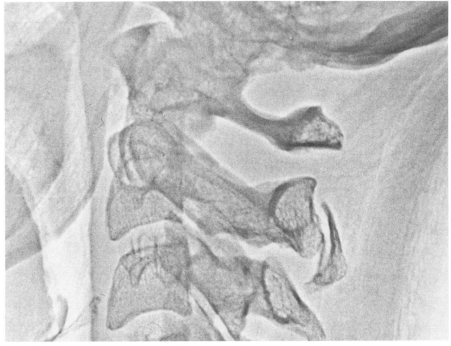

Figure 4–67. Ununited secondary ossification center (apophysis) of the spinous process of C-2 (xeroroentgenograph).

were isolated lesions in our cases. Clinically, one patient had a transitory weakness in one upper limb.[46]

Spinous processes usually fracture close to the spinolaminar line (Fig. 4–66). The fracture edges are jagged and may be comminuted with distraction between fracture fragments.

These fractures must be differentiated from nuchal ligament ossification and an unfused secondary ossification center (apophysis) of the spinous process (Fig. 4–67). The latter have corticated margins and are situated posterior to the spinolaminar line.

REFERENCES

1. Breasted, J. H.: The Edwin Smith Surgical Papyrus. Chicago, University of Chicago Press, 1930.
2. Werne, S.: Studies in spontaneous atlas dislocation. Acta. Orthop. Scand., Suppl. 23, 1957.
3. Fielding, J. W.: Dynamic anatomy and cineradiography of the cervical spine. In The Cervical Spine. Edited by R. W. Bailey. Philadelphia, Lea & Febiger, 1974.
4. Hohl, M., and Baker, H. R.: The atlantoaxial joint, roentgenographic and anatomical study of normal and abnormal motion. J. Bone & Jt. Surg., 46-A:1739, 1964.
5. Penning, L.: Functional Pathology of the Cervical Spine. Baltimore, Williams & Wilkins, 1968.
6. Braakman, R., and Penning, L.: Injuries of the Cervical Spine. London, Excerpta Medica, 1971.
7. Evarts, C. M.: Traumatic occipito-atlanto dislocation. Report of a case with survival. J. Bone & Jt. Surg., 52-A:1653, 1970.
8. Blackwood, N. J.: Atlanto-occipital dislocation: case of fracture of the atlas and axis, and forward dislocation of the occiput on spinal column, life being maintained for 34 hours and 40 minutes by artificial respiration, during which laminectomy was performed upon third cervical vertebra. Ann. Surg., 47:654, 1908.
9. Gabrielsen, T. O., and Maxwell, J. A.: Traumatic atlantooccipital dislocation; with case report of a patient who survived. Amer. J. Roentgenol., 97:624, 1966.
10. Farthing, J. W.: Atlantocranial dislocation with survival: a case report. N. Carolina M. J., 9:624, 1948.
11. Page, C. P., Story, J. L., Wissinger, J. P., and Branch, C. L.: Traumatic atlantooccipital dislocation. Case report. J. Neurosurg., 39:394, 1973.
12. Powers, B., Miller, M. D., Kramer, R. S., Martinez, S., and Gehweiler, J. A.: Traumatic anterior atlanto-occipital dislocation. J. Neurosurg., 4:12, 1979.
13. Bohlman, H.: The pathology and current concepts of cervical spine injuries; a critical review of 300 cases. J. Bone & Jt. Surg., 54-A:1353, 1972.
14. Greig, D. M.: Clinical Observations on the Surgical Pathology of Bone. Edinburgh, Oliver & Boyd, 1931.

15. Fielding, J. W., Cochran, G. V. B., Lawsing, J. F., and Hohl, M.: Tears of the transverse ligament of the altas. A clinical and biomechanical study. J. Bone & Jt. Surg., 56-A:1683, 1974.
16. Sharp, J., and Purser, D. W.: Spontaneous atlanto-axial dislocation in ankylosing spondylitis and rheumatoid arthritis. Ann. Rheum. Dis., 20:47, 1961.
17. Jackson, H.: Diagnosis of minimal atlanto-axial subluxation. Brit. J. Radiol., 23:672, 1950.
18. Greenberg, A. D.: Atlantoaxial dislocations. Brain, 91:655, 1968.
19. Haralson, R. H., and Boyd, H. B.: Posterior dislocation of the atlas on the axis without fracture. J. Bone & Jt. Surg., 51-A:561, 1969.
20. Patzakis, M. J., Knopf, A., Elfering, M., Hoffer, M., and Harvey, J. P.: Posterior dislocation of the atlas on the axis. J. Bone & Jt. Surg., 56-A:1260, 1974.
21. Sassard, W. R., Heinig, C. F., and Pitts, W. R.: Posterior atlantoaxial dislocation without fracture. J. Bone & Jt. Surg., 56-A:625, 1974.
22. Jackson, R. H.: Simple uncomplicated rotary dislocation of the atlas. Surg. Gynec. Obstet., 45:156, 1927.
23. Greenley, P. W.: Bilateral (90 degrees) rotatory dislocation of the atlas upon the axis. J. Bone & Jt. Surg., 12:958, 1930.
24. Martel, W., and Tishler, J. M.: Observations on the spine in mongoloidism. Amer. J. Roentgenol., 97:630, 1966.
25. Englander, O.: Non-traumatic occipito-atlantoaxial dislocation. A contribution to radiology of the atlas. Brit. J. Radiol., 15:341, 1942.
26. Sullivan, A. W., and Rochester, N. Y.: Subluxation of the atlanto-axial joint: sequel to inflammatory processes of the neck. J. Pediat., 35:451, 1949.
27. Wittek, A.: Ein Fall von Distensionsluxation im Atlanto-epistropheal-gelenk. Münch Med. Wschr., 35:1836, 1908.
28. Watson-Jones, R.: Spontaneous hyperaemic dislocation of the atlas. Proc. Roy. Soc. Med., 25:586, 1932.
29. Hess, J. H., Bronstein, J. P., and Abelson, S. H.: Atlanto-axial dislocations unassociated with trauma and secondary to imflammatory foci in the neck. Amer. J. Child. Dis., 49:1137, 1935.
30. Op den Orth, J. O.: Atlantoepistropheale luxaties in voorachterwaartse richting zonder oorzakelijk trauma. J. Belge. Radiol., 46:221, 1963.
31. Fielding, J. W., and Hawkins, R. J.: Atlanto-axial rotatory fixation. Fixed rotatory subluxation of the atlanto-axial joint. J. Bone & Jt. Surg., 59-A:37, 1977.
32. Wortzman, G., and Dewar, F. P.: Rotary fixation of the atlanto-axial joint: rotational atlantoaxial subluxation. Radiology, 90:479, 1968.
33. Coutts, M. B.: Atlanto-epistropheal subluxations. Arch. Surg., 29:297, 1934.
34. Grisel, P.: Énucléation de l'atlas et torticollis naso-pharyngien. Presse Méd., 38:50, 1930.
35. Sherk, H. H., and Nicholson, J. T.: Fractures of the atlas. J. Bone & Jt. Surg., 52-A:1017, 1970.
36. Gehweiler, J. A., Duff, D. E., Martinez, S., Miller, M. D., and Clark, W. M.: Fractures of the atlas vertebra. Skeletal Radiol., 1:97, 1976.
37. Jefferson, G.: Fracture of the atlas vertebra. Report of four cases and a review of those previously recorded. Brit. J. Surg., 7:407, 1920.

38. Jefferson, G.: Remarks on fractures of the first cervical vertebra. *In* Selected Papers. London, Pitman Med. Publ. Co., 1960.

39. Boni, R.: Spora un raro caso di frattura del tubercolo anteriore dell'atlante. Radiol. Med., 43:1095, 1966.

40. Von Torklus, D., and Gehle, W.: The Upper Cervical Spine. New York, Grune & Stratton, 1972.

41. Kattan, J. R. (Ed.).: "Trauma" and "No-trauma" of the Cervical Spine. Springfield, Charles C Thomas, 1975.

42. Ramon-Soler, R.: Traumatisme insolite de l'atlas: fracture transversale de son arc antérieur. Rev. Chir. Orthop., 56:488, 1970.

43. Budin, E., and Sondheimer, F.: Lateral spread of the atlas without fracture. Radiology, 87:1095, 1966.

44. Abel, M.: Occult Traumatic Lesions of the Cervical Vertebrae. St. Louis, Green, 1971.

45. Miller, M. D., Gehweiler, J. A., Martinez, S., Charlton, O. P., and Daffner, R. H.: Significant new observations on cervical spine trauma. Amer. J. Roentgenol., 130:659, 1978.

46. Martinez, S., Morgan, C. L., Gehweiler, J. A., Powers, B., and Miller, M. D.: Unusual fractures and dislocations of the axis vertebra. Skeletal Radiol., 3:206, 1979.

47. Howarth, M. B., and Petrie, J. G.: Injuries of the Spine. Baltimore, Williams & Wilkins, 1964.

48. Schaaf, R. E., Gehweiler, J. A., Miller, M. D., and Powers, B.: Lateral hyperflexion injuries of the cervical spine. Skeletal Radiol., 3:73, 1978.

49. Amyes, E. W., and Anderson, F. M.: Fracture of the odontoid process. (Report of 63 cases). Arch. Surg., 72:377, 1956.

50. Anderson, E., Forsyth, H. F., Davis, C. H., and Nashold, B. S.: Dislocation of the atlas on the axis. The value of early fusion of C1, C2 and C3. J. Neurosurg., 15:353, 1958.

51. Russin, L. D., and Guinto, F. C.: Multidirectional tomography in cervical spine injury. J. Neurosurg., 45:9, 1976.

52. Binet, E. F., Moro, J. J., Marangola, J. P., Hodge, C. J.: Cervical spine tomography in trauma. Spine, 2:163, 1977.

53. Fielding, J. W.: Disappearance of the central portion of the odontoid process. A case report. J. Bone & Jt. Surg., 47-A:1228, 1968.

54. Daffner, R. H.: Pseudofracture of the dens: Mach bands. Am. J. Roentgenol., 128:607, 1977.

55. Grogono, B. J. S.: Injuries of the atlas and the axis. J. Bone & Jt. Surg., 36-B:397, 1954.

56. Wood-Jones, F.: The ideal lesion produced by judicial hanging. Lancet, 1:53, 1913.

57. Schneider, R. C., Livingstone, K. A., Cave, A. J. E., and Hamilton, G.: "Hangman's fracture" of the cervical spine. J. Neurosurg., 22:141, 1965.

58. Gehweiler, J. A., Clark, W. M., Powers, B., Schaaf, R. E., and Miller, M. D.: Cervical spine trauma: the common combined conditions. Radiology, 130:77, 1979.

59. Seljeskog, E. L., and Chou, S. N.: Spectrum of the hangman's fracture. J. Neurosurg., 45:3, 1976.

60. Brashear, H. R., Venters, G. C., and Preston, E. T.: Fractures of the neural arch of the axis. A report of twenty-nine cases. J. Bone & Jt. Surg., 57-A:879, 1975.

61. Elliott, J. M. Rogers, L. F., Wissinger, J. P., and Lee, J. F.: The hangman's fracture. Fractures of the neural arch of the axis. Radiology, 104:303, 1972.

62. Garber, J. N.: Abnormalities of the atlas and axis vertebrae — congenital and traumatic. J. Bone & Jt. Surg., 46-A:1782, 1964.

63. Gehweiler, J. A., Martinez, S., Clark, W. M. and Stewart, G. C.: Spondylolisthesis of the axis vertebra. Am. J. Roentgenol., 128:682, 1977.

64. Minderhoud, J. M., Braakman, R., and Penning, L.: Os odontoideum — clinical, radiological, and therapeutic aspects. J. Neurol. Sci., 8:521, 1969.

65. Wollin, D. G.: The os odontoideum. Separate odontoid process. J. Bone & Jt. Surg., 45-A.:1459, 1963.

66. Giacomini, C.: Sull' esistenza dell' "os odontoideum" dell' uomo. Gior. d. R. Accad. di Med. di Torino, 49:24, 1886.

67. Frieberger, R. H., Wilson, P. D., and Nicholas, J. A.: Acquired absence of the odontoid process. J. Bone & Jt. Surg., 47-A:1231, 1965.

68. Fielding, J. W.: Os odontoideum: an acquired lesion. J. Bone & Jt. Surg., 56-A:187, 1974.

69. Gleason, I. O., and Urist, M. R.: Atlantoaxial dislocation with odontoid separation in rheumatoid arthritis. Clin. Orth., 42:121, 1965.

70. McRae, D. L.: The significance of abnormalities of the cervical spine. Am. J. Roentgenol., 84:3, 1960.

71. Lanier, R. R.: An anomalous cervicooccipital skeleton in man. Anat. Rec., 73:189, 1939.

72. Rowlan, L. P., Shapiro, J. H., and Jacobson, H. G.: Neurological syndromes associated with congenital absence of the odontoid process. AMA Arch. Neurol. & Psych., 80:286, 1958.

73. Degenhardt, K. H.: Missbildungen des Kopfes und der Wirhelsaule. *In* Humangenetik, Bd II, hsg. vo. P. E. Becker. Stuttgart, Thieme, 1964.

74. McRae, D. L.: Craniovertebral junction. *In* Radiology of the Skull and Brain. Edited by T. H. Newton and D. G. Potts. St. Louis, C. V. Mosby, Co., 1971.

75. McRae, D. L., and Barnum, A. S.: Occipitalization of the atlas. Amer. J. Roentgenol., 70:23, 1953.

76. McRae, D. L.: Bony abnormalities in the region of the foramen magnum: correlation of the anatomic and neurologic findings. Acta. Radiol., 40:335, 1953.

77. Hadley, L. A.: Atlantooccipital fusion, ossiculum terminale and occipital vertebra as related to basilar impression with neurological symptoms. Am. J. Roentgenol., 59:511, 1948.

78. Bharucha, E. P., and Dastur, H. M.: Craniovertebral anomalies. Brain, 87:469, 1964.

79. Green, H. L. H. H.: An unusual case of atlantooccipital fusion. J. Anat., 65:140, 1930.

80. Lombardi, G.: The occipital vertebra. Am. J. Roentgenol., 86:260, 1961.

81. List, C. F.: Neurologic syndrome accompanying developmental anomalies of occipital bone, atlas and axis. Arch. Neurol. & Psych., 45:577, 1941.

82. Holsten, D. R.: Eine besondere Form von Defektbildung in hintere Atlasbogen. Forschr. a. d. Geb. d. Röntgenstrahlen u. d. Nuklearmedizin, 108:541, 1968.

83. Oestreich, A. E., and Young, L. W.: The absent cervical pedicle syndrome: a case in childhood. Amer. J. Roentgenol., 107:505, 1969.

84. Eismont, F. J., and Bohlman, H. H.: Posterior atlanto-occipital dislocation with fractures of the atlas and odontoid process. Report of a case with survival. J. Bone & Jt. Surg., 60-A:397, 1978.

Chapter 5

TRAUMATIC LESIONS OF THE LOWER CERVICAL SPINE

"If thou examinest a man having a crushed vertebra in his neck...his falling head downward has caused that one vertebra crush into the next one...he is unconscious of his two arms and his two legs..."

The Edwin Smith Surgical Papyrus. Circa 17th Century B. C.

FRACTURES OF VERTEBRAL BODIES

Miller et al.[1] report that in their series of 400 patients with recognized fractures and/or dislocations of the cervical spine, 30 per cent sustained vertebral body fractures. Two-thirds of these fractures involved the lower three cervical vertebrae.

The C-4 vertebral body was least involved, while C-6 and C-7 were most frequently fractured. On the other hand, *isolated* vertebral body fractures occurred at all levels of the cervical spine with equal incidence. Such isolated lesions accounted for 11 per cent of the patients in Miller's series.

Classification

Vertebral body fractures may be divided into four types: (1) margin fractures, (2) burst (comminuted) fractures, (3) uncinate process fractures, and (4) lateral wedge fractures.

Margin Fractures

Fractures of the vertebral body margins usually occur at the anterosuperior or an-

teroinferior aspects of the body (Figs. 5–1 to 5–5). They may result from either hyperflexion or hyperextension forces associated with compression or disruption.[2, 3]

In this section, we will consider only minimal chip or wedge fractures. In these cases, the posterior portion of the vertebral body is not displaced backward into the vertebral canal, and thus the patients are usually neurologically intact. Fracture-dislocations may be found in the "Dislocations and Fracture-Dislocations" section of this chapter.

Margin fractures, such as those shown in Figures 5–1 to 5–5, are not difficult to diagnose. The hardest fractures of a vertebral body to diagnose are the simplest type. An accurate diagnosis, therefore, requires as much information as possible. This is where the significant signs of trauma, especially the soft tissue abnormalities, can be of aid. Soft tissue changes should increase the index of suspicion of an underlying fracture; in the absence of soft tissue changes, except when the clinical findings are formidable, the suspicion of fracture will decline. The reader is cautioned, however, that in some cases these valuable soft tissue abnormalities may not be manifest for hours or days after injury. If a fracture is suspected clinically, and if the plain films are normal, then tomography may be of value.[4, 5]

Probably the greatest source of error in

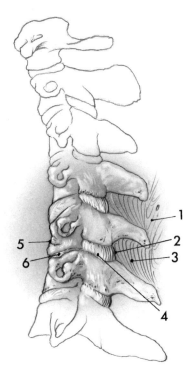

Figure 5–1. Wedge compression fracture of C-5 (5). The disk bordering the fracture (6) may be injured. Other structures shown: 1 = nuchal ligament; 2 = ligamentum flavum; 3 = interspinal ligament; 4 = articular capsule of the apophyseal joint.

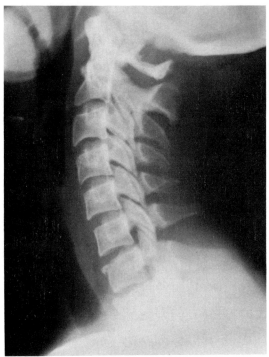

Figure 5–2. Fracture of the anterosuperior margin of the body of C-7. The fragment is displaced slightly ventral. There is minimal displacement of the prevertebral fat stripe. Mechanism of injury: hyperflexion compression.

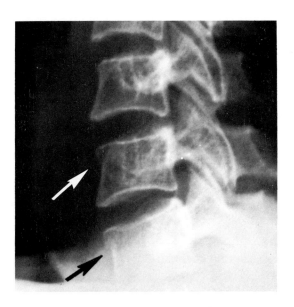

Figure 5–3. Hyperflexion compression fractures of the superoanterior margins of the bodies of C-6 and C-7 (arrows). There is retrotracheal soft tissue swelling indicating hemorrhage and/or edema.

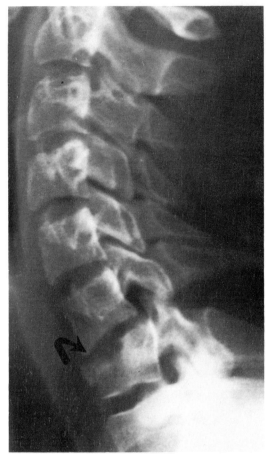

Figure 5–4. Hyperflexion compression fracture of the anterosuperior margin of C-7. Note the decrease in height of the C-6 intervertebral disk space (curved arrow), the widened interspinous space and acute kyphotic hyperangulation at the C-6/C-7 level. This patient has a hyperflexion sprain (momentary dislocation) in addition to the vertebral body fracture.

interpreting radiographs of the injured cervical spine is overdiagnosis of a vertebral body fracture, especially in patients with spondylosis deformans (Fig. 5–6). After the formation of osteophytes, the vertebral bodies are elongated in anteroposterior diameter and are tapered anteriorly. To the uninitiated these changes may be mistaken for fracture, even in the absence of soft tissue abnormalities.

Normal variants may mimic fractures on radiographs of the cervical spine. Patients will occasionally present with intercalary bones in the anterior longitudinal ligament or in the superficial fibers of the anulus fibrosus (Fig. 5–6); these may be mistaken for a fractured osteophyte. In our experience, osteophytes that fracture always take off the corner of an adjacent vertebral body as well.

Without benefit of a previous history, an anterior cervical fusion may be mistaken for a fresh fracture (Fig. 5–7). A slight decrease in the vertical height of the anterior surface of the C-5 or C-6 bodies is a commonly seen variation of the normal (Fig. 5–8) and should not be confused with a fracture. At times, a prominent "carotid tubercle" of C-6 may suggest a compression fracture or bulging intervertebral disk (Fig. 5–9). We have seen children diagnosed as having multiple fractures, when all the radiographs showed were the normal secondary ossification centers (apophyses) of the vertebral bodies (Fig. 5–10).

Burst (Comminuted) Fractures

These fractures are caused by a force applied to the vertex of the skull with the neck

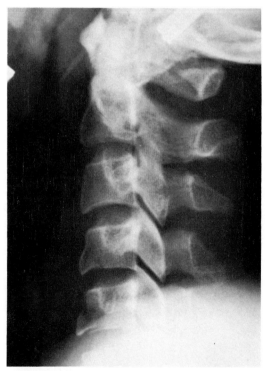

Figure 5–5. Fractures of the anteroinferior margins of the bodies of C-4 and C-5. Note the retropharyngeal soft tissue swelling and displacement of the prevertebral fat stripe secondary to hemorrhage and edema. Mechanism of injury: disruptive hyperextension.

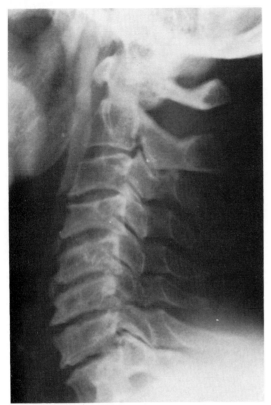

Figure 5–6. Spondylosis deformans of the cervical spine. The platyspondylia must be differentiated from compression fractures. The anterior soft tissues of the neck are normal. Note too the intercalary bones at the ventral aspect of the C-4 and C-5 intervertebral disk spaces.

held rigidly erect. The axial compressive force is transmitted to the lower cervical vertebral bodies. An adjacent intervertebral disk is driven into the vertebral body, which then bursts (Figs. 5–11, 5–12). If the posterior fragments are propelled into the vertebral canal, serious neurologic deficit may result from spinal cord compression.[6] (See the discussion about the type IV "teardrop" hyperflexion fracture-dislocation on page 252.)

Uncinate Process Fractures

The uncinate processes are present only on the C-3 through T-1 vertebral bodies. These bony, semilunar-shaped lips are located laterally on C-3 through C-6 vertebrae and posterolaterally on C-7 and T-1. More details about their development may be found in Chapter 1 (p. 7).

Two per cent of 400 patients in the Duke

series had fractures of the uncinate processes.[7] All of our patients sustained lateral hyperflexion injuries in traffic accidents. Clinically the patients may have neck pain, upper limb weakness, and radiculopathy.

Figure 5–13 shows an excellent example of an uncinate process fracture at T-1; another example is seen in Figure 5–14. Two varieties of uncinate fracture may be seen. The first type is a transverse fracture across the uncus with some distraction of the fragments (Fig. 5–13). In the second type, the uncinate process is fractured as well as the undersurface of the vertebral body above (Fig. 5–14). Similar fractures have been produced in cadavers by Abel.[8] These fractures

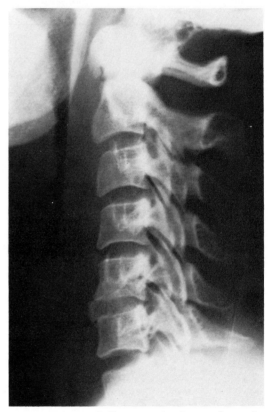

Figure 5–7. Following discharge from the hospital after an anterior cervical fusion at the C-5 intervertebral disk space, this patient was involved in an automobile accident. Because of the marked retropharyngeal soft tissue swelling and displacement of the prevertebral fat stripe, this patient was initially thought to have a vertebral body fracture. The history of prior surgery and comparison with postoperative films showed no change in the appearance of the cervical spine. Note that the graft is partially extruded from the C-5 disk space.

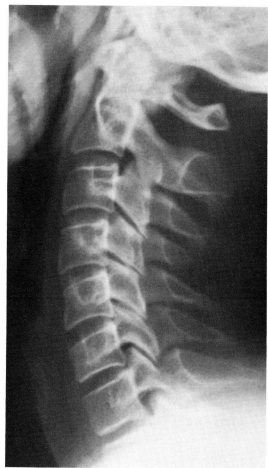

Figure 5–8. Normal lateral cervical spine. Note slight decrease in vertical height of the anterior surface of the C-6 vertebral body. This is a commonly seen variation of the normal and should not be confused with a fracture. Note that the soft tissue structures of the neck anteriorly are normal.

are easily overlooked on radiographs of the cervical spine.

The differential diagnosis of uncinate process fractures should include Mach bands produced by overlapping structures (Fig. 5–15) and congenital underdevelopment[7] (Fig. 5–16). The question often arises after an episode of cervical trauma as to whether asymmetry of the uncinate processes on the same vertebra is acute or congenital. Recall that the uncinate processes are not present at birth. They grow cranially during the first two decades of life, and, as they do, the undersurface of the vertebral body above bevels to accept them.[8] Therefore, if the short uncinate process is associated with a beveled vertebral body above,

the change is probably related to trauma; if the vertebral body above is square, the condition most likely represents congenital underdevelopment (Figs. 5–16, 5–17). Rarely, an unfused secondary ossification center of the uncinate process is seen on radiographs (Figs. 5–15, 5–18).[9-11]

Lateral Wedge-Type Vertebral Body Fracture

Less than 1 per cent of patients in the Duke series had lateral wedge-type fractures of a vertebral body[7] (Figs. 5–19, 5–20). This unusual fracture is thought to be

Text continued on page 199.

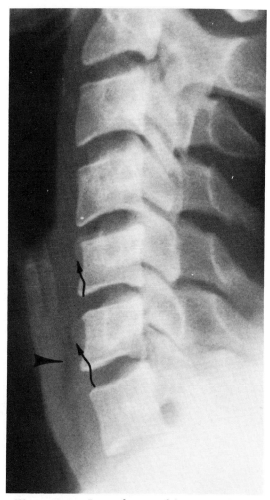

Figure 5–9. Lateral view of the cervical spine showing a prominent "carotid tubercle" of C-6 (lower curved arrow), and a prominent anterior tubercle of C-5 (upper curved arrow). The arrowhead shows the normal prevertebral fat stripe.

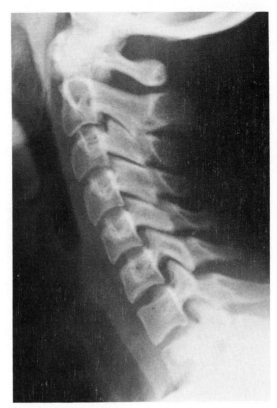

Figure 5–10. Lateral radiograph of the cervical spine in a child showing the normal secondary ossification centers (apophyses) at the anteroinferior margins of the bodies of C-3 to C-5.

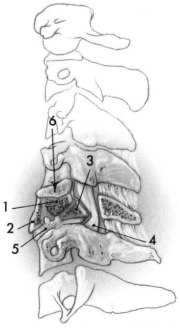

Figure 5–11. Burst (comminuted) fracture of a vertebral body. The C-5 vertebral body is comminuted (1); the anterior fragment is displaced forward (2), and the posterior fragment displaced backward into the vertebral canal (3). The spinal cord (4) may be crushed. The C-5 intervertebral disk is disrupted and may be extruded into the vertebral body (5). The direction of axial compressive force is shown at 6. These fractures usually occur with the Type IV "teardrop" hyperflexion fracture-dislocation. See Figures 5–78 to 5–82.

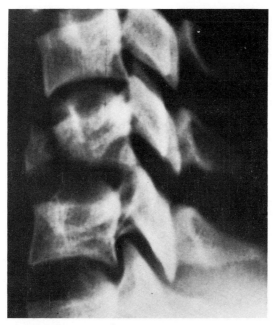

Figure 5–12. Burst (comminuted) fracture of the C-5 vertebral body. This patient has a Type IV "teardrop" hyperflexion fracture-dislocation. (See Figs. 5–78 to 5–82.)

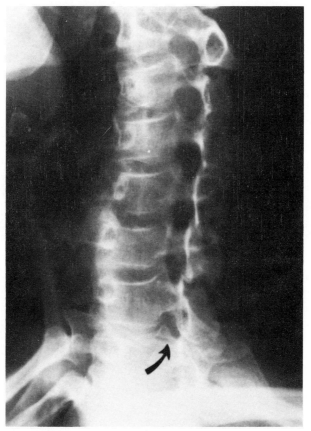

Figure 5–13. 45 degree oblique view of the cervical spine showing a transverse fracture across the uncinate process of T-1.

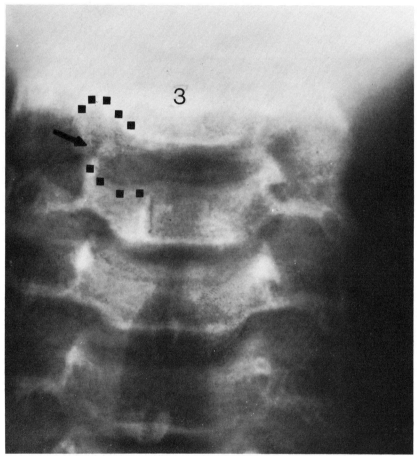

Figure 5–14. Fracture of the uncinate process of C-4 on the right (arrow). The fracture extends into the body (lower dots), and also involves the undersurface of the C-3 vertebral body above (upper dots).

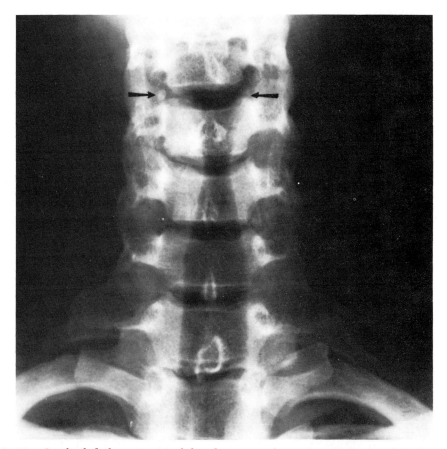

Figure 5–15. On the left there is a Mach band crossing the uncinate process of C-4 (arrow). On the right at the same level there is an unfused secondary ossification center (apophysis) of the uncinate process.

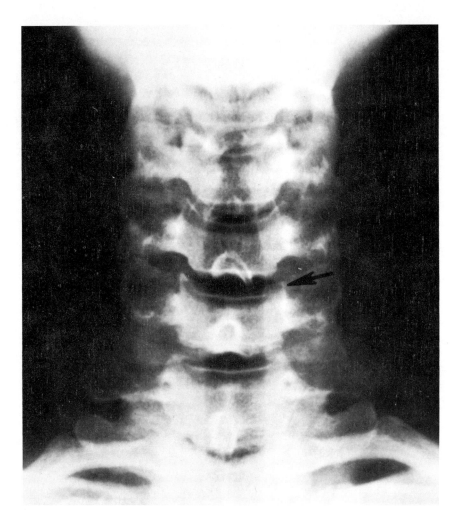

Figure 5–16. Congenital underdevelopment of the uncinate process of C-6 on the left (arrow). Note the squared off undersurface of the C-5 body on the left. Compare the two sides carefully. The right side is normal.

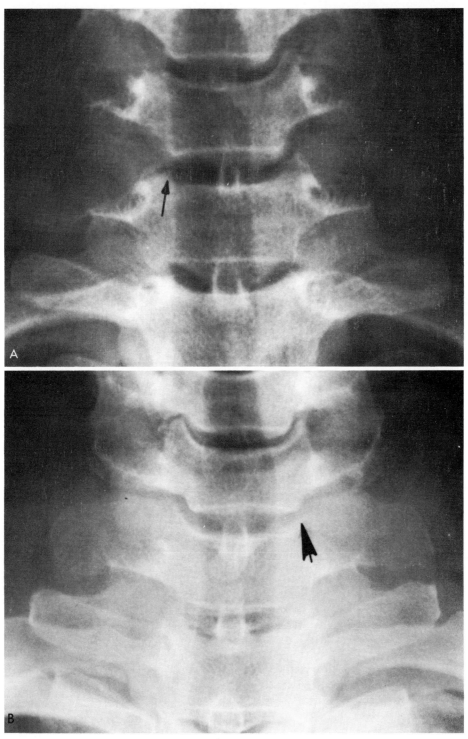

Figure 5–17. Underdevelopment of the uncinate processes. *A,* Short uncinate process of C-7 on the right (arrow) and squaring of the undersurface of the C-6 body immediately above. *B,* Similar changes on the left side in another patient.

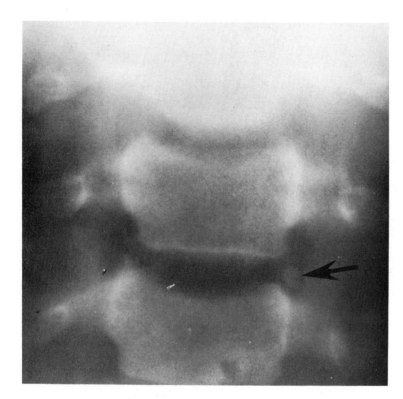

Figure 5–18. Frontal tomogram showing an ununited secondary ossification center (arrow).

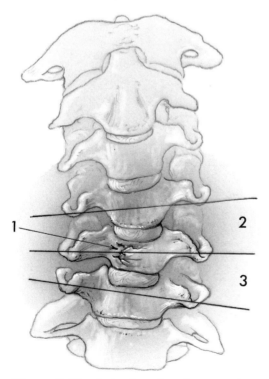

Figure 5–19. Lateral wedge fracture of C-5 (1). There is slight separation of C-5 from the body above and below (2, 3).

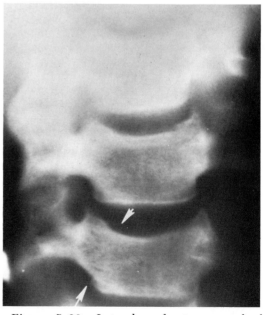

Figure 5–20. Lateral wedge-type vertebral body fracture in the lower cervical spine on the right (arrows). Mechanism of injury: lateral hyperflexion.

an injury of young patients with lateral hyperflexion trauma.[12] Selecki found experimentally that lateral hyperflexion forces applied to the adult cervical spine were converted to hyperextension injuries by the way in which the cervical spine is articulated. Thus we have found examples of lateral wedge fractures associated with vertebral arch fractures (Fig. 5–21). However, we have also found these unusual fractures associated with "teardrop" hyperflexion fracture-dislocations of the lower cervical spine (Fig. 5–22).

Since the lateral wedge-type vertebral body fracture rarely occurs as an isolated injury except in children or young adults, we would advise the reader to look for other fractures and dislocations on the radiographs (Figs. 5–21, 5–22). The lateral wedge fracture is best diagnosed on frontal views of the cervical spine.

VERTEBRAL ARCH FRACTURES

Classification and Incidence

The most common site of cervical spine fracture is the vertebral arch. *Fifty per cent* of all patients in the Duke series of 400 patients had vertebral arch fractures.[1] Table 5–1 lists the location and incidence of these fractures. Since many patients had more than one fracture, the total exceeds 50 per cent.

C-6 vertebral arch was the most vulnerable to fracture; 30 per cent of all arch fractures in the cervical spine occurred at this level. C-3 was the most protected, with only 8 per cent occurring at this level of the spine. These distribution patterns deviate significantly from the expected random pattern, and are most likely related to the mechanism of injury.

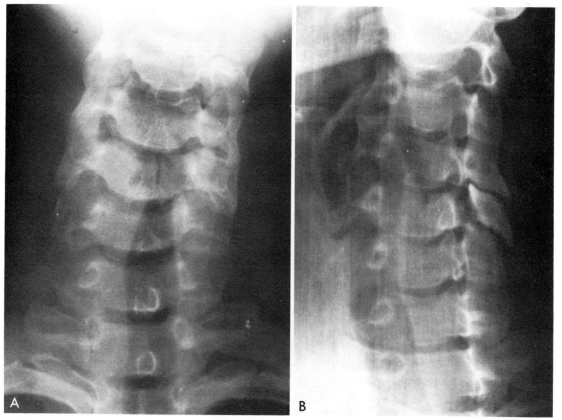

Figure 5–21. A, Frontal view showing sagittal and lateral wedge fractures of the body of C-5 on the left. B, The oblique view showing a fracture of the pedicle of C-5 on the left, distortion of the articular pillar of C-5 and rotation of the pillar into a more horizontal plane. Diagnosis: Type V-A hyperextension fracture-dislocation. Mechanism of injury: lateral hyperflexion converting to compression hyperextension.

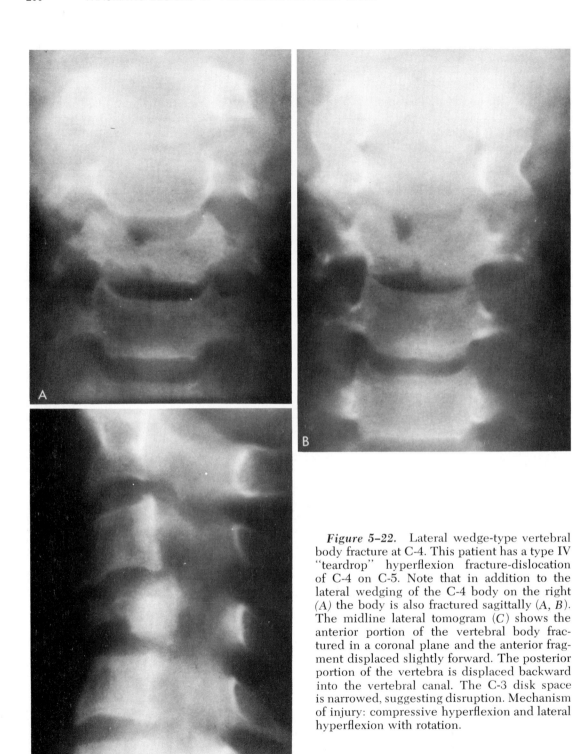

Figure 5–22. Lateral wedge-type vertebral body fracture at C-4. This patient has a type IV "teardrop" hyperflexion fracture-dislocation of C-4 on C-5. Note that in addition to the lateral wedging of the C-4 body on the right (*A*) the body is also fractured sagittally (*A, B*). The midline lateral tomogram (*C*) shows the anterior portion of the vertebral body fractured in a coronal plane and the anterior fragment displaced slightly forward. The posterior portion of the vertebra is displaced backward into the vertebral canal. The C-3 disk space is narrowed, suggesting disruption. Mechanism of injury: compressive hyperflexion and lateral hyperflexion with rotation.

TABLE 5–1. Vertebral Arch Fractures—
Location & Incidence*

LOCATION	INCIDENCE
Articular pillar	21%
Pedicle	13%
Lamina	13%
Spinous process	13%
Transverse process	2%

*The total exceeds 50%, since many patients had more than one fracture.

The physician must become familiar with the various types of vertebral arch fractures, as they are the most common fracture of the cervical spine. Incomplete filming of the patient accounts for the majority of misdiagnoses. We now routinely obtain six views of the cervical spine in our emergency room: (1) anteroposterior of the lower cervical spine, (2) AP of the atlas-axis through the open mouth, (3) cross-table lateral, (4) right and left 30 degree obliques, and (5) a vertebral arch view. To avoid injury to the spinal cord all views are made with the patient *supine*. If these six views prove to be *normal*, then the patient is placed erect for lateral and 45 degree oblique films. The reason for obtaining the erect films will become apparent in the "Dislocations and Fracture-Dislocations" section of this chapter.

Articular Pillar Fractures

Articular pillars are *not* lateral masses! In the lower cervical spine, from C-3 to C-7, the superior and inferior articular processes on each side are fused to form the rhomboid-shaped articular pillar. These pillars project laterally on each side from the junction of the pedicle and lamina (Figs. 5–23, 5–24).

In the Duke experience, the articular pillar was the most vulnerable to fracture (Table 5–1). Twenty-one per cent of the patients had a fracture here. Before we started to do vertebral arch views in all acutely traumatized cervical spines, many of these fractures went undetected on the initial screening radiographs. This was especially true in cases with *isolated* pillar fractures. The most common isolated fracture of the vertebral arch involved the articular pillar in 8 per cent of our total patient population. Forty-three per cent of these articular pillar fractures occurred at the level of C-6.[1]

We have observed three types of articular pillar fractures: (1) compression, (2) compression-distraction, and (3) displacement, with avulsion of an articular pillar fragment, oblique displacement, or comminution of the articular pillar fragments. The compression-distraction and displacement fractures pose little problem in diagnosis, as will be seen shortly. The most common is the compression fracture.

Most articular pillar fractures are caused by vehicular accidents. Compression and displacement fractures are thought to be the result of hyperextension-compression forces (Figs. 5–25, 5–27, 5–29). Abel produced compression-distraction fractures in cadavers by hyperextension-hyperflexion forces[8] (Figs. 5–26, 5–28).

Patients with articular pillar fractures complain of neck pain. On physical examination they may show limitation of motion, tenderness, sensory loss, and, most commonly, muscle weakness.[13]

Isolated *compression fractures* of the articular pillars present the greatest challenge to diagnosis. They are the subject of some medical controversy, for reasons that will become apparent below.[14] Several years ago, we studied 52 patients in conjunction with an orthopedic surgeon.[13] Thirty-eight patients sustained a neck injury from 3 months to 14 years prior to our evaluation, and 14 patients were injured less than 3 months before evaluation. In 77 per cent of these patients, a definite diagnosis of an articular pillar fracture was made. All of these patients had normal "routine" cervical spine radiographs. The patients were examined with a "complete" cervical spine series similar to that described by Abel.[8] The radiographic series included the following: (1) AP of the atlas-axis through the open mouth, (2) anteroposterior of the lower cervical spine, (3) laterals in neutral, flexion, and extension, (4) 45 degree right and left obliques, (5) 20 degree right and left obliques, (6) posteroanterior vertebral arch view, (7) right and left posterior oblique vertebral arch views, and (8) a semiaxial (Jackson) view of the atlas. A highly skilled technolo-

Text continued on page 206.

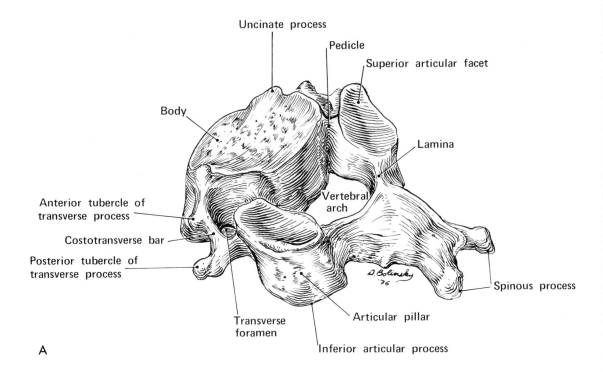

A

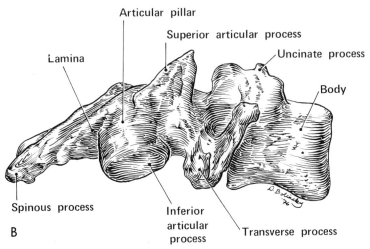

B

Figure 5–23. "Typical" cervical vertebra. *A*, Viewed from above and behind. *B*, Viewed from the side.

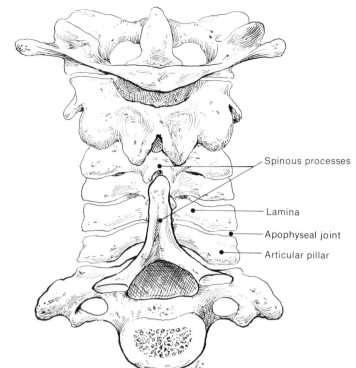

Figure 5–24. Drawing showing the structures visible on the verte-bral arch view.

Spinous processes

Lamina

Apophyseal joint

Articular pillar

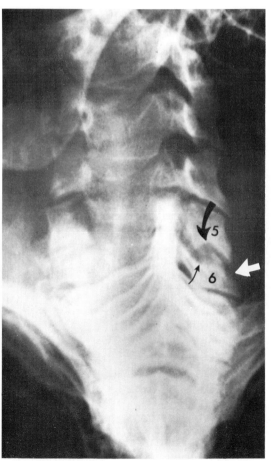

Figure 5–25. Fractures of the articular pillars of C-5 and C-6 on the left about the C-5/C-6 apo-physeal joint (arrows).

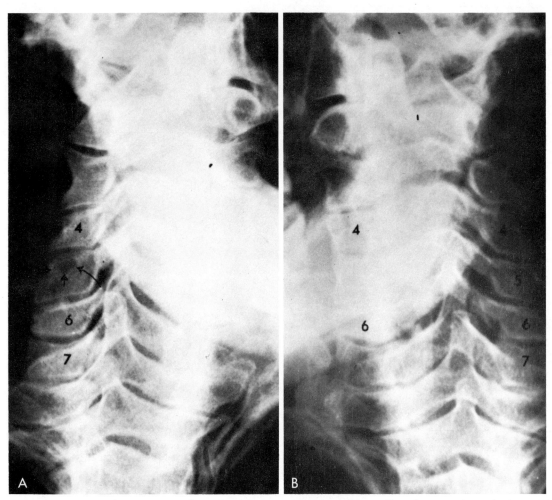

Figure 5–26. A, Compression-distraction fracture of the articular pillar of C-5 on the right (arrows). There is a large oval defect in the cancellous bone. The opposite normal side is seen in *B*.

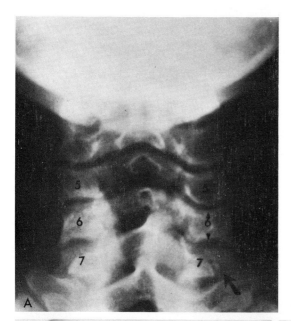

Figure 5-27. Articular pillar fractures at C-6 and C-7 on the left. Note the oblique fracture line coursing through the articular pillar of C-7 on the left in the frontal view (*A*) at the arrow. There is also central compression of the articular pillar of C-6 on the left. This is 3 mm less in vertical height than the C-6 pillar on the right. *B, C,* Oblique vertebral arch views. Note the large osseous defect in the pillar of C-7 on the left (arrow). Compare this with the normal appearance on the right.

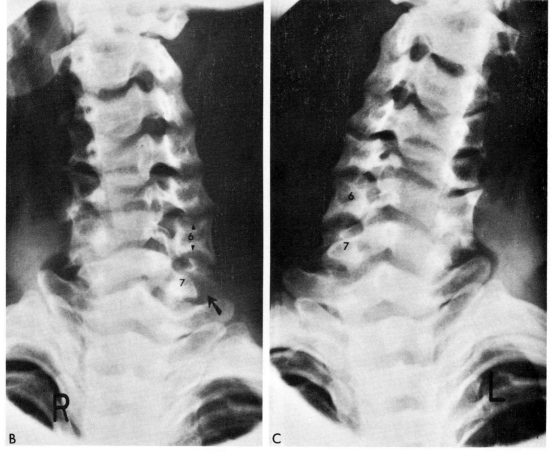

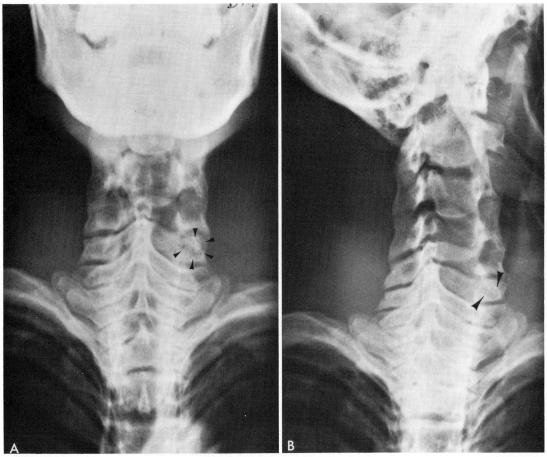

Figure 5–28. Compression-distraction fracture of the articular pillar of C-6 on the left (arrows). *A*, Frontal vertebral arch view. *B*, Oblique vertebral arch view.

gist could obtain this examination in about 45 minutes.

To the readers in the legal profession, we would like to emphasize that obtaining 13 views of the cervical spine in every acutely injured patient is impractical in any hospital in the world. There must be hard clinical evidence to justify the examination. In the series described above, patient selection was based on the following: (1) nondiagnostic plain films of the cervical spine and a "negative" workup, (2) the presence of motor weakness and electromyographic abnormalities (giant polyphasic potentials), (3) disability for longer than six months, (4) acute cases with severe pain, muscle weakness, and neurologic deficit that do not respond to conservative treatment.[13]

When clinically indicated, it is important to obtain all 13 projections of the cervical spine in order to fully visualize the mor-

phology of each vertebra. No single projection will reliably show the fracture for any given anatomic part of the cervical spine. While the vertebral arch view is ideal in one patient, it may not be the view that best demonstrates the fracture in another patient.

Displacement and compression-distraction fractures of articular pillars pose no problems in diagnosis. Displacement fractures course obliquely through an articular pillar, disrupting the cortex (Figs. 5–25, 5–29). Compression-distraction fractures appear as central radiolucencies within the cancellous bone of the pillar. The overall contour of the articular pillar may be distorted (Figs. 5–26, 5–28).

The most difficult diagnostic problem is the compression-type fracture (Figs. 5–27, 5–30). The radiologic appearance does not enable one to approximate the age of the fracture. It is also difficult to evaluate the in-

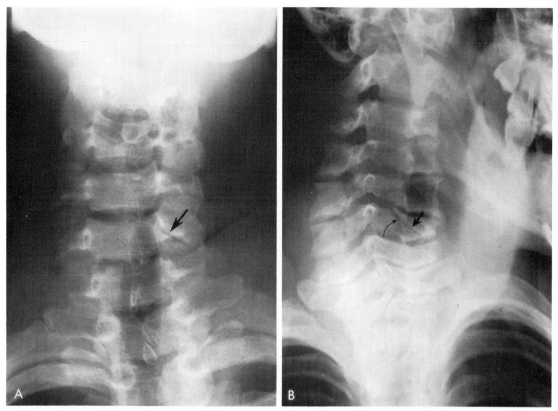

Figure 5–29. Oblique fractures of the C-6 articular pillar and lamina on the left. *A*, Frontal view. *B*, Oblique vertebral arch view. Note the spina bifidas at the cervicothoracic junction.

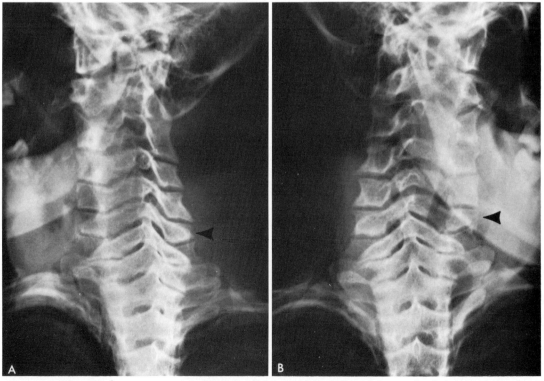

Figure 5–30. Wedge compression fracture of the articular pillar of C-6 on the left (arrows). *A*, Right oblique vertebral arch view. *B*, Left oblique vertebral arch view. Note the bony defect in the lateral aspect of the pillar (arrow).

ternal trabecular disorganization within the pillars. The problem is further compounded by the natural occurrence of articular pillar deformities in the lower cervical vertebrae. Abel[8] observed an increasing incidence of gross pillar deformity with age, ranging from no abnormality at less than one year of age to 51 per cent compression deformities above age 60. Abel suggests that these deformities are acquired. Vines, using 2 mm discrepancy in articular pillar height as a critical value in determining asymmetry, found unilateral compression to be common and unrelated to age or to the presence of associated degenerative changes. Thus he concluded that mere asymmetry of the articular pillars at the same level could not be used as a criterion of recent trauma. A definite fracture line with follow-up radiographs demonstrating healing changes are the only findings diagnostic of recent injury (Fig. 5–31). It is quite apparent that further research is needed into the subject of compression fractures of articular pillars.

Pedicle Fractures

Two-thirds of all pedicle fractures occur in the axis vertebra (C-2). In our experience, the axis is the only vertebra in the cervical spine that may sustain *isolated* unilateral pedicle fractures (Chapter 4).[15]

In the Duke series, 4 per cent of the patients had pedicle fractures in the lower cervical spine. The majority of these were in patients with type V hyperextension fracture-dislocations (p. 228). A few patients had pedicle fractures associated with locked articular facets. We found no isolated pedicle fractures in the lower cervical spine.

Lamina Fractures

In our series, lamina fractures occurred in 11 per cent of patients in the lower cervical spine. They were most often observed in C-5 and C-6 vertebrae; 26 per cent of all lamina fractures occurred at each level. Only 2 per cent of our total patient population had *isolated* lamina fractures (Fig. 5–32).

Lamina fractures may be caused by compressive hyperextension or hyperflexion forces. By far, the largest number of lamina

fractures is seen in patients with the Type V hyperextension fracture-dislocation (p. 228) (Fig. 5–55).

Isolated lamina fractures are usually best diagnosed on stereoscopic vertebral arch views or by tomography (Fig. 5–33). Occasionally they are seen on the other views of the cervical spine. These fractures course vertically or obliquely through the lamina. The greatest problem in differential diagnosis of lamina fractures arises from overlapping normal structures producing Mach bands. When in doubt, tomography is invaluable in diagnosis.

Spinous Process Fractures

The overwhelming majority of spinous process fractures occur in the lower cervical vertebrae. In our series, 13 per cent of the patients had fractures of the spinous processes, and of that total two-thirds occurred at C-6 and C-7.[1] Howarth and Petrie also found spinous process fractures to be common in the lower cervical spine.[16] Two per cent of our cases had *isolated* spinous process fractures.

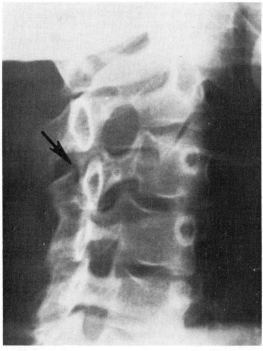

Figure 5–31. Fractured articular pillar at C-3 on the right (arrow). The pillar is also compressed.

radiographs taken to exclude hyperflexion sprain (p. 228).

On lateral radiographs, spinous process fractures occur near the spinolaminar line (Fig. 5–34). The edges of the fracture are jagged and not corticated. On frontal views of the cervical spine, a radiolucent line is observed and the dorsal fragment is displaced (Fig. 5–34 B).

Fractures of the spinous processes must be distinguished from nuchal ligament ossification and unfused apophyses. Nuchal ligament ossification occurs dorsal to the tip of the spinous process (Fig. 5–35). Unfused secondary ossification centers (apophyses) of the spinous process have smooth, corticated margins and are located well away from the spinolaminar line (Fig. 5–36). If in doubt as to whether a patient has an unfused apophysis or a fracture, follow-up radiographs may show callus formation if a fracture has occurred.

Transverse Process Fractures

Only 2 per cent of patients in the Duke series[1, 7] had fractures of the transverse processes; 1 per cent were *isolated* fractures. All but one case in that series involved

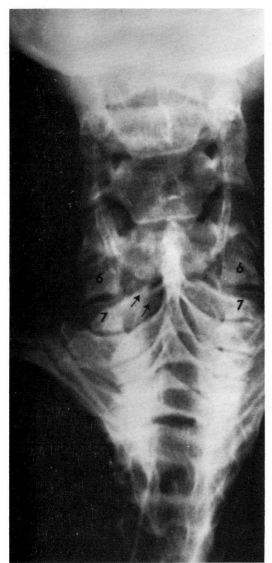

Figure 5–32. AP vertebral arch view showing an isolated oblique lamina fracture at C-7 on the right (arrows).

Spinous process fractures may result from direct or indirect violence. When produced by indirect violence, these fractures have been referred to as "clay-shoveler's fracture." They result from repeated stress caused by the pull of the trapezius and rhomboid muscles on the spinous processes. Similar fractures are caused by sudden hyperflexion of the neck in traffic accidents.[2] Spinous process fractures are also seen in patients with hyperflexion or hyperextension fracture-dislocations. When possible clinically, all patients with spinous process fractures should have erect lateral

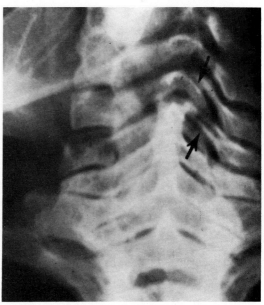

Figure 5–33. Lamina fractures at C-5 and C-6 on the left (arrows). These fractures are well visualized on this vertebral arch view.

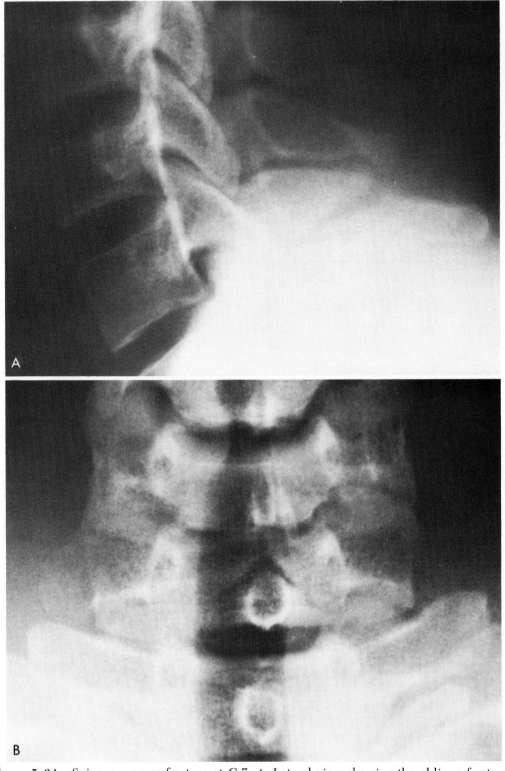

Figure 5–34. Spinous process fracture at C-7. *A*, Lateral view showing the oblique fracture. *B*, Frontal view.

Figure 5–35. Nuchal ligament ossification. *A*, Lateral view. *B*, Frontal view (arrow).

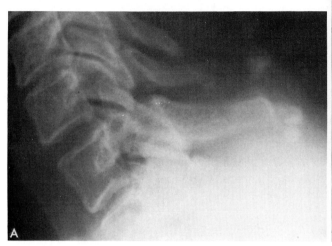

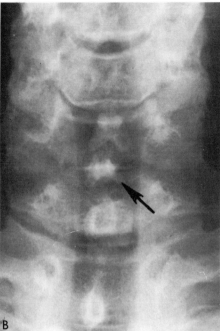

C-7 vertebra (Figs. 5–37, 5–38). The exception was a patient with a fracture at C-6 who also had an ipsilateral C-7 transverse process fracture. Abel[8] has described and illustrated transverse process fractures of the atlas.

The majority of patients with these fractures were involved in broad-side automobile accidents. Most of the cases had unilateral skull or facial trauma. Brachial plexus injuries were common, and this probably resulted from the close proximity of the nerve roots to the transverse processes. Other fractures of the vertebral arch were also present in the majority of cases. This is probably the result of lateral hyperflexion injuries in adults converted into hyperextension.[12]

Transverse process fractures are thought to be produced by forced lateral bending of the cervical spine, which results in avulsion of the transverse process by the pull of attached muscles and ligaments.[8]

As with all fractures produced by lateral hyperflexion, the diagnosis cannot be made on lateral radiographs of the cervical spine. Frontal and oblique views are usually required for accurate diagnosis. Tomography may sometimes be the only method of detecting these lesions.

Fractures of the transverse process are primarily unilateral, tend to be vertically or obliquely oriented, and occur commonly at the junction of the mid and distal two thirds[7] (Figs. 5–37, 5–38) of the transverse process.

The only things to consider in the dif-

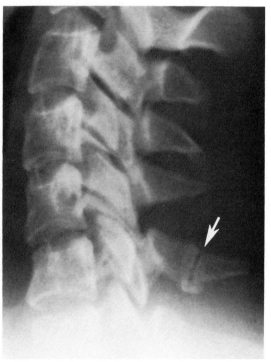

Figure 5–36. Unfused secondary ossification center (apophysis) of the spinous process of C-6. There was no history of prior injury to the head or neck.

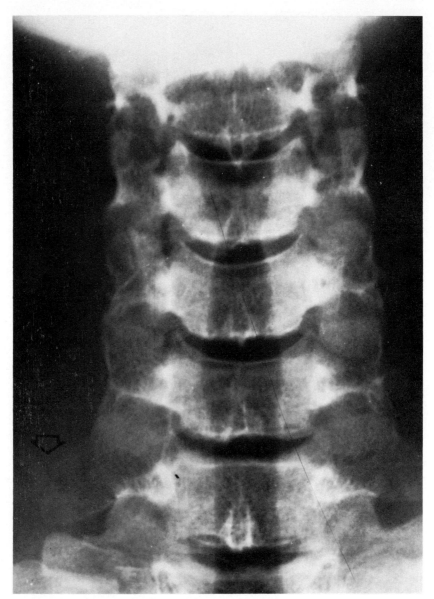

Figure 5–37. Oblique fracture of the transverse process of C-7 on the right (arrow). Note the jagged edges.

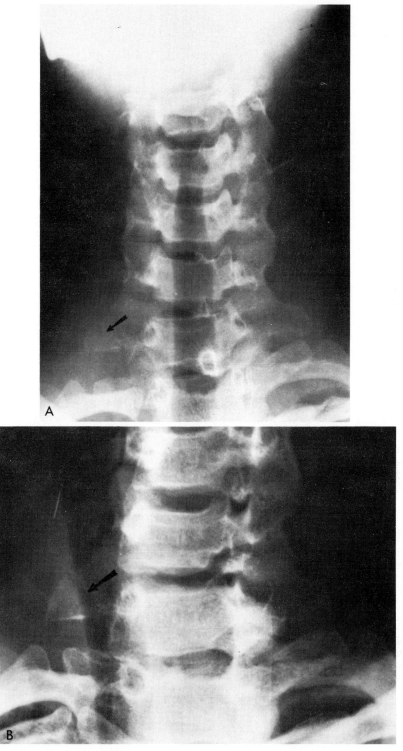

Figure 5–38. Fracture of the transverse process of C-7 on the right (arrow). In addition the head of the first rib is dislocated inferiorly. *A,* Frontal view. *B,* Oblique view.

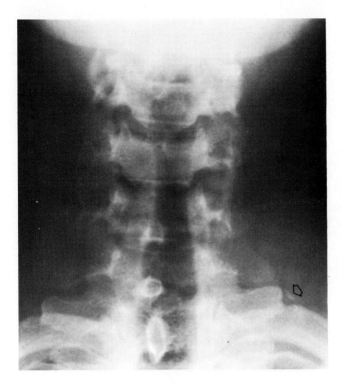

Figure 5–39. Unfused secondary ossification center (apophyses) of the transverse process of T-1 on the left. Note that the apophysis has smooth corticated margins rather than jagged edges.

ferential diagnosis of transverse process fractures are adjacent calcified vascular flecks, rudimentary cervical ribs, and an unfused secondary ossification center (apophysis) of a transverse process. The latter has smooth corticated margins, rather than jagged edges (Fig. 5–39).

TABLE 5–2. Classification of Hyperextension Fracture-Dislocations[17, 18] (Incidence of each type)

TYPE	PERCENT OF PATIENTS
I. Posterior fracture-dislocation of the dens	3
II. Traumatic spondylolisthesis of the axis (hangman's fracture)	7
III. Hyperextension sprain (momentary dislocation) with fracture	<1
IV. Hyperextension fracture-dislocation with fractured articular pillar	10
V. Hyperextension fracture-dislocation with comminuted vertebral arch	4

DISLOCATIONS AND FRACTURE-DISLOCATIONS

Summarized in Tables 5–2 and 5–3 are the hyperextension and hyperflexion fracture-dislocations of the entire cervical spine.[17, 18] These two conditions make up the two most common groups of traumatic lesions of the cervical spine. Dens fractures and "hangman's fractures" have been considered previously in Chapter 4. The other six conditions will be considered here.

TABLE 5–3. Classification of Hyperflexion Fracture-Dislocations[18] (Incidence of each type)

TYPE	PERCENT OF PATIENTS
I. Anterior fracture-dislocation of the dens	7
II. Hyperflexion sprain (momentary dislocation) with fracture	1
III. Locked articular facets with fracture	6
IV. "Teardrop" fracture-dislocation	5

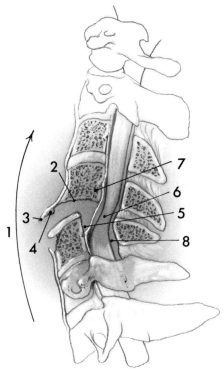

Figure 5–40. Hyperextension sprain with fracture caused by a disruptive hyperextension mechanism (1). The intervertebral disk is torn from the caudal end-plate of C-4 (2); the anterior longitudinal ligament is ruptured (3) and avulsion fracture of the anterosuperior margin of the body of C-5 is seen at 4; the posterior longitudinal ligament is widely separated from the body of C-5 (5); and the spinal cord (6) is pinched between the posterior inferior margin of the body of C-4 (7) and the laminae (8) of C-5.

Hyperextension Sprain (Momentary Dislocation)

Taylor and Blackwood, in a 1948 paper, discussed hyperextension sprain in a patient with severe neurologic findings of cervical cord damage, yet who had normal radiographs of the cervical spine.[19]

In the Duke series of 400 patients, 2 per cent had hyperextension sprains; half of these had associated fractures. Our cases were primarily caused by falls and traffic accidents

The mechanism of these injuries is a disruptive hyperextension force. The articular and spinous processes are forced together and, acting as a fulcrum, cause rupture of the anterior longitudinal ligament and intervertebral disk. As shown schematically in Figs. 5–40 and 5–41, the disk is bisected

or avulsed from the adjacent vertebral body along with a small fragment from the anterosuperior margin of the subjacent vertebral body. At times, instead of a disk disruption, the vertebral body may be fractured horizontally, or there may be no fracture[20] (Fig. 5–42). The cervical spine above the site of disk rupture or vertebral body fracture continues to move posteriorly, carrying the spinal cord with it. The posteroinferior margin of the dislocated vertebral body and the leading edge of the laminae of the vertebra below pinch the cord between them. On recoil of the neck a spontaneous reduction usually occurs, since there can be no articular facet locking. Thus the initial radiographs may appear entirely normal (Fig. 5–43). This is the Taylor-Blackwood, or traumatic pincers, mechanism of injury; Braakman and

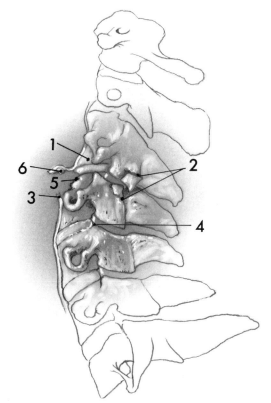

Figure 5–41. Hyperextension sprain with fractures. There is retrolisthesis of the body of C-3 on C-4 (1); rarely there may be fractures of adjacent articular pillars (2); the anterior longitudinal ligament is ruptured (3); the posterior longitudinal ligament may or may not be ruptured (4); the C-3 intervertebral disk is detached from the end-plate (5); and there is an avulsion fracture of the anterosuperior margin of the body of C-4 (6).

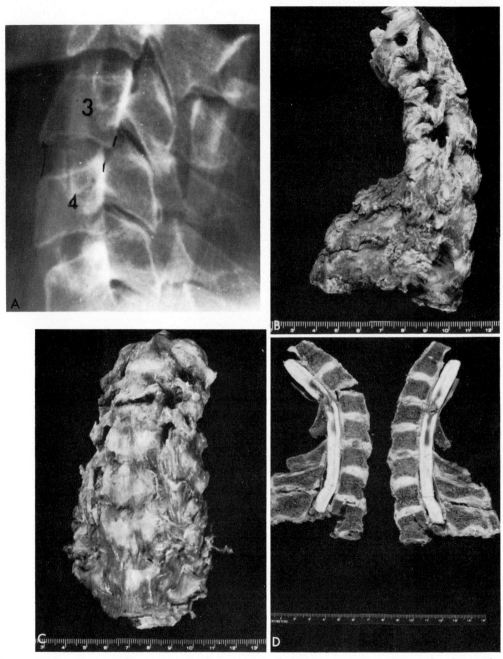

Figure 5-42. Hyperextension sprain (momentary dislocation). *A*, Initial lateral radiograph in patient involved in an automobile accident. There is slight widening of the C-3 intervertebral disk space (curved arrow) and retrolisthesis of C-3 on C-4. The patient was quadraplegic. *B-D*. Anatomic specimen of the same patient showing disruption of the anterior longitudinal ligament, C-3 intervertebral disk and central hematomyelia spreading upward to C-2/3 and downward to C-5. Note that the atlas is not included in this specimen.

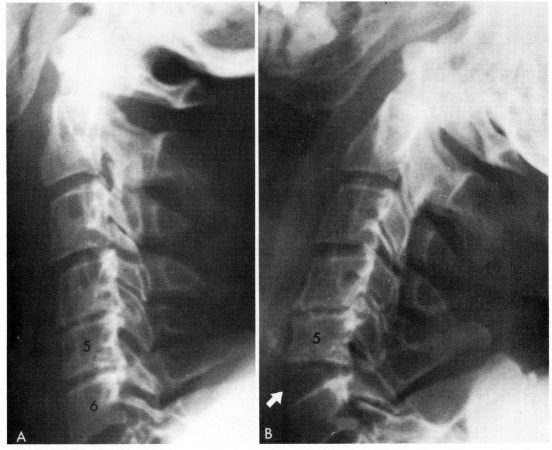

Figure 5–43. Hyperextension sprain (momentary dislocation). This patient presented with an acute central cord syndrome following an automobile accident. *A,* Cross-table lateral view showing changes of spondylosis deformans in the lower cervical spine, widened retropharyngeal soft tissue space, and slight retrolisthesis of C-5 on C-6. *B,* Extension lateral view showing gapping of the C-5 intervertebral disk space and retrolisthesis of C-5 on C-6. Note the nuchal ligament ossification behind the spinous process of C-7.

Penning have termed it a hyperextension sprain.[2]

In 1961 Taylor reported a case of cervical cord injury without postmortem evidence of any cervical spine trauma.[21] After evaluating myelographic studies on cadavers, he postulated that anterior bulging of the ligamentum flavum may result in spinal cord compression during extension of the neck. Patients with spondylosis deformans and a constitutionally small vertebral canal seem especially prone to such neurologic injury.

Clinically, the patient may exhibit an anterior, central, or complete cord compression syndrome; other patients will be neurologically normal.

The roentgen diagnosis of hyperextension sprain is often difficult unless the phy-

sician fully appreciates the clinical history and physical findings. Although the lateral cervical spine radiograph may seem normal on a cursory glance, there are often valuable signs — for example, retropharyngeal soft tissue swelling, displacement of the prevertebral fat stripe, or anterior widening of one or more intervertebral disk spaces — of significant cervical trauma (Figs. 5–42 to 5–45). An avulsion fracture adjacent to a widened intervertebral disk space is commonly encountered.

Miller et al., reporting upon the Duke experience with cervical spine trauma, noted no instances of *isolated* disk injuries.[1] Since that paper, we have observed two patients with transitory spinal cord damage. The routine six supine views of the cervical

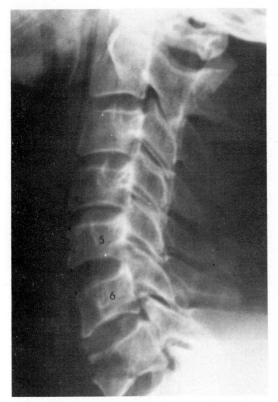

Figure 5–44. Hyperextension sprain and fracture. Cross-table lateral view showing retropharyngeal soft tissue swelling and gapping of the C-5 and C-6 intervertebral disk spaces and oblique fracture of the anteroinferior margin of the body of C-7. This patient had an acute central cord syndrome that developed after he was severely beaten about the face.

spine and the tomograms were normal. With gentle extension, however, lateral radiographs of the cervical spine demonstrated vacuum phenomena and slight anterior widening of intervertebral disks at the levels of hyperextension injury (Figs. 5–46, 5–47). A similar experience has been noted by Wheeler.[22] It now seems clear that in the appropriate clinical setting, dynamic lateral radiographs are indicated. Extreme caution should be exercised in performing these views so as not to further damage the spinal cord.

Hyperextension Fracture-Dislocation With Fractured Articular Pillar (Type IV)

This is the most common *combined* injury of the cervical spine. Ten per cent of the pa-

tients in the Duke series had this lesion.[17, 18] Automobile accidents and falls caused the majority of these injuries.

Forsyth, in a 1964 paper, provided the hypothesis of the mechanism of injury for this type IV lesion and for the type V hyperextension fracture-dislocation.[23] Hyperextension and compression forces applied to the head cause it to move in an arc. The head moves sequentially backward and downward (Fig. 5–48). It seems probable that the anterior longitudinal ligament either remains intact or ruptures late in the trauma. As the head and neck move into extension, the applied forces are on the downward segment of the arc. The force is applied to the articular and spinous processes, and finally to the pedicles and laminae (Fig. 5–48 *B*). As with the pillar fractures, the force that is still acting through an arc is free to displace the vertebral body anteriorly. The intervertebral disk beneath the involved vertebra is disrupted also (Fig. 5–48 *C*). Since the overwhelming majority of articular pillar fractures are unilateral, the presence of a concomitant rotary force is implied. The reader should be aware that these fracture-dislocations often occur at two adjacent levels.

In the type V hyperextension fracture-dislocation, the vertebral arch is comminuted.

Clinically our patients were usually neurologically normal, although a few had minor muscle weakness, and a few had severe neurologic deficit.

The reader must be cautioned at the outset that if only lateral radiographs of the cervical spine are obtained, gross errors in diagnosis may ensue. To accurately diagnose these conditions, frontal, lateral, and oblique radiographs must be obtained, since this lesion and unilateral locked articular facets may look identical on lateral radiographs (Figs. 5–49, 5–50).

On the *lateral* radiograph there are several pertinent observations to be made: anterolisthesis of the involved vertebra on the one below, slight rotation of the vertebra involved with respect to those caudal to it, diminished height of the intervertebral disk space below, and, on occasion, a triangular-shaped fractured articular pillar may be seen[3] (Figs. 5–49 *A*, 5–52 *A*, 5–53 *A*).

The *frontal* view shows the spinous process of the involved vertebra at or very near

Text continued on page 225.

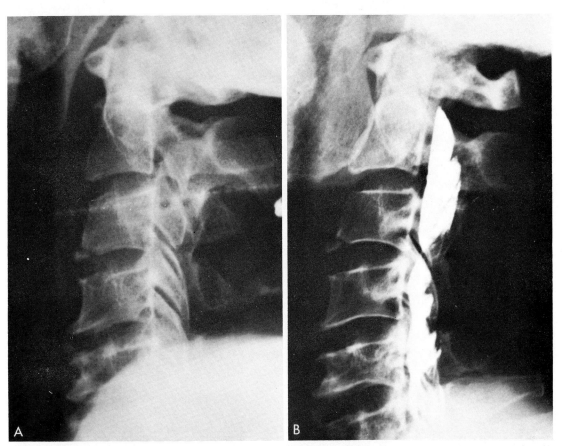

Figure 5–45. Hyperextension sprain with fracture. *A,* Initial cross-table lateral made through a hard collar. Note the retropharyngeal soft tissue swelling and a fracture of the anteroinferior margin of the body of C-3. Changes of spondylosis deformans are noted in the lower cervical spine. The patient at the time of filming had an acute central cord syndrome. *B,* Prone cross-table lateral obtained at the time of myelography. Note again the retropharyngeal soft tissue swelling and the fracture of the anterior-inferior margin of the C-3 body. With slight extension the C-3 intervertebral disk space widens abnormally. Extradural filling defect is noted at the level of the C-3 disk.

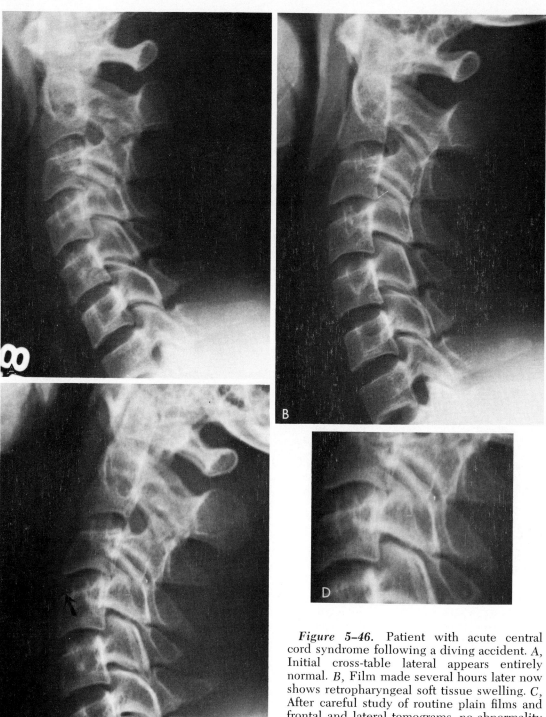

Figure 5–46. Patient with acute central cord syndrome following a diving accident. *A,* Initial cross-table lateral appears entirely normal. *B,* Film made several hours later now shows retropharyngeal soft tissue swelling. *C,* After careful study of routine plain films and frontal and lateral tomograms, no abnormality could be detected. A gentle lateral extension view (*C*) was then obtained. This demonstrated a vacuum sign in the lower aspect of the C-3 intervertebral disk space ventrally (arrow). *D,* closeup of *C.*

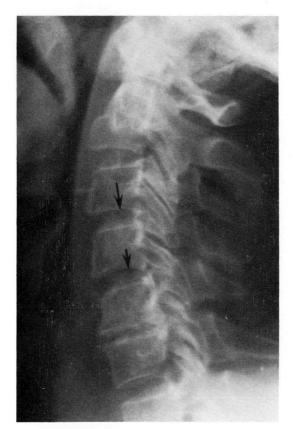

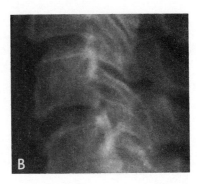

Figure 5–47. Isolated disk injury at the C-3 and C-4 intervertebral disk spaces. Patient sustained a hyperextension injury and had an acute central cord syndrome. Note the vacuum phenomenon at the injured disk levels (arrows). Changes of spondylosis deformans are noted at the C-5 intervertebral disk level. *B*, Closeup of the C-3 and C-4 disks.

A

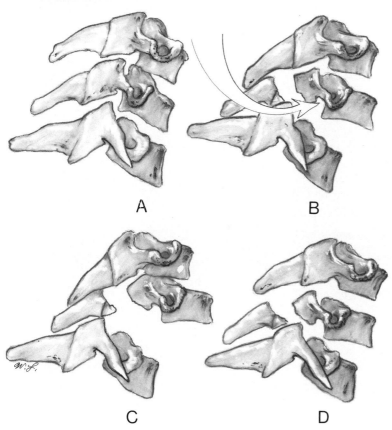

A B

C D

Figure 5–48. Type IV hyperextension fracture-dislocation with fractured articular pillar—mechanism of injury. *A*, Normal, prior to injury. *B*, Hyperextension and compressive forces applied to the head cause it to move in an arc. The head moves sequentially backward and downward. The anterior longitudinal ligament either remains intact or ruptures late in the trauma. As the head and neck move into extension, the applied forces are on the downward segment of the arc. The force is applied to the articular and spinous processes, and finally to the pedicles and laminae. As the articular pillar fractures, the force that is still acting through the arc is free to displace the vertebral body anteriorly. *C*, Disrupted also is the intervertebral disk beneath the involved vertebra. *D*, After the force passes, the fractured vertebra is displaced forward on the one below and the subjacent intervertebral disk is narrowed. Compare with Figure 5–78 (Type IV "teardrop" hyperflexion fracture-dislocation).

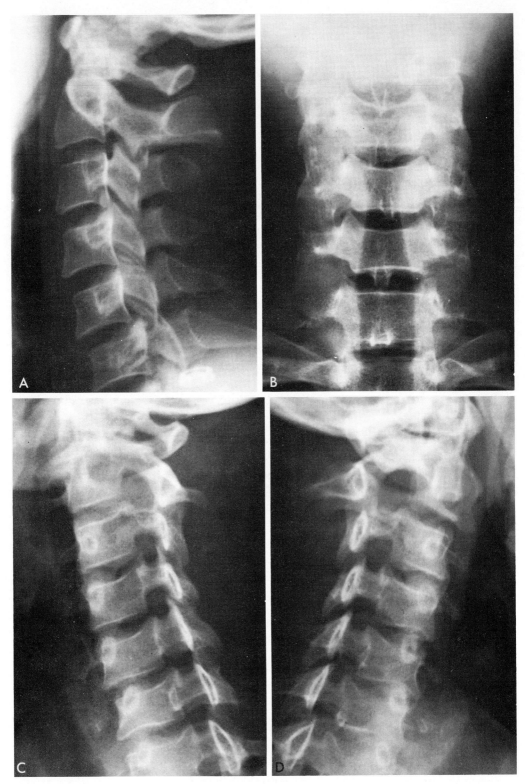

Figure 5–49.

See legend on the opposite page.

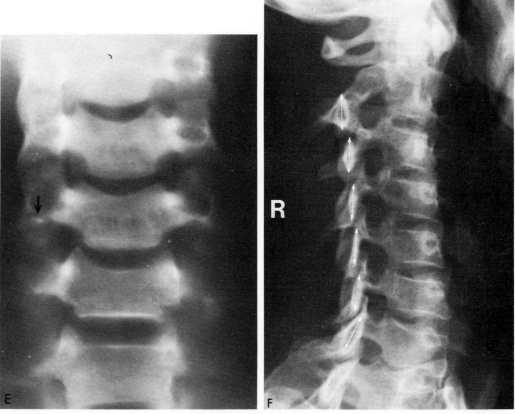

Figure 5–49.   Type IV hyperextension fracture-dislocation. *A,* Lateral view showing anterolisthesis of C-5 on C-6, slight rotation of the C-5 vertebra and those cranial to it, and narrowing of the C-5 intervertebral disk space. *B,* Frontal view shows the spinous process of C-5 displaced slightly to the left of midline. Note the transverse process fracture of C-7 on the right. *C* and *D,* 45 degree oblique views reveal anterolisthesis of C-5 on C-6, distortion of the C-5/6 intervertebral foramina, and loss of laminal imbrication at C-5/6 bilaterally. *E,* Frontal tomogram showing a horizontal fracture of the articular pillar at C-5 on the right (arrow). *F, Imbrication* (L., overlapping, like shingles on a roof). Arrows have been placed on the axis of each lamina on this *normal* patient's right side. Note how they normally overlap like shingles on a roof.

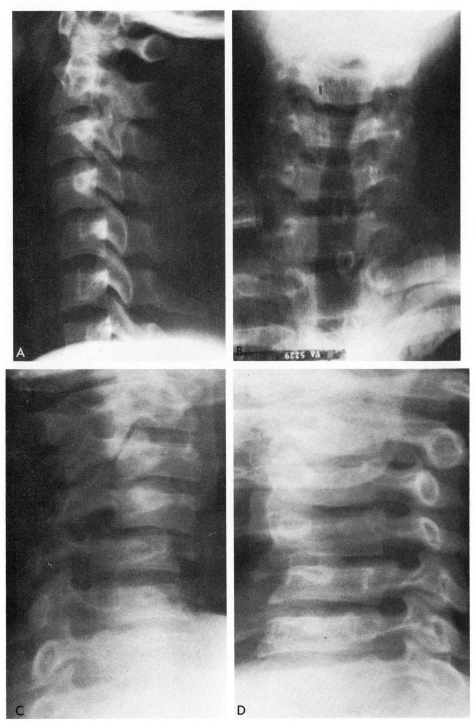

Figure 5–50. Unilateral articular facet locking. *A,* Lateral view showing anterolisthesis of C-4 on C-5, narrowing of the C-4 intervertebral disk space, and rotation of the C-4 vertebra and those craniad to it. *B,* Frontal view on which ink lines have been placed upon the spinous processes of C-4 through C-7. Note the deviated spinous process of C-4 to the patient's right, indicating unilateral facet locking. *C* and *D,* 30 degree trauma obliques made with the patient *supine.* There is unilateral articular facet locking of C-4 on C-5 on the right (C). Note the anterolisthesis of the C-4 vertebra, and marked distortion of the C-4/5 intervertebral foramina.

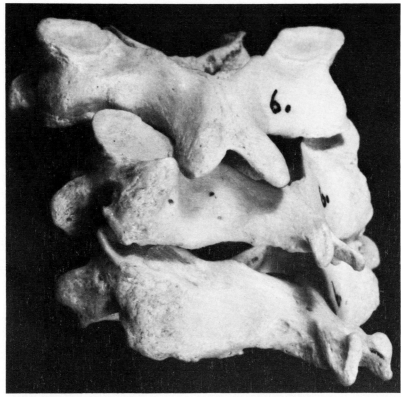

Figure 5–51. Unilateral facet locking. Gross lower cervical vertebrae photographed obliquely from behind to show unilateral facet locking and the marked deviation of the spinous process of the locked vertebra *toward* the side of locking.

the midline (Figs. 5–49 *B,* 5–52 *B,* 5–53 *B*). On occasion the articular pillar fracture may be observed on frontal views.

Oblique radiographs show anterolisthesis of the involved vertebra on one or on both sides. The degree of vertebral body displacement will determine the degree of intervertebral foraminal distortion between the vertebra in question and the one below. The degree of anterolisthesis will also determine the loss of imbrication (L. *imbricatus*, overlapping, like shingles on a roof) (Fig. 5–49 *F*) of the lamina unilaterally, and in some cases bilaterally (Figs. 5–49 *C,* 5–52 *C,* 5–53 *C*). There is no facet locking. In most cases, an articular pillar fracture is demonstrated on the oblique views; however, in some cases vertebral arch views, 20 degree oblique views, or tomography is required for diagnosis (Figs. 5–49 *E,* 5–53 *E*).

Type IV hyperextension fracture-dislocation and unilateral articular facet locking are often confused on lateral radio-

graphs (compare Figs. 5–49 and 5–50, 5–51). Time and again we have seen a physician look at the lateral radiograph of the cervical spine, note anterolisthesis of one vertebra on that below and make a diagnosis of facet locking. The reader should be aware that the type IV hyperextension fracture-dislocation is two and one-half times as common as unilateral facet locking, in our experience. To distinguish the two conditions frontal and oblique radiographs are mandatory. In cases of unilateral facet locking, the frontal view will show the spinous process of the involved vertebra to be significantly displaced from the midline *toward* the side of locking (Fig. 5–50 *B*). The oblique radiographs will show the facet locking; the inferior articular process of the involved vertebra sits in front of the superior articular process of the vertebra below. (Fig. 5–50 *C*). Compare the radiographic changes with the gross vertebral specimen shown in Fig. 5–51.

In accordance with accepted anatomic no-

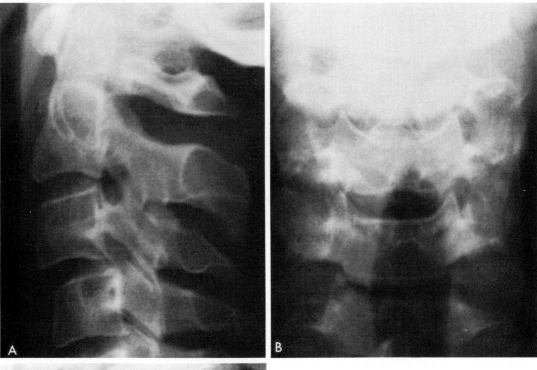

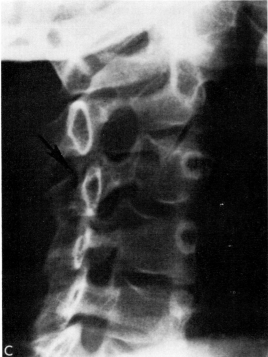

Figure 5–52. Type IV hyperextension fracture-dislocation. *A,* Lateral view showing anterolisthesis of C-3 on C-4, rotation of C-3 and those vertebrae cranial to it, and narrowing of the C-3 intervertebral disk space. *B,* Frontal view shows all of the spinous processes in the midline. *C,* Oblique view reveals anterolisthesis of C-3 on C-4, distortion of the C-3/4 intervertebral foramen, loss of imbrication of the laminae at C-3/4, and a fractured articular pillar at C-3 (arrow).

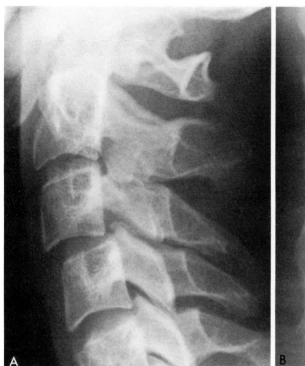

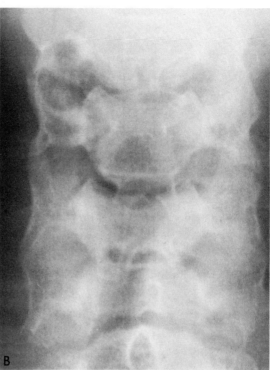

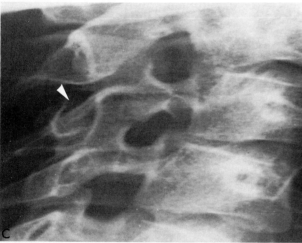

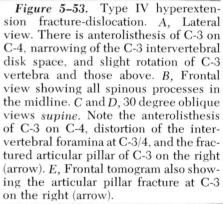

Figure 5–53. Type IV hyperextension fracture-dislocation. *A*, Lateral view. There is anterolisthesis of C-3 on C-4, narrowing of the C-3 intervertebral disk space, and slight rotation of C-3 vertebra and those above. *B*, Frontal view showing all spinous processes in the midline. *C* and *D*, 30 degree oblique views *supine*. Note the anterolisthesis of C-3 on C-4, distortion of the intervertebral foramina at C-3/4, and the fractured articular pillar of C-3 on the right (arrow). *E*, Frontal tomogram also showing the articular pillar fracture at C-3 on the right (arrow).

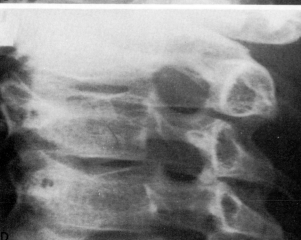

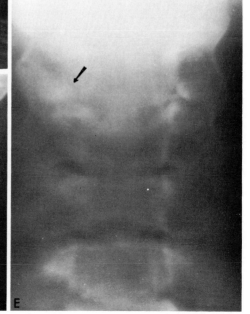

tation, we have used the term "interlocking" for the *normal* relationship of the articular surfaces of the apophyseal joints.

Hyperextension Fracture-Dislocation With Comminution of the Vertebral Arch (Type V)

In the Duke experience, this group of combined traumatic conditions accounted for 4 per cent of all our patients. It is equal in incidence to unilateral articular facet locking, and the two conditions are easily confused unless lateral, frontal, and oblique radiographs are obtained.

We recognize two distinct types: (1) those cases with fractures of an articular pillar, pedicle, and lamina, and with rotation of the fractured articular pillar into a more horizontal plane (Fig. 5–54); and (2) those with severe comminution of the vertebral arch of the involved vertebra. The latter are quite rare; we have two such cases in our files (Figs. 5–57, 5–58).[17]

The roentgen changes in the type V-A hyperextension fracture-dislocation are similar to the type IV condition, with only minor additions. In Figures 5–55 A and 5–56 A note the following changes: anterior displacement of the injured vertebra, narrowing of the intervertebral disk space below and rotation of the vertebral column from the level of dislocation cranially. A lamina fracture may be observed.

The spinous process of the involved vertebra is at or near the midline in the *frontal* view (Figs. 5–55 B, 5–56 B). Distinct pedicle, lamina, and articular pillar fractures are noted. The fractured articular pillar is characteristically rotated into a more horizontal plane. This rotation permits visualization of the facets of the pillar. Compare the two sides of the vertebra at the same level to appreciate this change fully. This significant change is best seen on a true anteroposterior view of the lower cervical spine rather than on one taken with the tube angled 20 degrees cephalad.

Oblique radiographs show the fractured pedicle, lamina, and articular pillar on one side. Again the rotated articular pillar is seen. Loss of imbrication of the laminae is observed, and there is distortion of the intervertebral foramina reflecting the degree of anterolisthesis of the body. (Figs. 5–55 C, 5–56 C).

Those patients with severe comminution of the vertebral arch bilaterally (type V-B) should not be difficult to diagnose. There is marked anterolisthesis of the involved vertebral body on that below (Figs. 5–57 to 5–59). Our own patients with this lesion were quadriplegic, but a similar case report by Pitman et al. showed the patient to be neurologically normal.[24]

Hyperflexion Sprain (Momentary Dislocation)

Hyperflexion sprain has been defined as a temporary and partial luxation (dislocation) of the apophyseal joints following traumatic hyperflexion, with concomitant rupture of the posterior ligaments and joint capsules between two or more vertebrae (Figs. 5–60 to 5–62). The injury results in a typical kyphotic hyperangulation of the cervical spine.[2, 25]

Approximately 2 per cent of the patients in our series of 400 patients had a hyperflexion sprain; half had associated fractures. Interestingly, Braakman and Penning also found in their series that this condition was uncommon. They explained this on the basis of the strength of the posterior ligaments of the cervical spine. A major disruptive force is required to rupture these ligaments; therefore, in most cases articular facet locking will result instead.[2, 25]

Traffic accidents were responsible for the majority of our injuries. In adults, hyperflexion sprains occurred primarily in the lower cervical spine. Younger patients sustained these injuries most often at C-2/C-3 and C-3/C-4 levels.[25]

The mechanism of injury is disruptive hyperflexion of the cervical spine (Fig. 5–63). If a severe blow is delivered to the occiput of the skull from below, the spinous processes are separated, with overstretching of the posterior ligaments. If the force continues, the posterior ligaments are torn at one or two levels, the capsules of the apophyseal joints are disrupted, and the articular facets lose contact and override. As the force passes, the cervical spine springs back toward its normal position. Articular facet locking may occur at this time, or a hyperflexion sprain may ensue (Fig. 5–60). Note in the schematic drawing how the posterior ligaments are disrupted along with the apophyseal joint capsules and the subjacent in-

Text continued on page 236.

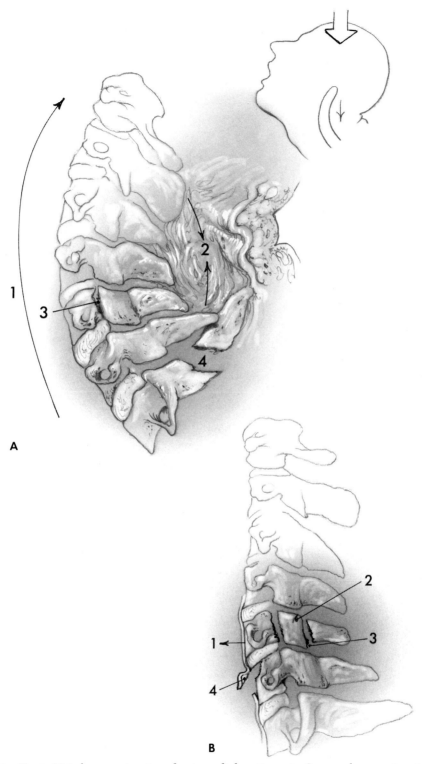

Figure 5-54. Type V-A hyperextension fracture-dislocation. *A,* Severe hyperextension of the cervical spine (1); approximation of the vertebral arches (2); fractures of the articular pillar and pedicle of C-5 (3); and a fractured spinous process of C-7 (4). *B,* After the force passes, there is anterolisthesis of C-5 on C-6 (1); the articular pillar of C-5 is fractured and rotated (2) and there is a fracture of the lamina (3); an avulsion of the superoanterior margin of C-6 vertebral body may be present (4) and the anterior longitudinal ligament ruptured.

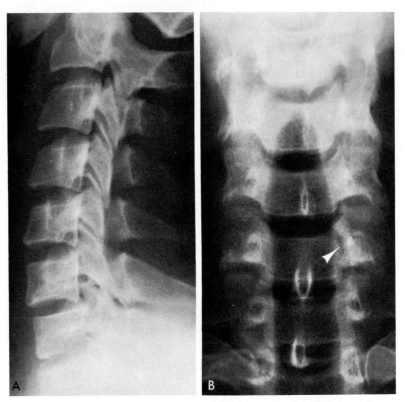

Figure 5–55. Type V-A hyperextension fracture-dislocation. *A,* Lateral view shows anterolisthesis of C-6 on C-7, narrowing of the C-6 intervertebral disk, rotation of the C-6 vertebra and those above, and a lamina fracture at C-6. *B,* Frontal view. The spinous process of C-6 is near the midline, pedicle and lamina fractures are present on the left, and there is slight rotation of the C-6 articular pillar fracture on the left. The rotation of the pillar is better demonstrated on straight AP views of the cervical spine.

Illustration continued on opposite page

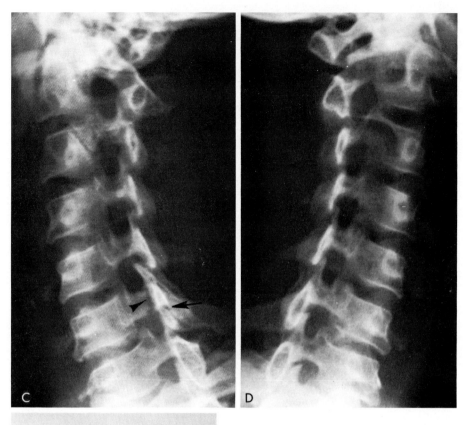

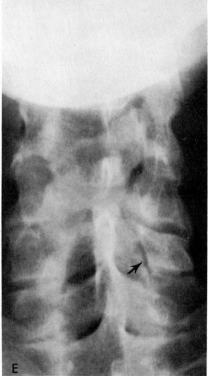

Figure 5–55 Continued. *C,* 45 degree oblique view. Note the pedicle (arrowhead) and lamina fractures (arrow), and the wedged and rotated C-6 articular pillar on the left. *D,* Opposite normal 45 degree oblique view for comparison. *E,* AP vertebral arch view nicely shows an oblique fracture of the C-6 lamina on the left (arrow), and the compressed C-6 articular pillar.

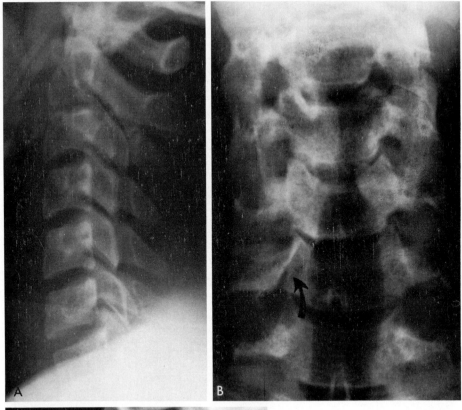

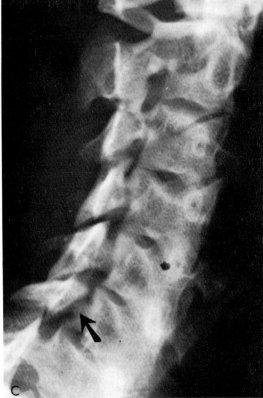

Figure 5–56. Type V-A hyperextension fracture-dislocation. *A,* Lateral view. There is anterolisthesis of C-6 on C-7, narrowing of the C-6 intervertebral disk space, and wedging of one articular pillar. *B,* Frontal view showing the pedicle fracture (arrow) at C-6 on the right. Note the rotated articular pillar into a more than normal horizontal plane permitting visualization of its facets. *C,* Oblique view shows the rotated articular pillar at C-6 on the right and a fractured pedicle (arrow). Lamina fractures may be seen only on vertebral arch views or tomography.

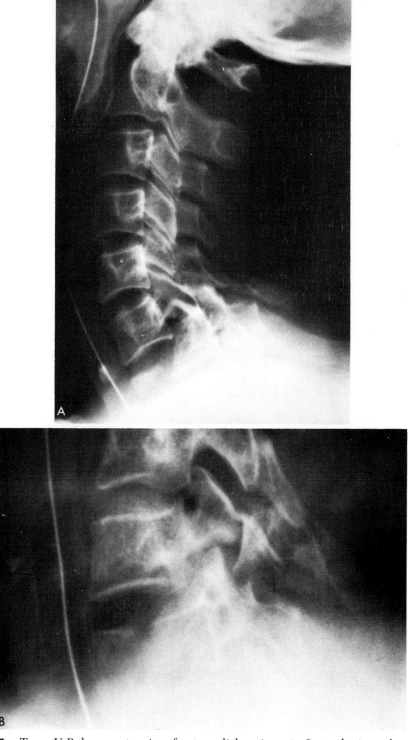

Figure 5-57. Type V-B hyperextension fracture-dislocation. *A,* Lateral view showing antero-listhesis of C-6 on C-7, and comminution of the vertebral arch of C-6. There is also a fracture of the body of C-7. *B,* Closeup after attempted reduction.

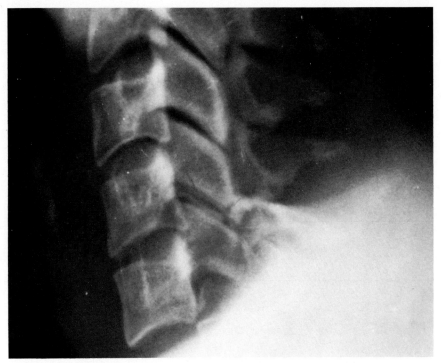

Figure 5–58. Type V-B hyperextension fracture-dislocation. Lateral view showing anterolisthesis of C-6 on C-7, and comminution of the vertebral arch of C-6.

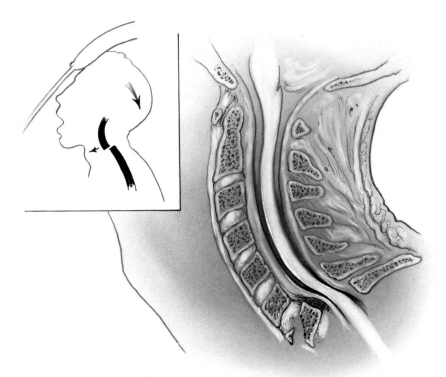

Figure 5–59. Drawing in sagittal section to show a type V-B hyperextension fracture-dislocation with a complete cord lesion.

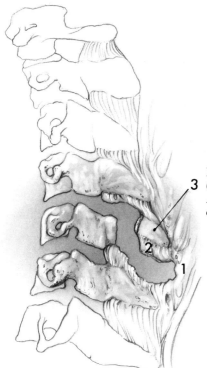

Figure 5-60. Hyperflexion sprain (momentary dislocation). Rupture of the supraspinal (supraspinous) and interspinal (interspinous) ligaments as shown at 1 and 2 respectively. Avulsion of the spinous process of C-5 (3). Note the widening of the apophyseal joints at the levels of injury.

Figure 5-61. Hyperflexion sprain (momentary dislocation). Rupture of the nuchal ligament at 1, and interspinal ligament (3), apophyseal joint capsule (2), ligamentum flavum (4), and posterior longitudinal ligament (5). There is widening of the apophyseal joint (6), and compression of the intervertebral disk (7).

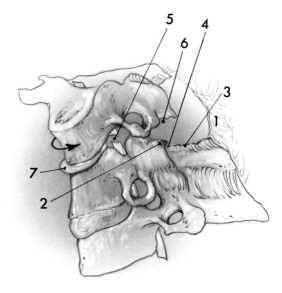

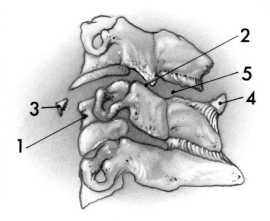

Figure 5-62. Hyperflexion sprain with fracture. There is disruption of the apophyseal joint capsules (2), and interspinal ligaments (5). Vertebral body (1, 3), and spinous process (4) fractures are also present.

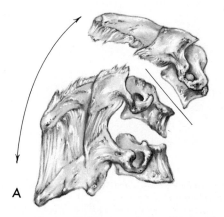
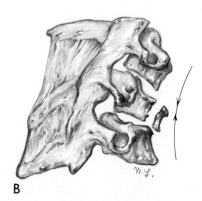

Figure 5–63. A, Disruptive hyperflexion injury with rupture of the posterior ligaments and apophyseal joint capsules. This injury may result in a hyperflexion sprain or locked facets. B, Compressive hyperflexion injury with intact ligaments posteriorly. Since the normal intervertebral disks are usually resistant to compression, the compressive force is primarily expended on the vertebral body.

tervertebral disk (Figs. 5–60, 5–61). A localized kyphotic hyperangulation will be present at the level of ligamentous injury.[26] Roaf has stated that there must be some element of rotation acting to produce posterior ligament tears.[27] Combinations of forces such as disruptive hyperflexion and compression may result in the picture seen in Figure 5–62. A fractured spinous process may be an indication of posterior ligamentous disruption (Figs. 5–60, 5–62, 5–65).

Patients may complain of neck pain, and some will have neurologic deficits. Associated fractures include those of spinous processes and subjacent vertebral bodies (Fig. 5–65).

The reader is cautioned that the roentgen diagnosis of a hyperflexion sprain is not made on a supine cross-table lateral radiograph of the cervical spine. The characteristic kyphotic hyperangulation of the spine may be apparent only on erect lateral radiographs (Figs. 5–64 to 5–66). An *erect lateral* radiograph of the cervical spine is mandatory in all cases of neck trauma before the patient leaves the Radiology Department for home.

A characteristic feature of the hyperflexion sprain is disappearance of the kyphotic hyperangulation when the neck is fully extended. This extension may be achieved only by hanging the unsupported head over the table edge (Figs. 5–64, 5–66). When the

patient is erect, attempted voluntary extension of the neck may not reduce the hyperangulation unless the gravitational center of the skull passes posterior to the longitudinal axis of the injured vertebra.[2, 25]

Once again the reader is directed to the significant signs of cervical spine trauma (Chapter 3). Patients with hyperflexion sprain usually show multiple signs — for example, intervertebral disk space narrowing, and widening of apophyseal joint spaces, and of the interspinous space. If there is an associated compression fracture of a vertebral body, one expects to see widening of the retropharyngeal or retrotracheal spaces, and displacement of the prevertebral fat stripe. Remember, however, that these soft tissue changes may not be manifest immediately after injury; they may require hours or days to appear.

It is better to reserve the diagnosis of *hyperflexion sprain* for a pure ligamentous injury without associated fractures of the cervical vertebrae. When cervical fractures coexist, the injury becomes a *fracture-dislocation* (Type II – Table 5–3).

An erroneous diagnosis of hyperflexion sprain may be avoided by noting several conditions in which there is only minimal loss of the usually smooth cervical lordotic curvature. The appearance may be a variation of normal.[28] On a cross-table lateral radiograph in an unconscious patient, the action of gravity unopposed by the normal

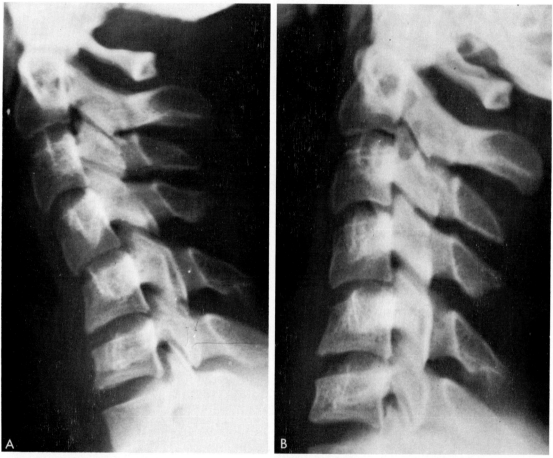

Figure 5-64. Hyperflexion sprain (momentary dislocation). *A*, Erect lateral showing an acute kyphotic hyperangulation of the cervical spine at C-4/5. This could not be changed with attempted extension of the neck. *B*, Cross-table hanging head lateral view showing reduction of the kyphotic hyperangulation.

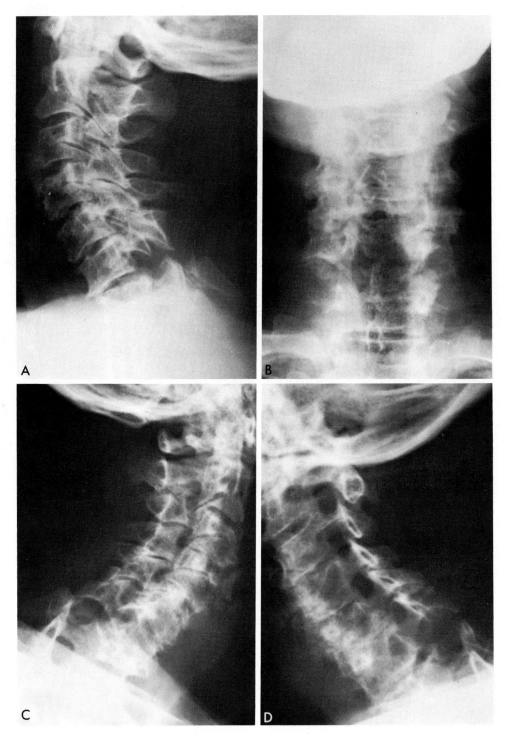

Figure 5–65. Hyperflexion sprain (momentary dislocation) with fracture. *A,* Erect lateral showing an acute kyphotic hyperangulation at C-6/7. Note the gapping of the apophyseal joints and the fractured spinous process of C-6. There is no facet locking. *B,* Frontal view. *C, D,* 45 degree obliques show the intervertebral foraminal widening and the disrupted apophyseal joints at C-6/7.

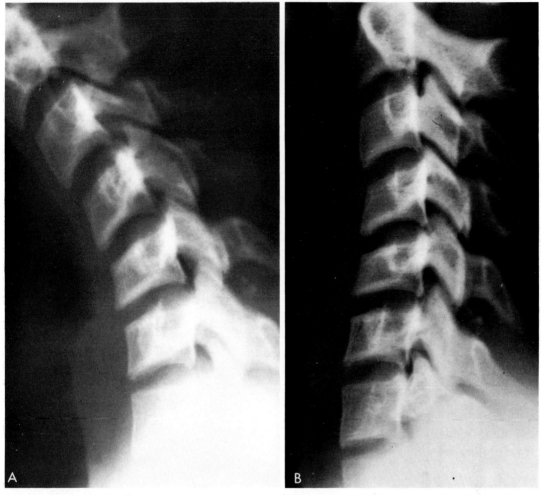

Figure 5–66. Hyperflexion sprain (momentary dislocation) with fracture of the C-5 lamina. *A*, Erect lateral view showing an acute kyphotic hyperangulation of the cervical spine at C-5/6, which could not be reduced with attempted extension while the patient was erect. *B*, Reduction of the kyphotic hyperangulation on a hanging head lateral view. Loss of lordosis was probably secondary to muscle spasm.

paraspinal muscle tone may cause reversal of curvature (Fig. 5–67). Patients with spondylosis deformans commonly have reversal of cervical lordosis. A wide range of normal motion is common between C-2, 3, and 4 vertebrae in young patients (Fig. 5–68). While this may reflect immature musculature in infants, in children it is usually due to improper positioning of the cervical spine. Following relatively minor trauma, reflex spasm of paraspinal musculature may result in an arcuate kyphotic deformity, as opposed to the abrupt kyphotic hyperangulation of a true hyperflexion sprain.[26]

Since the mechanisms of injury for a hyperflexion sprain and articular facet locking (hyperflexion dislocation) are almost the same, any patient with a kyphotic hyperangulation should have a routine film series of the cervical spine to exclude the possibility of facet locking.

Locked Articular Facets (Hyperflexion Dislocation)

In accordance with accepted anatomic notation, we use the term *interlocking* for the

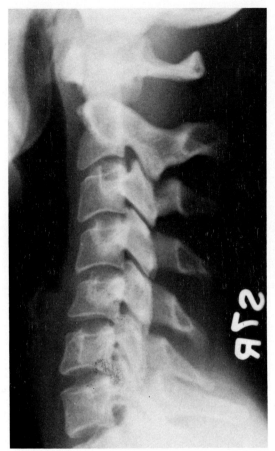

Figure 5-67. Reversal of the normal cervical lordotic curvature in an unconscious patient. Supine cross-table lateral view.

normal relationship of the articular surfaces of the apophyseal joints. The reader will find "interlocking" used for a dislocation in some of the medical literature.

Locked articular facets may not be diagnosed roentgenographically for a variety of reasons. Probably the most common cause of misdiagnosis is inadequate filming of the cervical spine (Fig. 5–69 *A*). The most frequent levels of articular facet locking are C-5/C-6 and C-6/C-7; 75 per cent of our cases occurred at those two levels.[1, 18] Therefore, all seven cervical vertebrae, and, ideally, the first thoracic vertebra, should be visualized (Fig. 5–69 *B–E*).

Failure of diagnosis may also result from failure to recognize the dislocation clinically.[29] The diagnosis of locked facets may not be made for weeks, months, or even years after the acute trauma.[2, 29]

Miller et al. reported that 13 per cent of all patients in our series had articular facet locking;[1] 6 per cent had facet locking with an associated fracture (Type III hyperflexion fracture-dislocation).[18] Bilateral facet locking exceeded unilateral facet locking by more than 2 to 1.

Locked articular facets are caused by a variety of injuries suffered in falls, in contact sports, and in vehicular accidents.

The mechanism of injury in bilateral facet locking is disruptive hyperflexion. Unilateral facet locking is apparently caused by simultaneous disruptive hyperflexion and rotation.[2, 30] If a severe force is exerted upon the occipital region of the skull from below, there is wide separation of the spinous processes, resulting in rupture of the ligamentous bonds and the intervertebral disk. The articular facets lose contact and override. In springing back, after the causative force has passed, the inferior articular processes become locked bilaterally in front of the superior articular processes of the vertebra below (Figs. 5–69 to 5–71). At postmortem examination there will be ruptures of the nuchal ligament, interspinous ligament, articular capsule, ligamentum flavum, and the intervertebral disk[2] (Fig. 5–72). Occasionally, pieces of the ruptured intervertebral disk are found within the vertebral canal.[31, 32]

Articular facet locking may occur without any associated fractures. However, in our series, we found that 28 per cent of the patients had a concomitant vertebral body fracture (Fig. 5–72), and another 28 per cent had an associated vertebral arch fracture (Fig. 5–69). These are correctly termed *hyperflexion fracture-dislocations* (Type III – Gehweiler et al.)[18]

Patients with facet locking may complain of neck pain and stiffness, with or without neurologic deficits. Since there is greater narrowing of the vertebral canal with bilateral facet locking, the neurologic deficits are more severe with bilateral than with unilateral locked facets.[2, 18] It is the fortunate patient who sustains a concomitant fracture of the vertebral arch of the dislocated vertebra. The fracture may produce additional space for the spinal cord. Patients with spondylosis deformans or a congenitally narrowed vertebral canal have the most severe neurologic deficit.[2]

While the roentgen diagnosis of locked articular facets may be suggested on lateral radiographs of the cervical spine, many

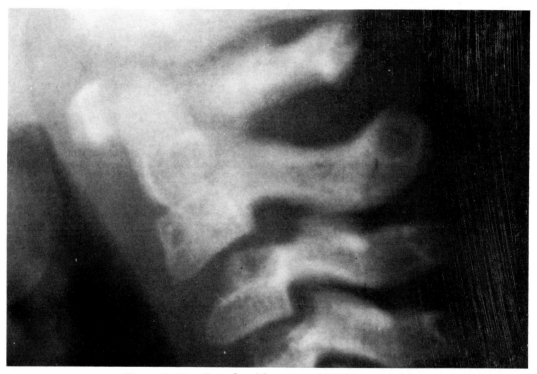

Figure 5–68. Pseudosubluxation of C-2/3 in a child.

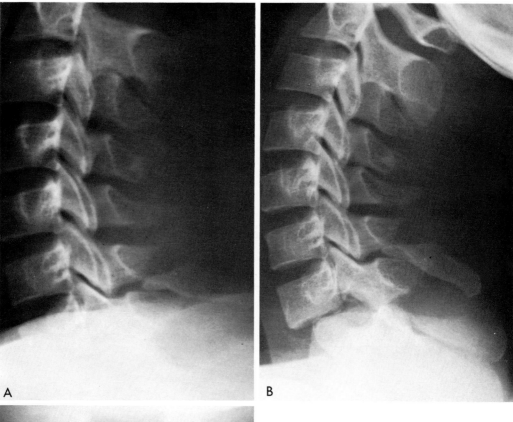

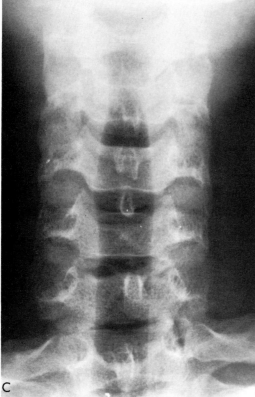

Figure 5–69. Bilaterally locked facets. *A,* Initial cross-table lateral showing fractures of the spinous processes of C-6 and C-7. The C-7 vertebra is inadequately visualized. *B,* Repeat lateral view made after pulling down steadily on the patient's arms. There is anterior displacement of C-7 on T-1, bilaterally locked facets and C-7 intervertebral disk space narrowing. *C,* Frontal view. Because of the spinous process fractures, it is difficult to evaluate displacement.

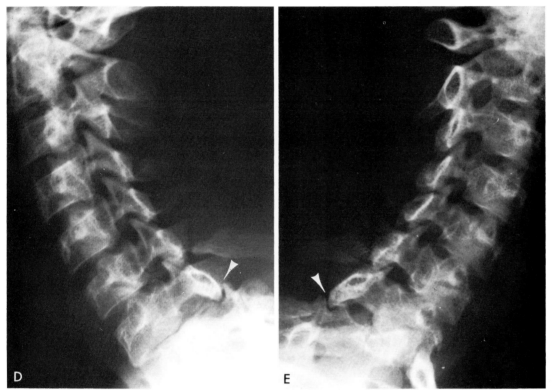

Figure 5–69 *Continued.* *D, E,* 45 degree oblique views clearly show the bilateral facet locking of C-7 on T-1 (arrows).

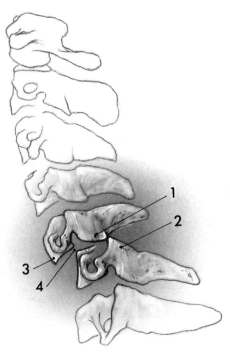

Figure 5–70. *Bilateral* facet locking. The inferior articular processes of C-5 (1) are locked on the superior articular processes of C-6 (2). The body of C-5 (3) is displaced anteriorly on the C-6 vertebra and the intervertebral disk (4) is narrowed.

errors in diagnosis occur because of inadequate filming. Remember that locked facets and certain hyperextension fracture-dislocations (types IV and V) of the cervical spine may look identical on lateral radiographs (see pp. 218–228).

Using the *lateral* radiograph alone, a practice that we strongly discourage, an educated "guess" of unilateral or bilateral facet locking may be made.[17, 18] The degree of displacement (anterolisthesis) of the dislocated vertebra is less than one-half of the anteroposterior width of the end-plate of the vertebra below in unilateral facet locking; with bilateral locking, the displacement is greater than one-half of the width of the end-plate of the vertebral body below (Figs. 5–70 to 5–76).[6] With unilateral facet locking, the dislocated vertebra and those cranial to it are rotated, and the intervertebral disk space subjacent is narrowed, indicating a disk injury. A concomitant fracture of a vertebral body or arch should be sought. (Fig. 5–69).

On the *frontal* view note the position of the spinous process of the dislocated vertebra (Figs. 5–69, 5–73, 5–74). With unilateral facet locking, the spinous process will be significantly deviated from the midline and point *toward* the side of lock (Figs. 5–73, 5–74, 5–76). If the dislocation is bilateral, the spinous process of the dislocated vertebra remains in or near the midline (Fig. 5–69). The reader must be *cautioned*, however, that in the presence of a fractured spinous process of the dislocated vertebra, these signs may not hold.

Two further points should be made about the appearance of facet locking on the frontal radiographs. With unilateral facet locking, the intervertebral disk space and the intervertebral foramen on the side of the dislocation will appear widened (Figs. 5–73, 5–76).

Text continued on page 251.

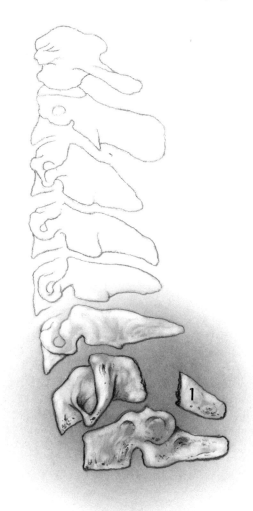

Figure 5–71. Type III hyperflexion fracture-dislocation. There is bilateral facet locking of C-7 on T-1 and a fracture of the spinous process of C-7 (1). Compare with Figure 5–69.

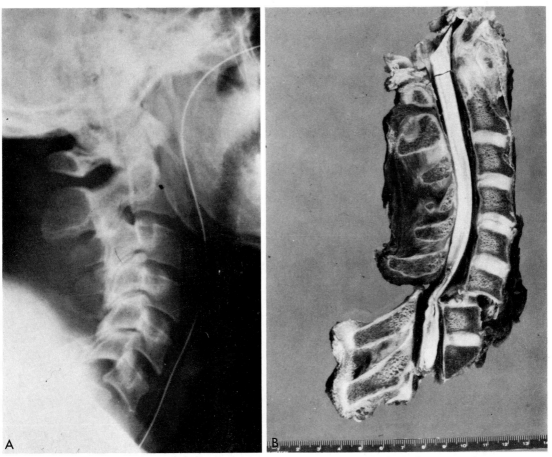

Figure 5–72. Bilateral facet locking of C-6 on C-7. A, Cross-table lateral view made just prior to death. Note the tiny fracture of the C-7 body. B, Postmortem sagittal section shows the anterior displacement of C-6 on C-7, disruption of the C-6 intervertebral disk, adjacent ligaments, and extensive hematomyelia.

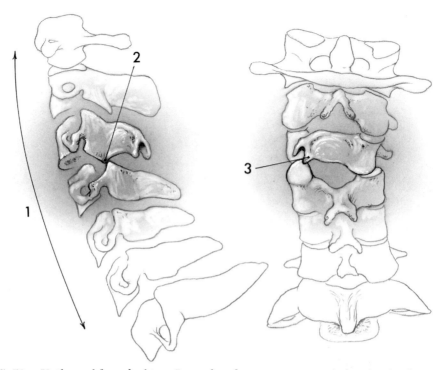

Figure 5–73. *Unilateral* facet locking. Lateral and posterior views (schematic). There is typically soft tissue edema and hemorrhage anteriorly (1). The inferior articular process of C-3 on the left is locked in front of the superior articular process of C-4 (2). At 3, the spinous process of C-3 is deviated *toward* the side of locking.

Figure 5–74. Unilateral articular facet locking. *A,* Lateral view showing anterolisthesis of C-4 on C-5, narrowing of the C-4 intervertebral disk space, and rotation of the C-4 vertebra and those craniad to it. *B,* Frontal film made with a poorly centered grid. Vertical lines have been placed on the spinous processes from C-4 through C-7; note the displacement of the C-4 spinous process toward the patient's right indicating that the locking at C-4/C-5 is on the right side. *C* and *D,* 30 degree trauma obliques clearly show the unilateral articular facet locking of C-4 on C-5 on the right (C). Observe the anterolisthesis of C-4 on C-5 causing loss of *imbrication* between the C-4 and C-5 laminae on each side, and the marked distortion of the C-4/C-5 intervertebral foramina.

See illustration on opposite page.

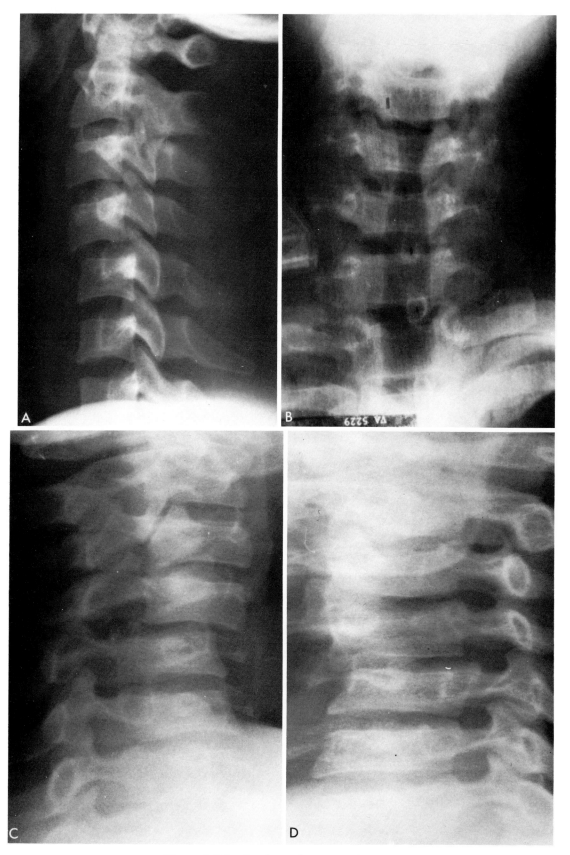

Figure 5–74. *See legend on opposite page.*

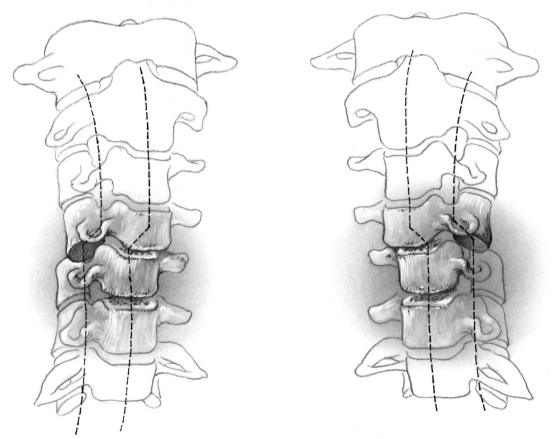

Figure 5–75. Bilateral locked facets (schematic). In patients with bilateral facet locking, the borders of the vertebral canal (dotted lines) will be disrupted at the level of locking (C-4 on C-5). Always trace out the boundaries of the vertebral canal on all views of the cervical spine.

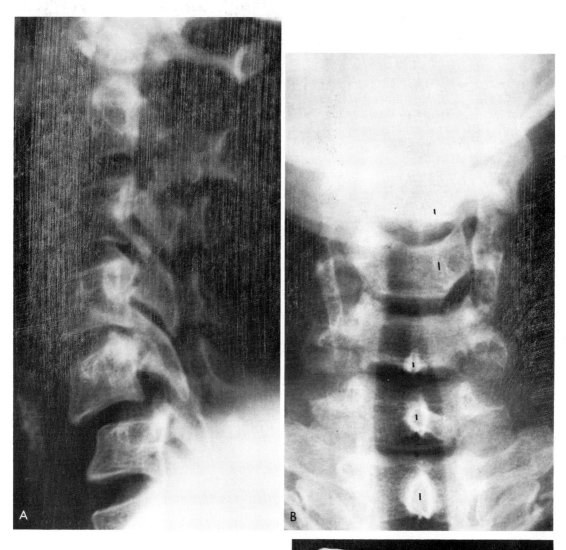

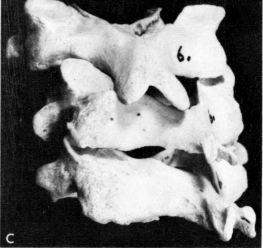

Figure 5–76. Unilateral articular facet locking. *A*, Lateral view showing anterior displacement of C-5 on C-6, narrowing of the C-5 intervertebral disk space, and rotation of the C-5 vertebra and those above. *B*, Frontal view (vertical lines have been placed on the spinous processes), showing the deviated spinous process of C-5 toward the patient's left side or the side of facet locking. *C*, Gross specimen of lower cervical vertebra with unilateral facet locking. Note the marked deviation of the spinous process toward the side of locking on the left.

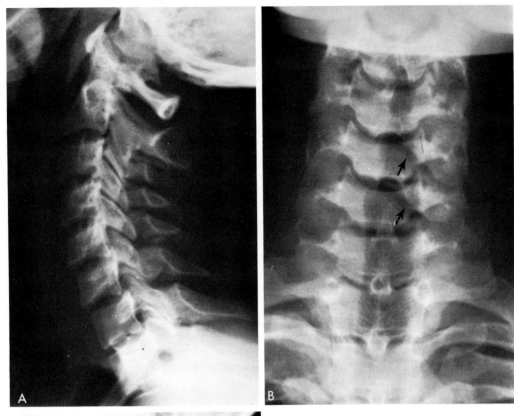

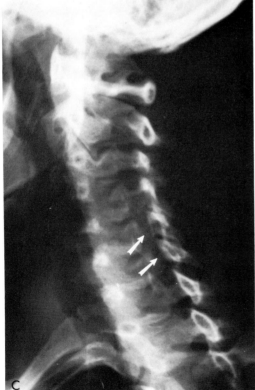

Figure 5–77. Type V-A hyperextension fracture-dislocation. *A,* Lateral view showing anterolisthesis of C-5 on C-6, and C-6 on C-7, narrowing of the C-5 and C-6 intervertebral disk spaces, and rotation of the C-6 vertebra and those above. Lamina fractures are also seen at C-5 and C-6. *B,* Frontal view clearly shows the C-5 and C-6 lamina fractures on the left (arrows). The tilted articular pillars are probably not appreciated because of the 20 degree cranial angulation used to make this radiograph. *C,* Oblique view. Note the tilted articular pillars of C-5 and C-6, and the pedicle fractures (arrows).

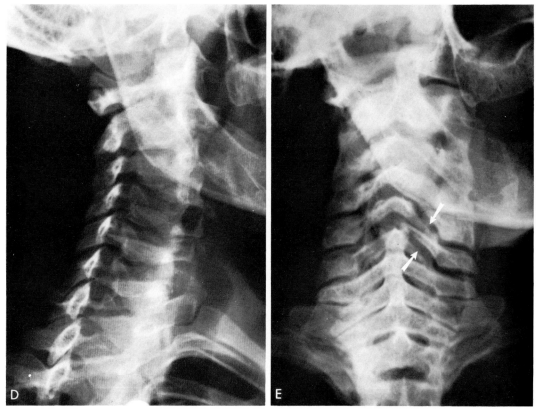

Figure 5–77 Continued. *D*, Opposite oblique for comparison. *E*, Vertebral arch view to see the oblique lamina fractures at C-5 and C-6 on the left (arrows).

In cases of bilateral facet locking, the distance between the spinous process of the dislocated vertebra and that below will usually be increased.

Oblique radiographs show articular facet locking, either unilateral or bilateral (Figs. 5–69, 5–74). What you are seeing on the radiographs is exactly what we have illustrated in Figures 5–75 and 5–76 C. The inferior articular process of the dislocated vertebra rests in front of the superior articular process of the vertebra below. Note the appearance of the laminae on the side of locking; the normal imbrication between the laminae of the dislocated vertebra and the one below is lost. That is exactly what may be seen on the oblique radiographs. Imbrication is lost unilaterally on the side of the unilateral locking and bilaterally in cases of bilateral articular facet locking (Figs. 5–69, 5–74). Consider this point in a different manner. On the oblique radiographs, always try to trace out the borders of the vertebral canal at each level. Note in Fig-

ures 5–69, 5–74, and 5–75 that there is an abrupt shift at the level of the dislocation.

It cannot be emphasized too strongly to the reader that the diagnosis of articular facet locking should not be attempted from lateral radiographs alone. Certain hyperextension fracture-dislocations (Type IV and V — Gehweiler) look identical to unilateral facet locking on the lateral radiograph (Figs. 5–49, 5–52, 5–53. and 5–77). Distinction between these different conditions is not merely an academic exercise! The ability to characterize the different patterns of trauma, their varied clinical courses, and the expected pathologic change permits a rational approach to therapy.

Both the hyperextension fracture-dislocations cited above and unilateral facet locking, on *lateral* radiographs, show anterior displacement of the involved vertebra on that below, narrowing of the intervertebral disk space beneath, and rotation of the involved vertebra with the cervical vertebral column above. In those cases of hyperextension fracture-dislocation with bilateral facet locking, the spinous process of the involved vertebra is at or is very near the midline (Figs. 5–69, 5–77) in the *frontal* views. With unilateral facet locking, the spinous process is significantly displaced from the midline toward the side of facet locking (Figs. 5–73, 5–74, 5–76). Oblique views will clearly differentiate type IV-V hyperextension fracture-dislocations from unilateral facet locking. Articular facet locking is not present in patients with hyperextension fracture-dislocations. In both conditions there may be vertebral body or vertebral arch fractures.[17, 18]

"Teardrop" Hyperflexion Fracture-Dislocation

Five per cent of all patients in the Duke series had "teardrop" hyperflexion fracture-dislocations (Type IV — hyperflexion fracture-dislocation — Gehweiler).[18] This condition is frequently caused by falls, diving, and traffic accidents. The clinical picture is quite variable: some patients are neurologically normal, while others may be quadriplegic. The degree of neurologic deficit seems to depend upon the extent of retrolisthesis of the involved vertebra.

Figure 5–78 shows the probable mechan-

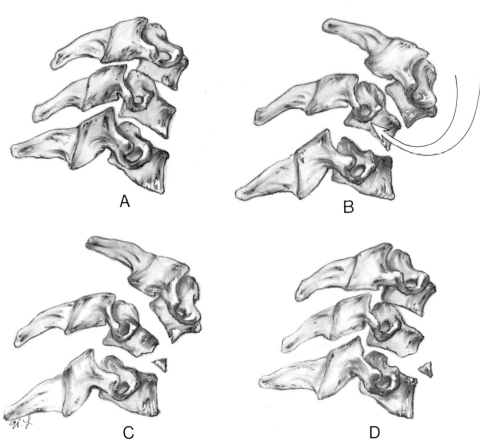

Figure 5–78. Type IV "teardrop" hyperflexion fracture-dislocation — mechanism of injury. *A,* Normal, prior to injury. *B,* The hyperflexion compressive force moves the cervical spine in an arc. At the level of injury, the vertebra is displaced posteriorly, causing disruption of the apophyseal joint capsules and the posterior portion of the intervertebral disk below. Either the anterior or the anteroinferior margin of the involved vertebra is fractured (*C*). The fragment resembles a "teardrop." *D,* After the force passes, the fractured vertebra remains displaced posteriorly on the vertebra below.

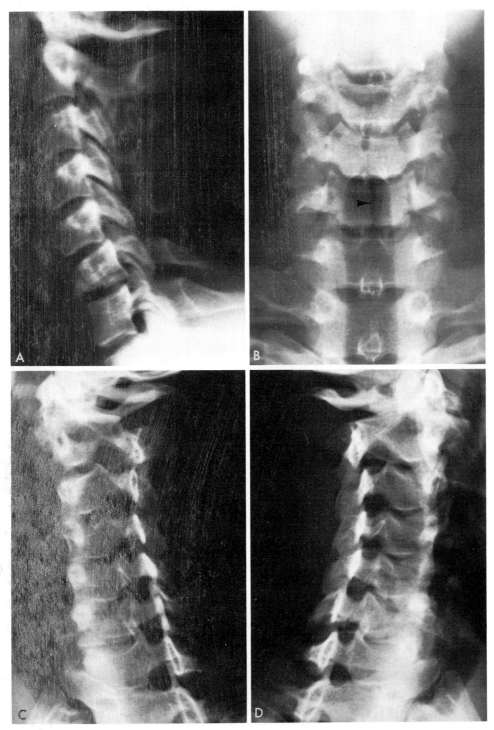

Figure 5–79. Type IV "teardrop" hyperflexion fracture-dislocation. *A,* Lateral view. The anterior margin of C-6 is fractured and displaced anteriorly, and the remainder of that vertebra is flexed on the adjacent vertebrae and displaced posteriorly. The C-5 and C-6 intervertebral disk spaces are diminished in height. *B,* Frontal view. There is a sagittal fracture (arrow) of the C-6 body. *C, D,* Oblique views showing posterior displacement of the C-6 vertebra, and loss of laminal imbrication at C-5/6 and C-6/7.

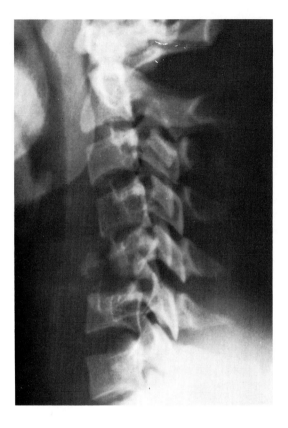

Figure 5–80. Type IV "teardrop" hyperflexion fracture-dislocation. The lateral view shows the anterior fracture of the C-5 vertebral body, which is displaced forward. Note the flexion of the remainder of the C-5 vertebra on the vertebra above and below, and the widening of the C-5/6 apophyseal joints.

ism of injury: hyperflexion compression. The force acting on the spine moves it in an arc (Fig. 5–78 B). At the level of the injury, the vertebra is displaced posteriorly, causing disruption of the apophyseal joint capsules and the posterior portion of the intervertebral disk below. Either the anterior or the anteroinferior margin of the involved vertebral body is fractured (Fig. 5–78 C). The smaller fragment, which resembles a "teardrop," is displaced anteriorly. After the force passes, the fractured vertebra remains displaced posteriorly on the vertebra below (Fig. 5–78D).[2, 6] In a few cases, the vertebral arch is fractured by pull of the posterior ligaments.[3, 18]

All of our cases showed strikingly similar, quite characterisitc changes. In the *lateral* radiograph, the anterior margin fragment is displaced anteriorly (Figs. 5–78 to 5–82). The remaining portion of the vertebra is flexed on the adjacent vertebrae and displaced posteriorly. The intervertebral disk space below is narrowed, indicating an injury. Note that the sagittal diameter of the vertebral canal of the level in question is unaffected, since the vertebral arch is not often fractured. We have mentioned earlier

that the apophyseal joint capsules are disrupted. This change may be manifested on the initial radiographs or when the patient is in traction (Fig. 5–80). Indirect signs of cervical trauma other than apophyseal joint widening may also be observed, for example, retropharyngeal and retrotracheal soft tissue widening and displacement of the prevertebral fat stripe.

Frontal views always show a sagittal fracture of the vertebral body, which may be midline or off-center (Figs. 5–79, 5–81). Frequently this vertebral body is wedged laterally on one side, suggesting that a rotational force was also acting along with the compressive hyperflexion force.

Retrolisthesis of the involved vertebra is clearly visible on *oblique* radiographs. Retrolisthesis usually causes two distinctive findings: loss of imbrication between the laminae of the involved vertebra and those of the vertebra beneath, and distortion of the intervertebral foramina above and below (Fig. 5–79). Apophyseal joint widening may also be observed.

The reader should be aware that the "teardrop" hyperflexion fracture-dislocation results in *posterior* displacement of the

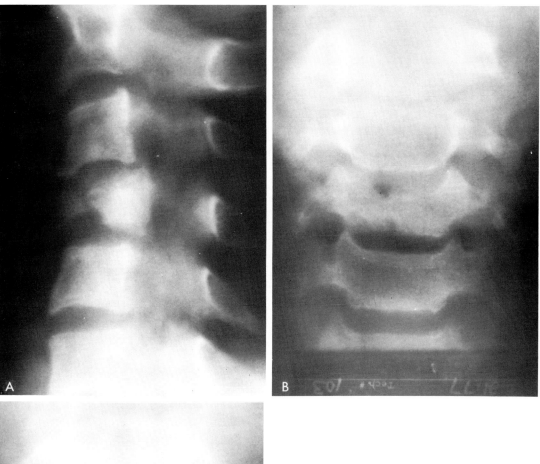

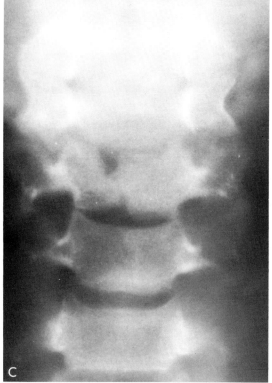

Figure 5–81. Type IV "teardrop" hyper-flexion fracture-dislocation. *A*, Lateral tomo-gram. There is displacement of the posterior portion of the C-4 body and the vertebral arch. The anterior portion of the body is frac-tured and slightly displaced forward. *B, C*, Frontal tomograms. The C-4 body is fractured in a sagittal plane and wedged laterally on the right.

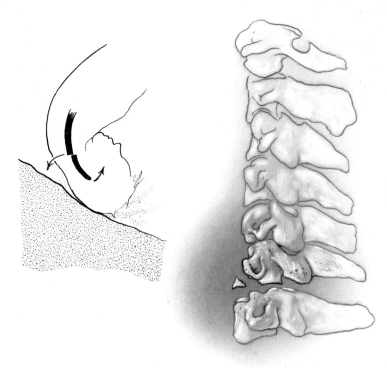

Figure 5–82. Type IV "teardrop" hyperflexion fracture-dislocation—mechanism of injury.

major portion of the involved vertebra. Many times such an appearance is called a *hyperextension* injury; such a misunderstanding may result in incorrect treatment. The reader might find it productive at this time to review the mechanism of injury for the type IV and V hyperextension fracture-dislocation (p. 218–228) in order to firmly establish the distinction between these lesions and the "teardrop" hyperflexion fracture-dislocation.

REFERENCES

1. Miller, M.D., Gehweiler, J. A., Martinez, S., Charlton, O. P., and Daffner, R. H.: Significant new observations on cervical spine trauma. Am. J. Roentgenol., *130*:659, 1978.
2. Braakman, R., and Penning, L.: Injuries of the Cervical Spine. London, Excerpta Medica, 1971.
3. Whitley, J. E., and Forsyth, H. F.: The classification of cervical spine injuries. Am. J. Roentgenol. 83:633, 1960.
4. Binet, E. F., Moro, J. J., Marangola, J. P., and Hodge, C. J.: Cervical spine tomography in trauma. Spine, 2:163, 1977.
5. Russin, L. D., and Guinto, F. C.: Multidirectional tomography in cervical spine injury. J. Neurosurg., 45:9, 1976.
6. Schneider, R. C., and Kahn, E. A.: Chronic neurologic sequelae of acute trauma to the spine and spinal cord. The significance of acute flexion or teardrop cervical fracture-dislocation of the cervical spine. J. Bone. & Jt. Surg., *38-A*:985, 1956.
7. Schaaf, R. E., Gehweiler, J. A., Powers, B., and Miller, M.D.: Lateral hyperflexion injuries of the cervical spine. Skeletal Radiol., *3*:73, 1978.
8. Abel, M. S.: Occult traumatic lesions of the cervical spine. Crit. Rev. Clin. Radiol. and Nucl. Med., 7:469, 1975.
9. Köhler, A., and Zimmer, E. A.: Borderlands of the Normal and Early Pathologic in Skeletal Roentgenology, 3rd Ed.. Translated and edited by S. P. Wilk. New York, Grune & Stratton, 1968.
10. Jackson, R.: The Cervical Syndrome. Springfield, Charles C Thomas, 1966.
11. Schmorl, G., and Junghanns, H.: The Human Spine in Health and Disease, 2nd American Ed.. Translated and edited by E. F. Besemann. New York, Grune & Stratton, 1971.
12. Selecki, B. R., and Williams, H. B. L.: Injuries to the Cervical Spine and Cord in Man. Australian Medical Association, 1970.
13. Allen, B.: Personal communication.
14. Vines, F. S.: The significance of "occult" fractures of the cervical spine. Am. J. Roentgenol., *107*:493, 1969.
15. Martinez, S., Morgan, C. L., Gehweiler, J. A., Powers, B., and Miller, M. D.: Unusual fractures and dislocations of the axis vertebra. Skeletal Radiol., 3:206, 1979.
16. Howarth, M. B., and Petrie, J. G.: Injuries of the Spine. Baltimore, Williams & Wilkins, 1964.
17. Gehweiler, J. A., Clark, W. M., Powers, B., Schaaf, R. E., and Miller, M. D.: Hyperextension fracture-dislocations of the cervical spine. Medical Imaging, 3:12, 1978 (Abstract).
18. Gehweiler, J. A., Clark, W. M., Schaaf, R. E.,

Powers, B., and Miller, M. D.: Cervical spine trauma: the common combined conditions. Radiology, *130*:77, 1979.

19. Taylor, A. R., and Blackwood, W.: Paraplegia in hyperextension cervical injuries with normal radiographic appearances. J. Bone & Jt. Surg., *30-B*:245, 1948.

20. Marar, B. C.: Hyperextension injuries of the cervical spine. The pathogenesis of damage to the spinal cord. J. Bone & Jt. Surg., 56-A, 1655, 1974.

21. Taylor, A. R.: The mechanism of injury to the spinal cord in the neck without damage to the vertebral column. J. Bone & Jt. Surg., *33-B*:543, 1961.

22. Medical news: Will the real whiplash patient tip back his head? J. Amer. Med. Assoc., *238*:2341, 1977.

23. Forsyth, H. F.: Extension injuries of the cervical spine. J. Bone & Jt. Surg., *46-A*:1792, 1964.

24. Pitman, M. I., Pitman, C. A., and Greenberg, I. M.: Complete dislocation of the cervical spine without neurologic deficit. A case report. J. Bone & Jt. Surg., *59-A*:134, 1977.

25. Braakman, R., and Penning, L.: The hyperflexion sprain of the cervical spine. Radiol. Clin. Biol., 37:309, 1968.

26. Clark, W. M., Gehweiler, J. A., and Laib, R.: Significant signs of cervical spine trauma. Skeletal Radiol., 3:201, 1979.

27. Roaf, R.: A study of the mechanics of spinal injuries. J. Bone & Jt. Surg., *42-B*:810, 1960.

28. Juhl, J. H., Miller, S. M., and Roberts, G. W.: Roentgenographic variations in the normal cervical spine. Radiology, 78:591, 1962.

29. Braakman, R., and Vinken, P. J.: Old luxations of the lower cervical spine. J. Bone & Jt. Surg., *50-B*:52, 1968.

30 Braakman, R., and Vinken, P. J.: Unilateral facet interlocking in the lower cervical spine. J. Bone & Jt. Surg., *49-B*:249, 1967.

31. Schneider, R. C.: The syndrome of acute anterior spinal cord injury. J. Neurosurg., *12*:95, 1955.

32. Verbiest, H.: La chirurgie antérieure et latéral du rachis cervical. Neuro-chirurgie 16, Suppl. 2, 1970.

33. Beatson, T. R.: Fractures and dislocations of the cervical spine. J. Bone & Jt. Surg., *45-B*:31, 1963.

INJURIES OF THE THORACOLUMBAR SPINE

Chapter 6

ANTERIOR COMPRESSION FRACTURES AND RELATED DISORDERS

INTRODUCTION

The human spine may be regarded as a flexible bony pillar that performs three functions simultaneously: (1) The spine supports the combined weight of the head, arms, and torso in the upright position. (2) It allows a wide range of motion for the head, neck, and trunk of the body in all directions. (3) It encases the spinal cord and nerve roots in a durable cylinder of bone and protects them from injury all the while. This is truly a remarkable feat of engineering! (Fig. 6–1).

However, the spine is not without its limitations. The stress of heavy weight-bearing or of sudden compressive force may cause it to crumble. Violent wrenching or distortive forces applied to it may interrupt its continuity through fractures and/or dislocations of the vertebrae. But the gravest damage of all occurs with injury to the spinal cord that results from disruption of the vertebral arches, which when superimposed form a bony cylinder that surrounds and protects the cord.

Although the cervical, thoracic, and lumbar divisions of the vertebral column perform analogous functions, they differ in certain anatomic respects, affecting their reaction to injury. The bodies of the lumbar vertebrae are broader than those of the thoracic vertebrae both in their coronal and their sagittal dimensions; the thoracic bodies, in turn, are broader than those of the cervical vertebrae (Figs. 6–2, 6–3). The lumbar vertebrae are therefore able to tolerate greater weight-bearing, or axial compressive stress, than the smaller bodies above, because the force is distributed over a greater surface area.[15] In addition, the intervertebral disks increase in size (both in diameter and in thickness) from the cervical to the lumbar spine. This allows them to absorb far greater stresses in the lower spine than in the upper in their capacity as shock absorbers. A much greater force, then, is required to injure the lower spine than the upper.[8]

The thoracic spine normally has a slight forward curve, being dorsally convex and ventrally concave. Such a spinal curve is defined as *kyphosis*. The cervical and lumbar portions of the spine curve in the opposite direction, being dorsally concave and ventrally convex; this is defined as *lordosis*. A lateral curve, which is always abnormal when viewed from in front or behind, is a *scoliosis*. These curvatures are accentuated by axial compressive forces, which in turn influence the nature of the resultant vertebral injury (Fig. 6–1).

The thoracic spine is relatively rigid, being restricted and held in its forward curvature by the rib cage and thoracic muscles. The cervical and lumbar spine, however, enjoy a much wider range of motion, the cervical spine most of all. The lumbar spine, although not protected by the rib cage, is solidly buttressed by the thick paraspinal musculature surrounding it, and anteriorly by the abdomen and its muscles. The cervical spine lacks these mechanical supports and, as we have seen, pays a price for its

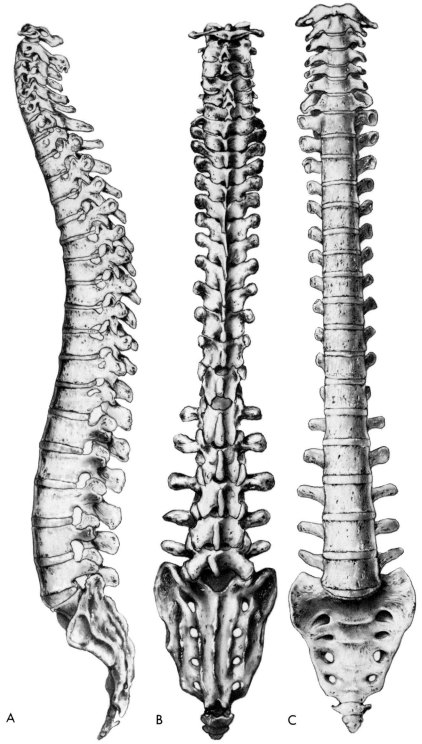

Figure 6–1. The normal vertebral column. *A*, Lateral aspect: The thoracic curve, or *kyphosis*, is concave anteriorly (to the left), while the cervical and lumbar curves above and below (*lordoses*) are convex anteriorly. *B*, Posterior aspect: The spinous processes are aligned in the midline; the laminae and articular processes overlap, or imbricate, like tiles on a roof. *C*, Anterior aspect: The intervertebral disks are placed between the vertebral bodies, where they function as buffers or shock absorbers for spinal movements and mechanical stresses.

added mobility in its increased vulnerability to injury.

ANTERIOR COMPRESSION FRACTURES OF THE VERTEBRAL BODIES

Incidence

Fractures of the vertebral bodies increase in incidence progressively with age. There are two reasons for this: (1) vertebral bone mineral content and elasticity decrease with age, making the bodies increasingly brittle and susceptible to fracture; and (2) the nucleus pulposus of the intervertebral disk becomes increasingly dehydrated with age. This water loss reduces the elasticity of the nucleus and of the disk as a whole, which in turn reduces its efficacy as a shock-absorbing mechanism and increases the degree of trauma to the vertebrae themselves.

Spinal contusions without fractures or dislocations are quite common. Lob found them to constitute 64 per cent of all acute spinal injuries in his series of 443 cases.[8] Clinically, such patients complain of pain, and exhibit swelling, tenderness, restricted

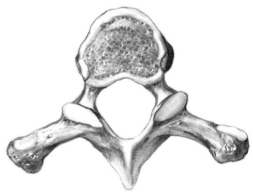

Figure 6–2. A thoracic vertebra, superior aspect. The bodies and arches of the thoracic vertebrae, although broader and stouter than those of the cervical vertebrae, are less so than the lumbar vertebrae. The ribs exert a stabilizing effect upon the thoracic spine (note rib facets on either side of the vertebral body), which is lacking in the cervical and lumbar regions.

motion, and ecchymosis of the injured portion of the back, but no abnormalities are found on the radiographs.[8]

Of all the vertebral injuries that result in detectable radiographic abnormalities, isolated anterior compression fractures of the vertebral bodies constitute a majority in all ages. They result from flexion violence, in

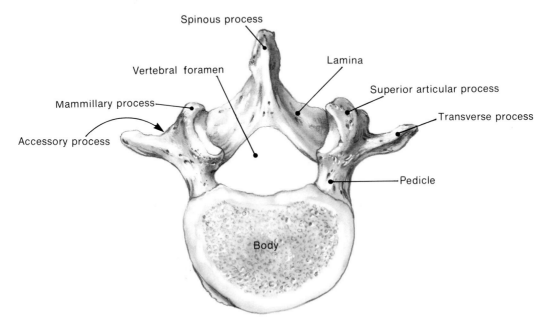

Figure 6–3. A lumbar vertebra, superior aspect. Note the broader body and stouter vertebral arch of the lumbar vertebra when compared with the thoracic. This allows the lumbar vertebrae to tolerate greater weightbearing, or axial compressive stresses, than any other portion of the vertebral column, because the force is distributed over a greater surface area.

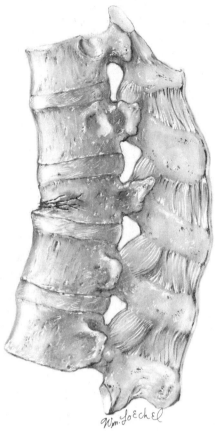

Figure 6-4. Anterior compression fracture. The anterior portion of a vertebral body has been fractured by compression injury, resulting in a wedge-shaped deformity of the vertebral body. Note that the vertebral arches and posterior intervertebral ligaments remain intact.

which the anterior portion of one or more vertebral bodies is fractured and deformed by compression injury. The vertebral arches and posterior intervertebral ligaments re-

main intact (Fig. 6–4). Occurring with greater frequency in elderly and osteoporotic patients, anterior compression fractures represent the preponderance of all vertebral injuries sustained in the sixth decade and beyond.

All forms of thoracolumbar spine injury, including anterior compression fractures, occur most frequently at the thoracolumbar junction, where the twelfth thoracic and first lumbar vertebral bodies sustain compression injuries more often than do any others. A second increase in incidence occurs at the cervicothoracic junction, although not as great as that noted at the thoracolumbar junction.[5] Occasionally, however, certain types of injury, such as those resulting from convulsions or electroshock therapy, show predilection for other levels of the thoracolumbar spine. In these cases, violent contractions of the thoracic and abdominal body muscles bring maximal compressive stresses to bear on the midthoracic vertebrae, between T-4 and T-8. These vertebrae, then, are most frequently fractured under such circumstances (Fig. 6–5).[15] Compression fractures that result from weakening of the bones and loss of elasticity of the intervertebral disks in the elderly are frequently noted in the upper thoracic spine (Fig. 6–6),[8] and an increased incidence of injuries in this region has been noted with vehicular trauma.[1]

Mechanism of Injury

By far, the greatest number of injuries involving the spine below the neck are sustained in a position of spinal flexion. This

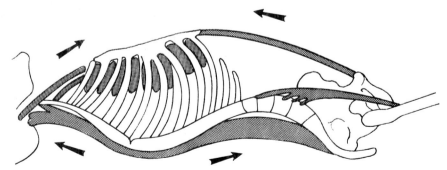

Figure 6-5. Mechanism of thoracic compression fractures in convulsive states. Marked, synchronous contraction of the somatic musculature occurs in convulsions, and with electroconvulsive therapy. The anterior muscles of the torso and the intercostal muscles of the ribs pull the midthoracic spine into sharp flexion. This is accentuated by the pull of the cervical and lumbar paraspinal muscles above and below, fixing those portions of the spine in lordosis. The outcome is often one of vertebral compression fractures occurring characteristically in the midthoracic region. (After Schmorl.)

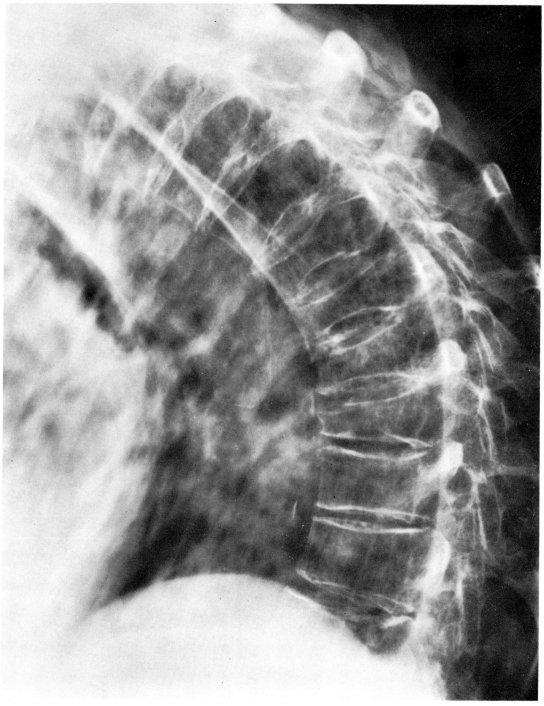

Figure 6–6. Upper thoracic compression fractures in osteoporosis. Multiple vertebral compression fractures have occurred in the upper thoracic spine of this elderly patient, producing a kyphotic or "round-back" deformity clinically. Severe osteoporosis is present, reflected in the overall loss of bone density, and in the heightened contrast between cortical and medullary bone substance.

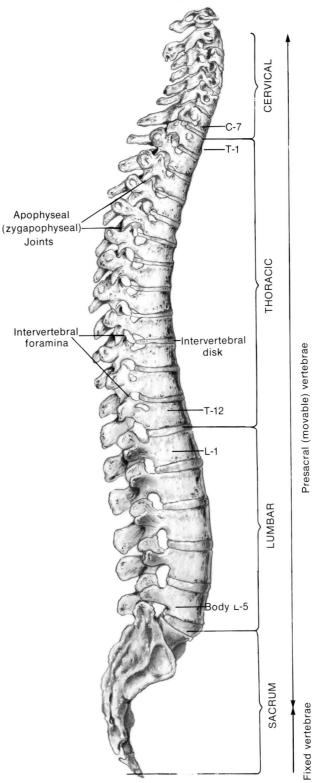

Figure 6–7. Articulated vertebral column. The vertebral column consists of an anterior column of vertebral bodies separated by intervertebral disks and a posterior column of a series of bony rings, the vertebral arches, aligned along the spinal cord and articulating with one another by the apophyseal joints. Whereas the anterior column consists of more yielding, cancellous bone, the posterior column is composed of relatively dense, incompressible cortical bone. The anterior column is thus more likely to collapse when compressed, converting an axial compressive force to a flexion injury.

position affords the body maximum protection against the threat of external injury, by covering up vulnerable areas such as the face, abdomen, and genitals. Spinal flexion is encouraged by the protective reflex of Magnus, in which a person will involuntarily bend forward in response to any unexpected touch on the head.[5]

Structural factors, too, increase the frequency with which flexion injuries of the spine are encountered. The spine may be considered to consist of two adjoining structural columns. The anterior column is made up of the vertebral bodies and intervertebral disks, alternating one above the other. The posterior column consists of a series of bony rings, the vertebral arches, aligned along the spinal cord and separated from each other by the apophyseal joints (Fig. 6–7). Examination of a skeleton, or of the individual vertebrae, will show that the vertebral bodies consist of compressible spongy, cancellous bone within thin cortical casings; the intervertebral disks are compressible, too. The vertebral arches and articular processes, on the other hand, are composed of dense, incompressible cortical bone. A compressive force applied to the vertebral column from top to bottom will force the softer anterior column to yield, while the more durable posterior column resists. An axial compressive force may thus be converted to a flexion injury, with wedging of the vertebral bodies and anterior displacement of the intervertebral disks between them. The fulcrum about which flexion occurs may be considered to pass through the nucleus pulposus of the disk in the coronal plane (Fig. 6–8). In the thoracic spine, this tendency toward flexion is enhanced by the normal kyphosis already present because of the thoracic cage.

The points of transition between the relatively immobile thoracic spine and the more flexible cervical and lumbar spine show the greatest predisposition to injury. More vertebral injuries occur at the thoracolumbar junction than at any other level of the spine (Fig. 6–9). The two vertebrae most frequently injured are the twelfth thoracic and the first lumbar. The eleventh thoracic and second lumbar vertebrae are less frequently injured; in general, the frequency of vertebral injuries continues to decrease with distance moved away from the thoracolumbar junction. Jefferson has likened the

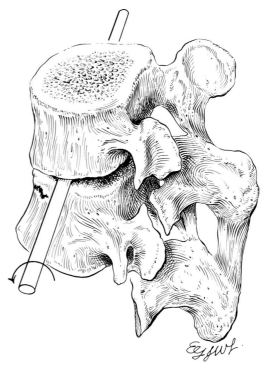

Figure 6–8. Axis of spinal flexion. The fulcrum about which flexion occurs passes through the nucleus pulposus of the intervertebral disk in the coronal plane. The vertebrae are compressed anterior to the fulcrum, but distracted posterior to it.

thoracolumbar spine in the flexed state to a parabola, with its apex at the thoracolumbar junction. Vertebral fracture is thus most likely to occur at the point of maximum bend.[5]

The incidence of vertebral injury shows another increase at the cervicothoracic junction, although not as great as that occurring at the other end of the thoracic spine.[5] Again, this represents a point of transition from the relative rigidity of the thoracic spine to the extreme mobility of the cervical spine.

Roaf[13] has made a valuable contribution to the understanding of the mechanics of spinal injuries by his work on cadaver spines. He observed a series of events occurring upon application of compressive forces to his specimens leading up to fracture by flexion deformity. In specimens with an intact nucleus pulposus within the intervertebral disk, he noted first a bulging of the vertebral end-plates about the nucleus pulposus into the vertebral body, accompanied by slight

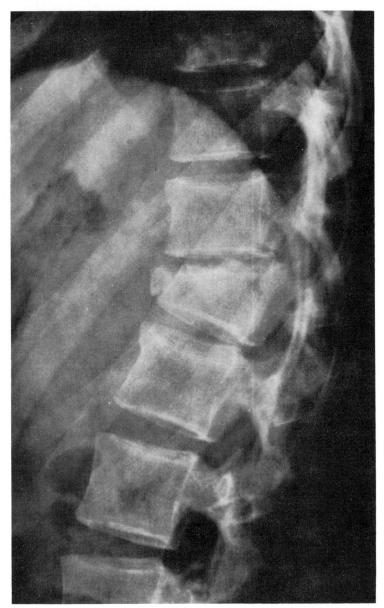

Figure 6–9. Thoracolumbar fracture-dislocation. The point of transition between the relatively immobile thoracic spine and the more flexible lumbar spine shows the greatest predisposition to injury. More vertebral injuries occur at the thoracolumbar junction than at any other level of the spine.

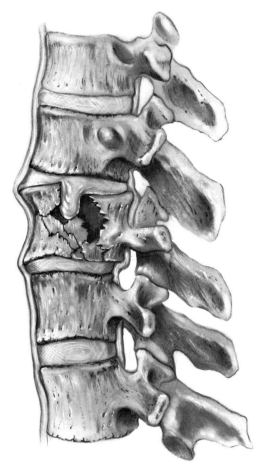

loss of disk turgor, and marked bulging of the anterior surface of the anulus fibrosus ensued "like the walls of a flat tire." Posterior bulging and displacement of the intervertebral disk in flexion injuries of the spine were noted to be negligible, and Roaf surmises that neurologic compression from herniation of the nucleus pulposus would be an unlikely complication of such an injury. Further escalation of pressure to the spine resulted in disintegration of the vertebral body and disruption of the vertebral arches and intervertebral ligaments posteriorly.

As motion in spinal flexion pivots about a fulcrum centered at the nucleus pulposus, the compression effect of a flexion injury is maximal at the anterior ends of the vertebral bodies. Initially, the intervertebral disk serves as a buffer in absorbing compressive force (see also p. 279); but when a critical level is exceeded, fracture of the vertebral body ensues. As the anterior aspect of the vertebral body is under the greatest stress, the first bony injury to result is a buckling of the anterior cortex (Fig. 6–11). With further compression, loss of anterior height of the

Figure 6–10. Vertebral body compression fracture. As pressure exerted by the nucleus pulposus on the vertebral end-plate mounts in compression injuries, the end-plate may crack, and substance from the nucleus may be extruded into the vertebral body. Escape of nuclear material from the confines of the intervertebral disk then results in a marked loss of disk turgor (disk above fracture.)

outward bulging of the anulus fibrosus anteriorly and laterally. Pressure from the end-plates indented by the nucleus pulposus expressed blood from the cancellous substance of the vertebral body, thus decompressing the vertebral body from the force of injury. Roaf considers this to be an important shock-absorbing mechanism in the injured spine. As the pressure exerted by the nucleus pulposus on the vertebral end-plate mounted further, the end-plate cracked, and substance from the nucleus pulposus was forced through the crack into the vertebral body (Fig. 6–10). Escape of nuclear material from the confines of the intervertebral disk then resulted in a marked

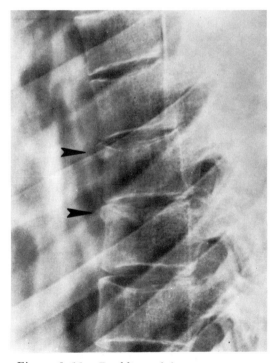

Figure 6–11. Buckling of the anterior cortex of a vertebral body. The first bony injury to be noted radiographically in anterior wedge compression fractures of the vertebral bodies is often a buckling, or torus, fracture of the anterior cortex (arrows).

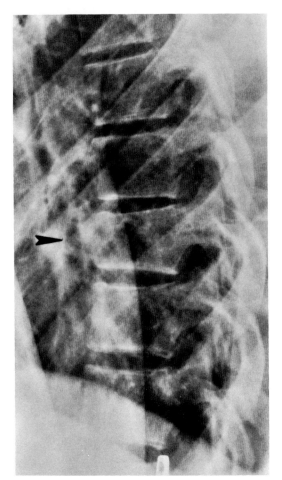

Figure 6–12. Slight loss of height in vertebral body compression fracture. Slight anterior loss of vertebral body height has occurred at T-9 vertebra as a result of a compression fracture (arrow). Such compression injuries may be subtle, and easily overlooked if the vertebral body heights anteriorly are not compared in cases of suspected vertebral injury.

Figure 6–13. Severe compression fracture of L-1 vertebral body. A severe compression fracture of L-1 vertebra has produced marked loss of height in the vertebral body, and disruption of the intervertebral disk spaces above and below.

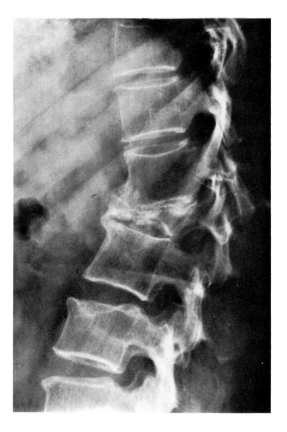

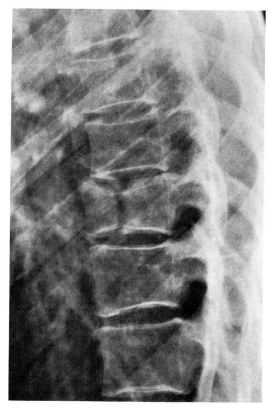

Figure 6–14. Coronal fracture of T-9 vertebral body. Nuclear material from the intervertebral disk above has indented the cranial endplate of T-9 vertebral body, and then has been forced through the thickness of the vertebral body to divide it into two halves, the result of an axial compression injury.

vertebral body follows (when compared with its posterior height). This gives a wedge-shaped appearance to the vertebral body on the lateral radiograph, which may range in severity from a barely perceptible injury (Fig. 6–12) to flattening and severe comminution of the body (Fig. 6–13).[13]

The intervertebral disks, too, are often injured in anterior compression fractures of the thoracolumbar spine. They are more resistant to compression than are the vertebral bodies, and isolated tears or ruptures of the intervertebral disk with intact vertebral bodies seem to be relatively infrequent occurrences (although the radiographic diagnosis is easily missed). In more severe injuries, however, the intervertebral disks are frequently torn. In these cases, the substance of the nucleus pulposus may herniate anteriorly, posteriorly, laterally, or through

a fractured end-plate into the vertebral body. Such herniations may be so extensive as to cleave the body vertically into two or more fragments (Fig. 6–14).

The mechanics of vertebral compression fractures differ somewhat between the upper thoracic spine and the lower thoracolumbar spine. The difference is due to variation in the thickness of the intervertebral disks, which are thin in the upper thoracic spine but become thicker below. The thinner upper thoracic disks are less effective in dispelling the force of spinal injury, being relatively stiff shock absorbers. As a result, the vertebral end-plates are less often fractured in compression injuries of the upper thoracic spine, and the compressed vertebral body assumes a true wedge-shape, with a slight infolding of the anterior cortex (Fig. 6–15 *A,C*).[8]

In the lower thoracolumbar spine, on the other hand, the thicker intervertebral disks play a greater role in dispelling the force of compression, which alters the nature of the vertebral body injury. The nucleus pulposus absorbs a greater share of the force, which it transmits in turn to the vertebral end-plates enclosing it, increasing the likelihood of end-plate fracture and the possibility of nuclear herniation into the vertebral body or elsewhere.

Where the intervertebral disks are thicker, and the vertebral bodies are consequently spaced further apart, increased gliding motion is facilitated at the apophyseal joints in flexion injuries of the spine, which is translated anteriorly to a shearing stress on the intervertebral disk. As the outermost fibers of the anulus fibrosus (Sharpey's fibers) are tightly bound to the rims of the vertebral end-plates, these bony rims are often avulsed as a result of the shearing force exerted on the disk, together with a greater or lesser fragment of the vertebral body itself (Fig. 6–15 *B, D*).[9]

Axial Compressive Injuries

Compression injuries of the spine are most often associated with flexion, as has been noted. At times, however, compressive injury may be applied in the long axis of a straightened spine to produce collapse of the vertebral bodies without flexion (Fig. 6–16). The effect on the vertebral body may be likened to jumping on top of a carton or

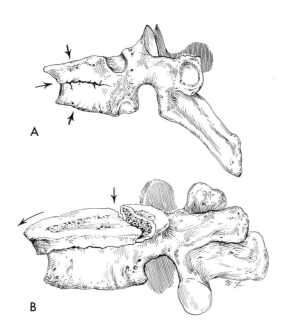

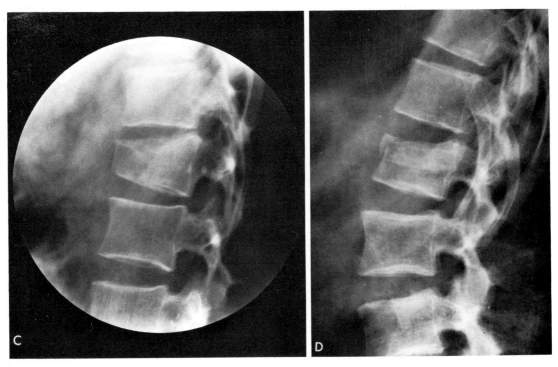

Figure 6–15. Upper and lower thoracolumbar compression fractures. *A*, Upper thoracic compression fracture. Note the wedged vertebral body shape with end-plates intact, occurring more commonly in the upper thoracic spine owing to thinner intervertebral disks. *B*, Lower thoracic and lumbar compression fracture. Shearing forces transmitted through the thicker intervertebral disks have fractured the cranial end-plate (vertical arrow) and displaced it anteriorly (curved arrow). This type of flexion fracture predilects the lower thoracic and lumbar spine, where the intervertebral disks are thicker. *C*, Lateral view of fracture Type A as it appears on the radiograph. (This fracture involves L-1; cf. also Fig. 6–6). *D*, Radiograph of fracture Type B.

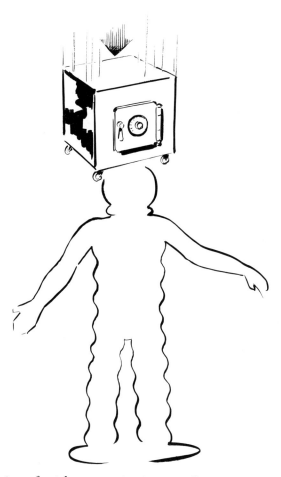

Figure 6–16. Mechanism of axial compressive injuries. Compressive injury may be applied to the long axis of a straightened vertebral column to produce collapse of the vertebral bodies without flexion. The vertebral bodies are flattened as their sides balloon outward and break.

overturned basket; the container is flattened as the sides balloon outwards and break (Fig. 6–17). Extensive herniation of the nucleus pulposus into the fractured vertebral body is common in this type of injury, and the body may be vertically cleft into two or more fragments by extruded nuclear material (Fig. 6–14). These vertebral collapse, or "burst," fractures are stable in that they are not associated with ligamentous disruption in hyperflexion or hyperextension; but posterior displacement of vertebral body fragments into the vertebral canal may injure the spinal cord nonetheless.

Stable and Unstable Thoracolumbar Spine Injuries

It should always be borne in mind that the difference between a stable anterior compression (flexion) injury and an unstable hyperflexion injury with disruption of the posterior ligament complex is but one of degree. Just as compression is produced anterior to the fulcrum about which the flexion injury pivots, so distraction is produced posteriorly between the vertebral arches at the same time. When enough force is exerted to distract the spinous processes and avulse the posterior intervertebral ligaments in addition to producing an anterior compression injury, then flexion becomes hyperflexion, and a clinically stable spinal injury is rendered *unstable*. This means that damage to the spinal cord and nerve roots may occur either at the time of the initial injury or as a result of injudicious handling of the patient thereafter. The distinction between stable flexion and unstable hyperflexion injuries is therefore of the utmost clinical significance.

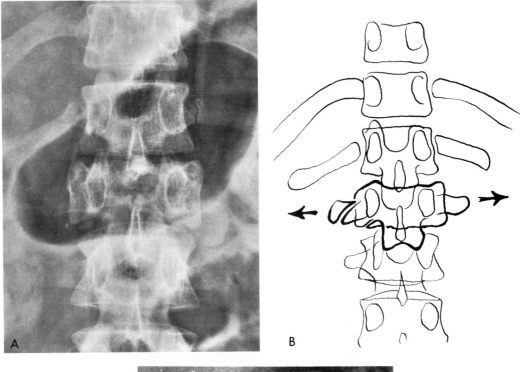

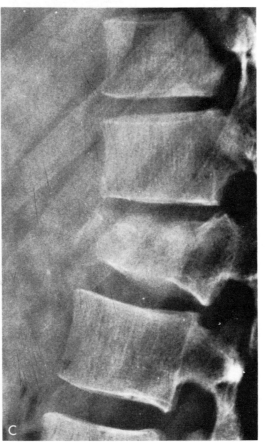

See legend on the opposite page.

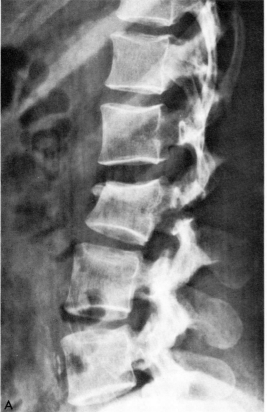
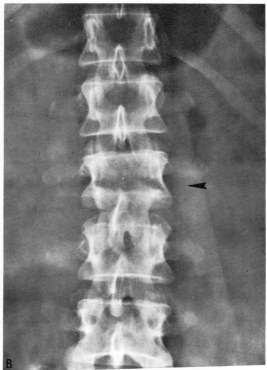

Figure 6–18. Unstable fracture-dislocation of L-2 vertebra. *A*, Lateral view: An anterior compression fracture of L-2 vertebral body is readily seen. Of more clinical significance, however, is the posterior widening between the L-1 and L-2 spinous processes, indicating an unstable spinal injury. The pedicles of L-2 have both been split in this seat-belt fracture-dislocation of the Smith type (see Chapter 7.) *B*, Frontal view: Note the widening of the L-1/2 interspinous interval and the horizontal fractures of the L-2 pedicles and transverse processes (arrow), producing an "empty vertebra" appearance. Such findings on a supine KUB film in an injured patient denote a severe spinal fracture-dislocation that should not be moved. (See Chapter 7.)

All apparent anterior compression injuries of the spine should be closely inspected both clinically and radiologically for any evidence of fracture, separation, or malalignment of the vertebral arches, indicating an unstable spinal injury (Fig. 6–18)[4, 11] *(see Chapter 7).*

Roentgen Diagnosis of Anterior Compression Fractures

The radiologic findings in anterior compression fractures of the vertebral bodies reflect the mechanical changes described above. They include:

Figure 6–17. Axial compression or "burst" fracture of L-1 vertebra. *A*, *B*, Frontal view and tracing exhibit decreased height but increased width (arrows) of L-1 vertebral body resulting from an axial compression, or "burst," fracture. *C*, Lateral view: The posterior cortex of the vertebral body has been ballooned into the vertebral canal, where spinal cord injury may result.

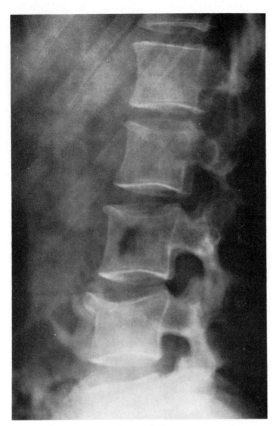

Figure 6–19. Buckling of the anterior cortex. Several lumbar vertebral bodies have been compressed, with the severity of injury progressing from above downward, to produce characteristic cortical deformities of the involved bodies. (See also Figs. 6–11, 6–15B, 6–20.)

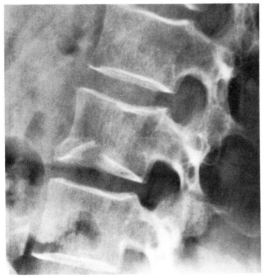

Figure 6–20. Buckling of the anterior cortex. Less commonly, buckling occurs inferiorly, as in this patient with caudal end-plate fracture resulting from upward nuclear displacement out of the intervertebral disk.

1. *Buckling of the anterior cortex* is the first and sometimes the only sign of vertebral body compression fracture. This may assume an inverted funnel-shape in the upper thoracic spine, but is more often a torus or step deformity of the upper anterior aspect of the vertebral body when it occurs about the thoracolumbar junction or in the lumbar spine (Figs. 6–11, 6–19, 6–20).
2. *Wedge deformity* of a fractured vertebral body is the consequence of anterior compression, with a loss of vertebral body height anteriorly in comparison with its posterior height. This results in a greater or lesser degree of kyphosis (Figs. 6–15 A,C; 6–21). Lateral wedging (Fig. 6–22) may produce scoliosis. It has been estimated that a 30 per cent or greater

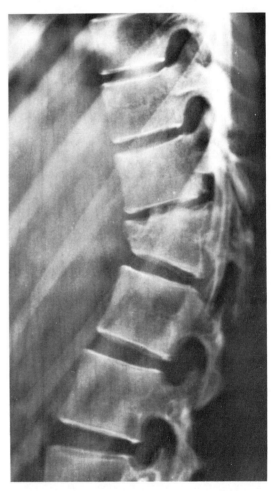

Figure 6–21. Wedge deformity of a fractured vertebral body. Wedge deformity is the consequence of anterior compression, with a loss of vertebral body height anteriorly. This results in a greater or lesser degree of kyphosis of the spine.

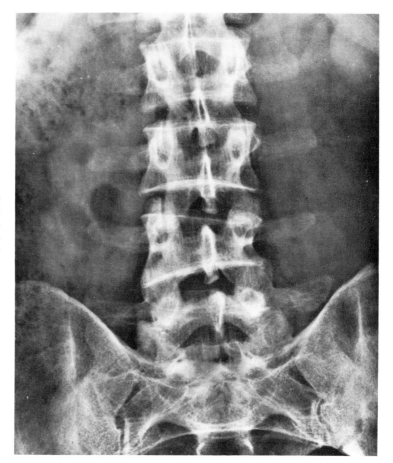

Figure 6–22. Lateral wedge deformity. Note this lateral compression fracture of L-4 vertebra. Lateral wedge deformity of a vertebral body may result in scoliosis.

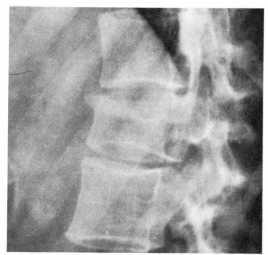

Figure 6–23. Zone of condensation. The zone of condensation appears as a band of increased bony density extending through the cancellous substance of a fractured vertebral body beneath the affected end-plate, and represents compaction of the trabecular elements of the spongiosa due to volume loss within the vertebral body. Note also buckling of the anterior cortex and slight wedge deformity of the injured vertebral body.

loss in anterior height is required before the deformity is readily apparent on conventional lateral radiographs of the spine. Other conditions may present a similar appearance (see "Differential Diagnosis," p. 286).

3. *The zone of condensation* of the fractured vertebral body appears as a band of increased bony density extending through the cancellous substance of the vertebral body beneath the affected endplate (Fig. 6–23). In a wedge deformity, the zone of condensation is more prominent anteriorly. Initially, the radiologic appearance of increased density is due to compaction of the trabecular elements of the spongiosa because of volume loss within the vertebral body. Later, endosteal callus formation appears in this zone with healing of the fracture, adding to the radiologic density and prolonging its duration in time.[8]

4. *Vertebral end-plate fractures*, resulting from pressure exerted through the nu-

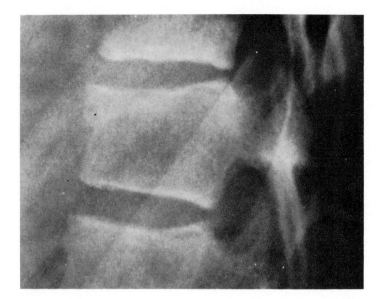

Figure 6–24. Vertebral end-plate fracture. Pressure exerted through the nucleus pulposus has cracked the cranial end-plate of T-12 vertebral body. Forward gliding of T-11 on T-12 vertebra then exerts shearing stress on the intervertebral disk between them, which in turn displaces the fractured end-plate of T-12 forward.

cleus pulposus, occur more frequently in the lower thoracic and lumbar spine than in the cervical or upper thoracic regions (Figs. 6–15 B,D; 6–24). The cranial end-plate is more often fractured than its caudal partner. This may be explained by two factors: (1) The surface of the cranial end-plate is comparatively flat, whereas that of the caudal end-plate is more deeply recessed, providing greater structural stability and resistance to compressive forces transmitted through the nucleus pulposus below the end-plate. As the cranial end-plate is flatter, it is structurally more vulnerable to injury by the nucleus. (2) Forward gliding of the upper vertebra over the lower one occurs in flexion injuries of the lower spine, subjecting the intervertebral disk to a shearing stress. Sharpey's fibers of the anulus fibrosus insert so strongly into the rims of the vertebral bodies that fracture of the ver-

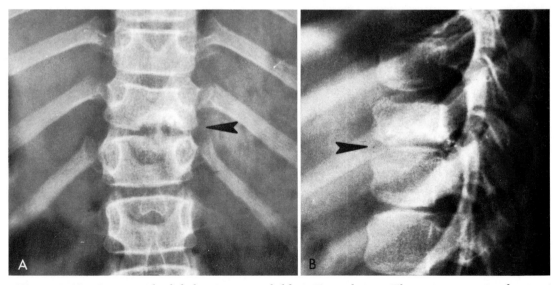

Figure 6–25. Intervertebral disk injury in a child. *A,* Frontal view: The patient sustained an accidental bullet wound through the spine at the T-11/12 level, passing through the intervertebral disk substance, and unfortunately, the vertebral canal as well (arrow). The adjacent vertebral end-plates were grooved in the process. *B,* Lateral view: Loss of height has resulted in the injured intervertebral disk (arrow).

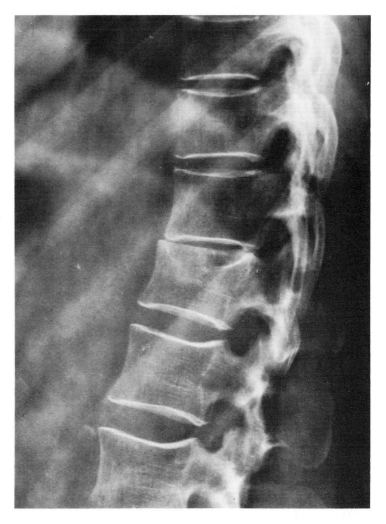

Figure 6–26. Intervertebral disk injury. A compression injury has driven intervertebral disk substance through the cranial end-plate of T-12 vertebra, resulting in end-plate infraction, collapse of the disk space, and malalignment of the vertebral bodies.

tebral body occurs before the fibers are avulsed. The bone beneath the cranial end-plate of the lower vertebra becomes the area of least resistance when the upper vertebra and disk are displaced anteriorly. The cranial end-plate then shifts anteriorly with the disk, resulting in an increased anteroposterior diameter of the cranial surface of the vertebral body compared with the caudal, when viewed on lateral projection.

5. *Intervertebral disk injury* is a common occurrence in spinal fractures, although it is infrequent as an isolated injury in acute trauma (Fig. 6–25). Such an injury results from tearing and disruption of the anulus fibrosus associated with herniation and loss of the nucleus pulposus. The intervertebral disk is a water-density structure on the radiograph, and cannot

be differentiated from other soft tissue structures around it. The roentgen findings in acute disk injury are therefore indirect, and must be presumed from the relative positions of the adjacent vertebral bodies.

The early signs of disk injury are an acute loss of height of the intervertebral disk space, and malalignment of the vertebral bodies at the level of injury (Fig. 6–26). Loss of disk space height is the result of herniation of the nucleus pulposus and collapse of the disk. Anterior herniation of the nucleus in flexion injuries occurs far more frequently than posterior herniation.[8] Malalignment of the vertebral bodies is often accompanied by displacement of the cranial end-plate of the body below, either forward or to one side.

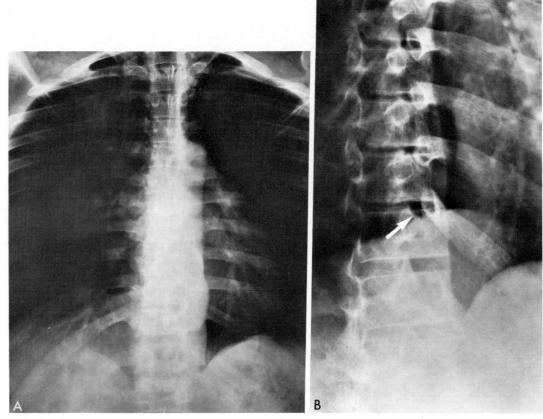

Figure 6-27. Paraspinal soft tissue injury. *A*, Frontal view: Note the lower left paraspinal soft-tissue mass representing hematoma in this man with a back injury. *B*, Right anterior oblique view: Traumatic avulsion of the left tenth rib from the vertebral column (arrow) is associated. (Courtesy of Dr. Raymond K. Luomanen, Memorial-Sloan Kettering Cancer Center, New York, N.Y.)

Narrowing of the disk space persists on subsequent films, for the injured intervertebral disk is unable to reconstitute itself by the mechanisms of healing available to it.[15] Later radiographic changes of disk injury include sclerosis and osteophyte formation of the adjacent vertebrae, as well as amorphous calcification within the substance of the disk (which may appear from one to eight months following injury).[8] These changes may become indistinguishable from those of degenerative joint disease with the passage of time.

6. *Paraspinal soft tissue injury.* When sufficient injury has been sustained by the spine to produce bone damage, considerable soft tissue injuries have also occurred, which are often of more clinical significance than the bone trauma.[8] Paraspinal soft tissue masses due to edema or hematoma formation are frequently observed with spinal compression fractures (Fig. 6-27).[14]

Associated Injuries

Although the majority of nuclear disk herniations occur anteriorly in flexion injuries, spinal cord or nerve root compression from posterior nuclear herniation may also occur, more frequently in the lower lumbar region with axial compression, or "burst," fractures. Disruption of the margins of the intervertebral foramina may produce nerve root compression, especially in more severe flexion injuries with vertebral displacement (Fig. 6-28). Such traumatic changes in the intervertebral foramina may be very difficult to discern on even the best quality radiographs.

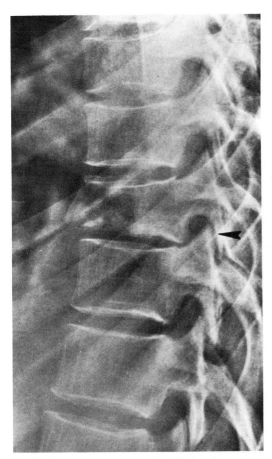

Figure 6–28. Compression of intervertebral foramen in vertebral body fracture. Posterior displacement of a vertebral body fragment at T-9 has compromised the intervertebral foramen (arrow). (Compare this foramen with the others above and below.)

Posterior displacement of a vertebral body fragment into the vertebral canal may compress the spinal cord or nerve roots. This most commonly occurs with axial compression, or "burst," fractures, with extensive disk herniation and fragmentation of the vertebral body (Figs. 6–29, 6–30, 6–31).

Abdominal ileus may occur with any spinal injury, the result of disturbance to the visceral autonomic nerves or ganglia from paraspinal soft tissue injury, edema, or hematoma (Fig. 6–32).

Healing of Vertebral Body Fractures

Fractures of the vertebral body heal by both endosteal and periosteal callus formation. Microscopically, extensive hemor-

rhage occurs within the fractured vertebral body about the broken trabeculae of the spongiosa. After several weeks, capillaries invade the fracture zone, and new bone deposition begins along some of the injured trabeculae, while others are resorbed. New trabeculae are formed that gradually bridge the fracture line through the vertebral body. Firm union normally requires from three to six months.[8]

Periosteal callus formation does not appear as soon, and is noted anteriorly only at the fracture site at first; later it spreads up and down along the anterior cortex as it becomes thicker. Endosteal resorption does not keep pace, however, and the result is considerable cortical thickening due to periosteal new bone at the fracture site. The steplike disturbance in the anterior cortical

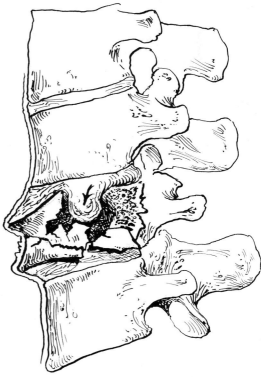

Figure 6–29. Axial compression or "burst" fracture. A severe "burst" fracture of a vertebral body has been sustained owing to a compression force from above acting parallel to the vertebral column. Severe comminution of the vertebral body has resulted, and nuclear material from the intervertebral disk above has been displaced into the body. A posterior body fragment has been pushed backward into the vertebral canal, but the posterior longitudinal ligament remains intact, and no damage to the posterior intervertebral ligaments has occurred, making this a clinically stable spinal injury.

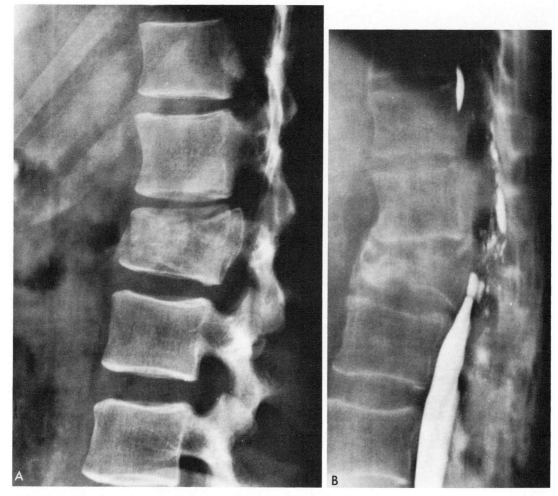

Figure 6–30. Posterior displacement of vertebral body fragments. *A,* Note the posterior displacement of a vertebral body fragment into the vertebral canal in this axial compression, or "burst," fracture of L-2 vertebra. *B,* Tomographic section of another case of axial compression or "burst" fracture. Posterior fragments of L-1 vertebral body have been displaced backwards to produce extradural cord compression outlined on myelography.

contour gradually smooths out over a period of three to five months, but cortical thickening from periosteal new bone accretion may persist for years afterward.[8]

Healing of vertebral fractures may be delayed by a number of factors. Generally, old age and poor health delay healing. Locally, a severe vertebral injury interrupting nutrient vessels to the bone and extensive herniation of nuclear disk material into the fracture may produce the same result. The zone of condensation and endosteal callus formation may disappear in three months with normal healing[8, 14] but in some cases may persist for years after the injury.[2] Restoration of vertebral body height following compression fracture is seldom ob-

served, and the cuneiform deformity remains (Fig. 6–33).

Excessive callus formation about the injured vertebral body may result, extending itself along the anterior longitudinal ligament in the manner of syndesmophyte formation, adhering broadly to the anterior surfaces of vertebral bodies above and below the level of injury (Figs. 6–34, 6–35). Degenerative osteophytes, which form only at the junction of the marginal ring with the vertebral body, present a different appearance, as they lack this broad base of origin.

The intervertebral disks, once torn, never heal satisfactorily nor quite regain their normal function. The disks are essentially avas-

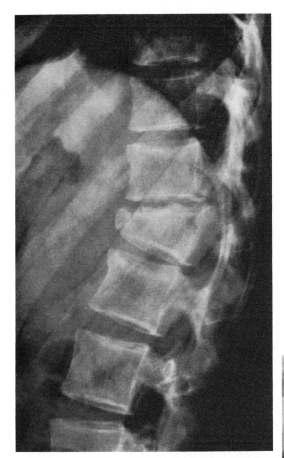

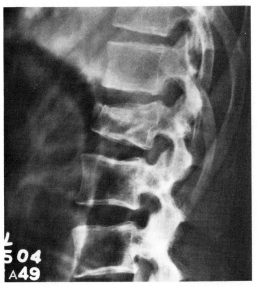

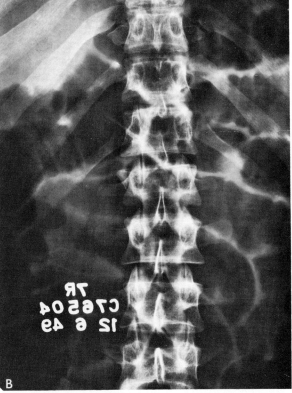

Figure 6–31. Posterior displacement of a vertebral body fragment in an anterior wedge compression injury. Such fragments may compress the spinal cord and nerve roots. If hyperextension of the spine is attempted to reduce the injury, the posterior body fragment may be driven further backward to aggravate spinal cord injury. Operative reduction may be indicated in such cases.[1]

Figure 6–32. Abdominal ileus with L-1 compression fracture. *A*, Lateral view. A wedge compression fracture of L-1 vertebral body has been sustained, with anterior displacement of the cranial endplate. *B*, Frontal view. The bowel gas pattern indicates intestinal ileus accompanying the spinal injury. Traumatic disturbance of visceral autonomic function may be produced by paraspinal soft-tissue injury, edema, or hematoma formation, resulting in intestinal ileus, bladder dysfunction, or splanchnic circulatory disturbances.

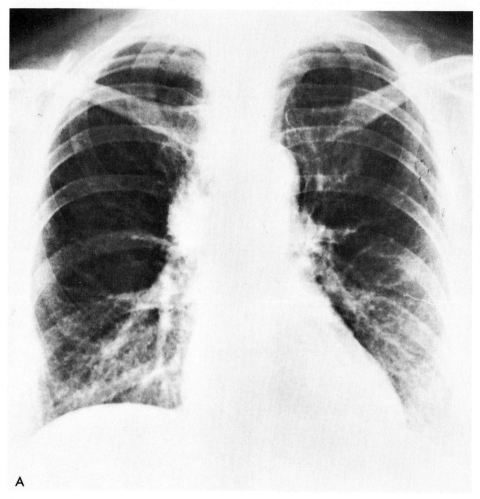

A

Figure 6–33. Compression fracture callus presenting as a paraspinal mass. A, PA chest film suggestive of right paraspinal mass.

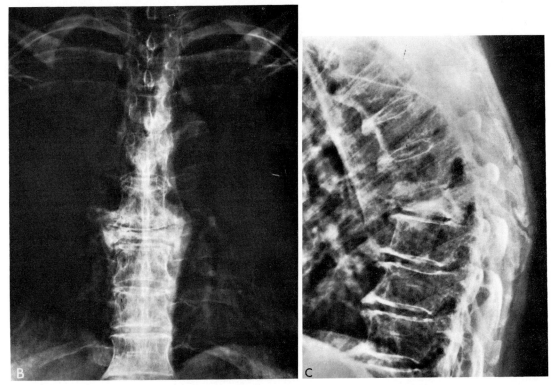

Figure 6–33 Continued. B, High kilovoltage views of the thoracic spine, revealing an old compression fracture of T-7 vertebra with paraspinal callus formation and soft tissue deformity. *C,* Lateral view, confirming the presence of a severe compression fracture of T-7 vertebra. (Note posterior calcification in the supraspinous ligament, resulting from organization of previous hematoma accompanying the fracture.)

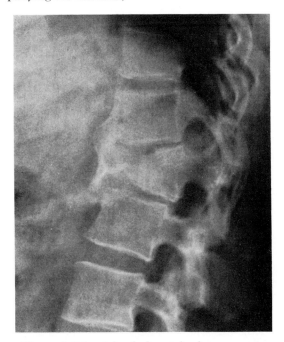

Figure 6–34. A healed vertebral compression fracture. Callus formation persists about the old compression fracture of L-1 vertebral body, extending along the anterior longitudinal ligament in the manner of syndesmophyte formation. The wedge-shaped deformity of L-1 body has not been corrected by healing.

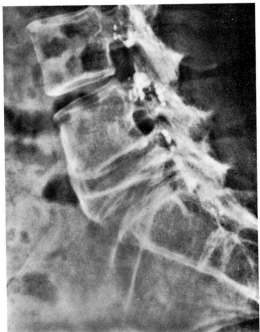

Figure 6–35. A healed axial compression fracture. Anterior callus formation signifies healing of this axial compression, or burst, fracture of L-5 vertebra. Vertebral body height was not restored. Posterior displacement of vertebral body fragments compressed the nerve roots of the cauda equina.

cular structures, and healing occurs only through invasion by capillaries and fibroblasts from outside the disk. With time, amorphous calcium deposits gradually appear within the intervertebral disk substance on the radiograph, together with degenerative changes of the adjacent vertebrae. In more severely injured intervertebral disk joints, complete bony ankylosis may result from healing.[15]

Telling the Age of a Vertebral Compression Fracture

Armed with the foregoing information, it is usually possible to tell from the radiograph whether a vertebral fracture is long-standing or of recent origin, but it is often difficult to be more precise. The injured vertebral body retains its wedge-shaped deformity, but the zone of condensation gradually disappears, and the buckle or step deformity of the anterior cortex becomes smooth with healing. Completion of changes requires a minimum of three months in the adult, and may well take longer. Soft tissue calcification and ossification about the vertebral fracture of course indicate duration of the injury. When recent origin of the fracture is questioned, radionuclide bone scanning may provide additional information. Such scans are positive in recent fractures undergoing active repair, but become negative when healing is complete.

Differential Diagnosis of Anterior Compression Fractures

Congenital Causes

DORSAL HEMIVERTEBRA. Ossification in the embryonic vertebral centrum normally proceeds from two centers, one situated dorsally and one ventrally within the primitive centrum.[15] Failure of the two ossification centers to fuse results in a coronally cleft vertebral body. If one ossification center fails to appear, a defective vertebral body results (Fig. 6–36). Ischemia of the tissues giving rise to the ossification center may explain its absence.[15] When the ventral ossification center fails to appear, a dorsal hemivertebra results, in which the ventral half of the body is congenitally absent. This

malformation is structurally unstable, and a kyphos rapidly forms with weight-bearing at the site of the dorsal hemivertebra. Presumably in response to the forces placed upon it, the dorsal hemivertebra assumes a wedge shape that may prove impossible to distinguish from a compression fracture (Fig. 6–37). If such a patient undergoes radiographic examination after recent spinal injury, comparison of these films with old films of the spine made prior to injury may be the only way to arrive at the correct diagnosis.

SAGITTALLY CLEFT "BUTTERFLY" VERTEBRA. Sagittal clefts in a vertebral body may persist from an earlier stage in the embryologic development of the vertebral centrum, when the primitive centrum is divided by remnants of the notochord and neurenteric canal into two sagittally opposed halves. Such a persistent sagittal cleft may result in a "butterfly" vertebra. This is easily identified on the anteroposterior radiographic view by the characteristic double triangles of the divided vertebral body, with their apices meeting in the midline to resemble the wings of a butterfly (Fig. 6–

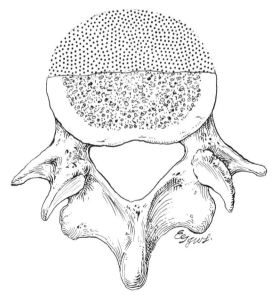

Figure 6–36. Dorsal hemivertebra. Two ossification centers arise in the primitive vertebral centrum. When the anterior ossification center fails to appear (stippled area on drawing), deficiency of the anterior portion of the adult vertebral body results. A kyphos of the spine results from structural instability, which in turn produces a wedge-shaped deformity of the dorsal hemivertebra on lateral view, resembling a compression fracture.

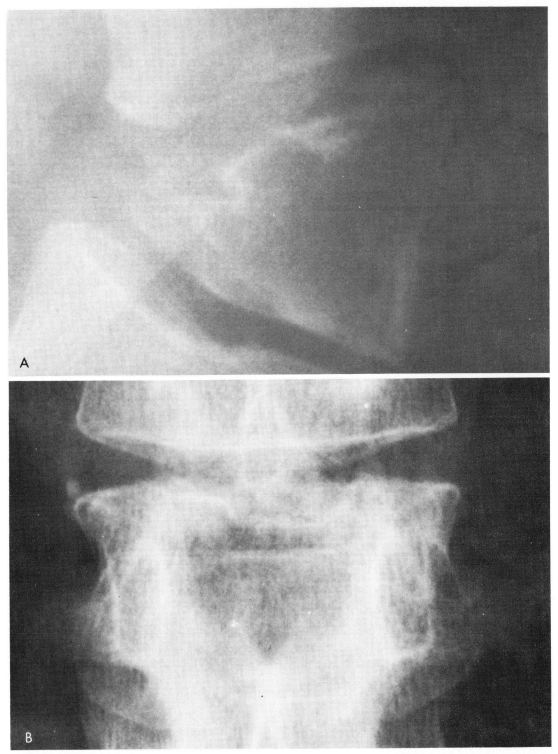

Figure 6–37. Dorsal hemivertebra. *A,* Lateral view. Note anterior deficiency in the vertebral body associated with wedge-shaped deformity. *B,* Frontal view of same vertebra.

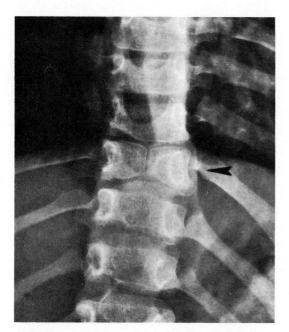

Figure 6–38. Sagittally cleft "butterfly" vertebra. Note the well-defined cleft passing sagittally through T-9 vertebral body (arrow at T-9 level). The contours of the body segments suggest the wings of a butterfly.

38). On the lateral view, however, this malformation may readily be mistaken for an old wedge compression fracture, or a dorsal hemivertebra as described above (Fig. 6–39). Sagittally cleft vertebrae have been observed to occur at every vertebral level in the spine, and they sometimes accompany other congenital malformations.

Tuberculosis

Tuberculous spondylitis, or tuberculous osteomyelitis of the spine, commonly originates within a vertebral body, and causes destruction of the body, collapse, and gibbus deformity at the affected level. The diseased body assumes a wedge shape similar to that occurring after trauma (Fig. 6–40). Of importance in arriving at the correct diagnosis are the following: (1) a clinical history of tuberculous infection; (2) other radiologic findings of tuberculosis, in the chest or elsewhere; (3) loss or destruction of adjacent intervertebral disks; (4) a prominent paraspinal soft tissue mass (cold abscess), especially if calcified; (5) involvement of multiple vertebral levels by anterior sub-

ligamentous spread of the infection; (6) anterior erosions of the vertebral body cortex; and (7) marked osteoporotic or osteosclerotic change in the affected area, indicating a greater disturbance of bone metabolism than would be expected in uncomplicated trauma.[15]

Pathologic Fracture

A spontaneous vertebral compression fracture without an adequate history of trauma should always arouse suspicion of a pathologic fracture, especially in the younger patient.[10] Further clinical investigation is warranted to ascertain the cause of the collapse. Available views of the spine should be studied for evidence of underlying osteoporosis, absence of pedicles, lytic destruction, or blastic bone involvement suggesting malignant disease (Figs. 6–41, 6–42). Less frequently, benign lesions of the vertebral bodies, such as hemangioma or giant cell tumor, may structurally undermine bone to produce compression fractures (Fig. 6–43). Complete collapse of one or more vertebral bodies in childhood suggests vertebra plana, eosinophilic granuloma, or Calvé's disease (Fig. 6–44). The most frequent malignancies metastatic to the spine originate from the bronchus, prostate, breast, kidney, and thyroid. Multiple myeloma, the lymphomas and leukemias are other common causes of malignant bone destruction in the vertebrae.

Intervertebral disk obliteration with destruction of adjacent vertebral end-plates always points toward infection, rather than neoplasm as the underlying cause of vertebral collapse.

Scheuermann's Disease

Moderate wedging of one or several vertebral bodies producing a kyphosis (often involving the lower thoracic spine) characterizes this disorder, initially affecting older children and adolescents. Narrowing of involved intervertebral disk spaces and multiple Schmorl's nodes are frequently seen. Sclerosis and irregularity of the vertebral end-plates differentiate Scheuermann's disease from other causes of wedging. Hypertrophic changes often ensue with age. The findings are usually characteristic (see p. 299).

Text continued on page 295.

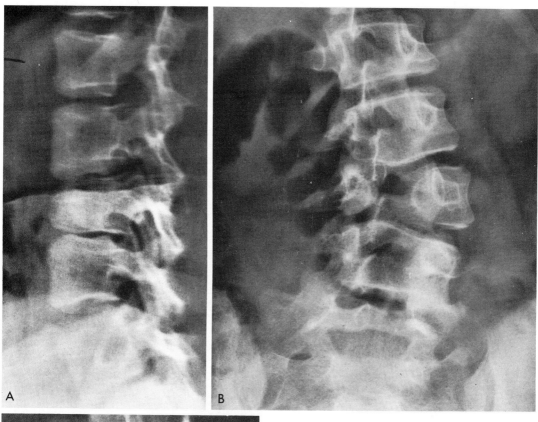

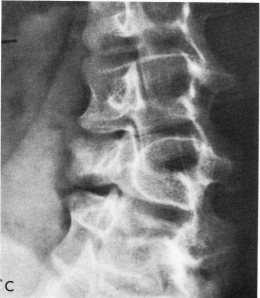

Figure 6–39. Sagittally cleft "butterfly" vertebra at L-3. *A,* On lateral view, loss of vertebral body height and anterior wedging suggest a compression fracture. *B,* On frontal view, sagittal deficiency identifies the "butterfly" malformation of the vertebral body. (The "wings" of the butterfly are not symmetric in this case.) *C,* Left anterior oblique views, again demonstrating the sagittal cleft. (Courtesy of Dr. Robert H. Freiberger, Hospital for Special Surgery, New York, N.Y.)

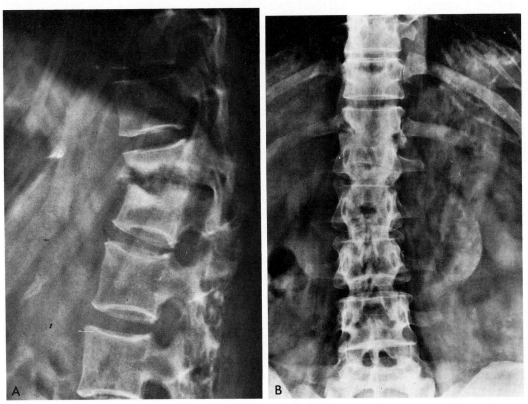

Figure 6–40. Tuberculous spondylitis. *A,* Lateral view: Wedge deformity of T-12 and L-1 vertebrae has resulted from tuberculous spondylitis. Note (1) destruction of the intervertebral disk space
and adjacent vertebral end-plates, (2) increased sclerosis of the bone adjacent to the destroyed disk,
and (3) soft-tissue calcification in an abscess anteriorly, indicating the correct diagnosis. *B,* Frontal
view: Disk destruction is again noted between T-12 and L-1 vertebrae, and a calcified abscess may be
seen on the left. (Courtesy of Dr. R. H. Freiberger, Hospital for Special Surgery, New York, N.Y.)

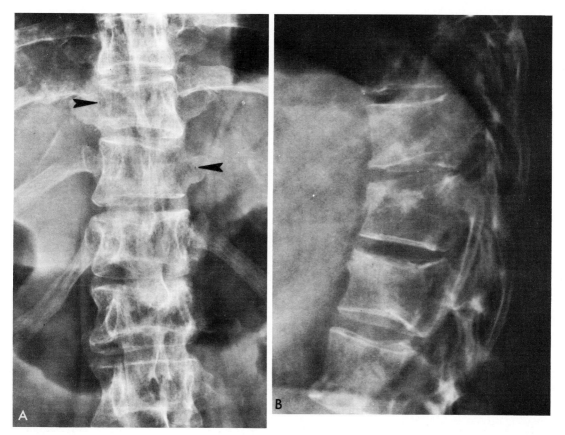

Figure 6–41. Pathologic vertebral fractures. *A,* Frontal view: Metastatic tumor deposits from breast carcinoma have produced considerable bone destruction. Note the absent pedicles (arrows) indicating vertebral arch involvement. *B,* Lateral view: Anterior wedge compression fracture of T-11 vertebral body is the result of metastatic disease in this instance.

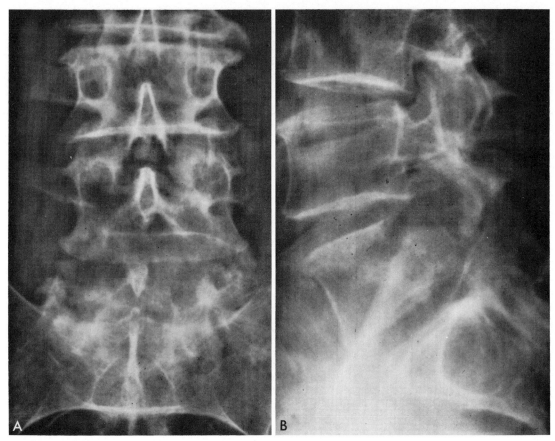

Figure 6–42. Metastatic vertebral destruction. *A*, Frontal view: Both pedicles of L-5 vertebra have been destroyed by metastatic carcinoma. *B*, Lateral view: The posterior aspect of L-5 vertebral body has been destroyed as well.

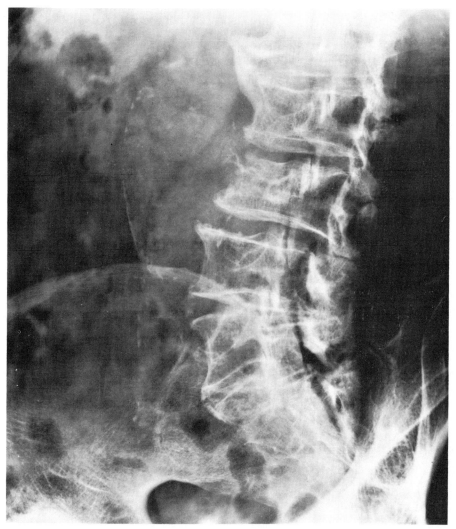

Figure 6–43. Erosion of L-3 vertebra by aortic aneurysm. The anterior cortex of L-3 vertebral body has been eroded by pulsation of an abdominal aortic aneurysm. Slight compression of the vertebral body has occurred as a result.

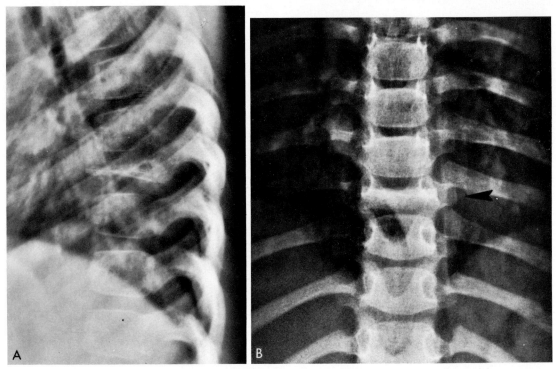

Figure 6–44. Vertebra plana (Calvé's disease). *A,* Lateral view: Almost complete collapse of T-9 vertebral body has resulted from Calvé's disease, or eosinophilic granuloma of bone, involving the body of T-9 in this child. The appearance of the fracture is characteristic of Calvé's disease in this age group. *B,* Frontal view: Vertebra plana has occurred at T-9 level (arrow). Note that the pedicles and vertebral arch are not grossly involved by the lesion.

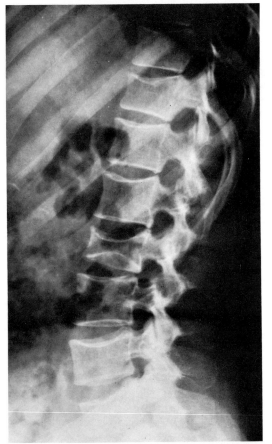

Figure 6–45. Multiple compression fractures in osteoporosis of the spine. Maximal compression injury has occurred at L-2 in this young man with axial osteoporosis. Note multiple biconcave disk deformities, a structural adaptation by osteopenic bone to resist vertical weight-bearing stresses.

*Other Congenital and Metabolic
Disorders*

Achondroplasia, the mucopolysaccharidoses, and many other types of dwarfism may exhibit vertebral deformities, wedging, or collapse. Diagnosis rests with identification of the clinical picture and the associated radiologic findings.

PATHOLOGIC FRACTURES OF THE VERTEBRAE

Pathologic fractures of the vertebrae commonly announce themselves as compression fractures of the vertebral bodies due to bone mineral loss with resultant mechanical instability (Fig. 6–45). Nicholas, Wilson, and Freiberger[10] reviewed 105 cases of verte-

bral compression fractures occurring in patients with no history of adequate trauma or known malignant bone disease. Osteoporosis was found to be the most common cause; malignant bone disease, rheumatoid arthritis treated with corticosteroids, and osteomalacia followed in that order (Fig. 6–46). The likelihood of finding underlying malignant bone disease in patients age 55 or older with vertebral compression fractures was approximately 20 per cent, whereas in patients younger than age 55 this likelihood rose to about 50 per cent. When compared with other conditions associated with pathologic fractures, malignancies metastatic to bone were noted to produce significantly fewer vertebral fractures in a given patient than were the others (bone destruction being focal rather than generalized).

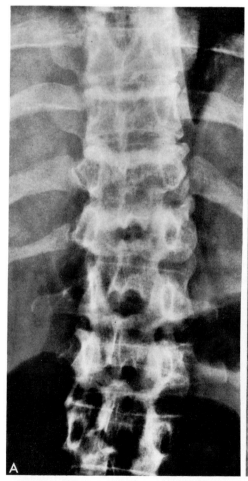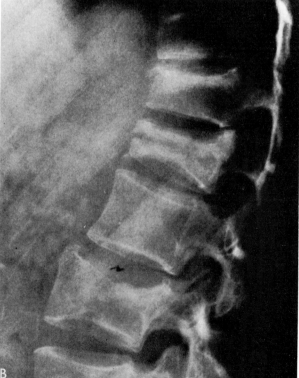

Figure 6–46. Steroid-induced compression fractures. *A,* Frontal view. Prolonged corticosteroid therapy has resulted in severe osteoporosis in this forty-year-old woman, which in turn has given rise to multiple vertebral compression fractures. *B,* Lateral view. Dense callus formation appears in the zones of condensation associated with compression, a characteristic feature of healing steroid-induced fractures.

KÜMMELL'S DISEASE (DELAYED POSTTRAUMATIC VERTEBRAL COLLAPSE)

Delayed posttraumatic vertebral collapse was first described by Kümmell in 1891.[6] Numerous cases were subsequently described in the French and German literature (syndrome de Kümmell-Verneuil, spondylitis traumatica). Kümmell originally described a rarefying process in the vertebral bodies of an injured patient occurring months after an episode of spinal trauma clinically inadequate to account for the findings. The patient remained relatively asymptomatic until rarefaction of the vertebra produced pain, collapse, and gibbus formation. Kümmell was unable to find evidence of bone suppuration to indicate tuberculosis, thickening of the bones to indicate syphilis, or proliferative changes to suggest deforming arthritis in the cases he examined. He concluded that the bone rarefaction in the spine represented a delayed inflammatory response to the injury ("traumatic spondylitis").[7] Many theories as to the cause of this were subsequently advanced, invoking nutritional, circulatory, and neurologic factors; premature weight-bearing; prolonged immobilization without exercise; traumatic necrosis; and fatigue fractures.[15]

The existence of this condition is controversial. Although well-documented cases occur in earlier writings, Kümmell's disease has become something of a rarity in both European and American literature of the last 40 years; whether this relates to the wider application of diagnostic radiology to the initially traumatized spine remains an open question. Schinz et al.[14] doubt the existence of Kümmell's disease and believe that any fracture of the spine that can be diagnosed later should have been immediately detectable after the initial injury with radiographs of adequate quality. Böhler[1] emphatically states he has never seen cases such as Kümmell describes; he is also of the opinion that significant trauma to the spine occurs at the time of the initial injury in instances of alleged Kümmell's disease. Schmorl[15] indicates that some of Kümmell's original cases were subsequently proved to represent tuberculous spondylitis. We agree with Morton[9] that the diagnosis should be avoided unless one is certain of the facts involved in the history.

SCHMORL'S NODES

Displacement or herniation of the nucleus pulposus may occur in any direction (Fig. 6–47). Penetration of the nucleus into the adjacent vertebral bodies results in the formation of *Schmorl's nodes*.

Normally, the cranial and caudal surfaces of the vertebral bodies are protected by hyaline cartilaginous plates, which completely cover the upper and lower surfaces of the vertebral body except for the marginal rims. These plates, together with the anulus fibrosus, confine the nucleus pulposus within the intervertebral disk.

Occasionally, under conditions of stress, gaps or fissures may develop in the hyaline cartilaginous plates. Fissures may occur in a number of locations: (1) along the course of the embryonic notochord where the cartilage may be thinned or indented; (2) the sites where the nutrient vessels that nourished the disk early in life leave scars in the cartilage after they degenerate; (3) at the junction of the cartilaginous plate with the bony marginal rim; or (4) at points of degeneration within the cartilage. Schmorl[15] gave these points the fanciful name "ossification pores." The cartilaginous plates may also be weakened and eventually breached by tumor, infection, or trauma.

Whatever the cause of cartilaginous plate weakening may be, these gaps permit the nucleus pulposus to penetrate into the vertebral body (Fig. 6–47). Bony trabeculae are absorbed about the displaced disk tissue. The cavity thus created permits more of the nucleus pulposus to enter the vertebral body. The pressure exerted within the vertebral body by the herniated nuclear tissue elicits a reaction from the surrounding bone, initially in the form of a cartilaginous casing about the disk tissue. Later, as ossification of the cartilaginous casing ensues, the characteristic radiographic findings of Schmorl's nodes appear (Fig. 6–48; see also Figs. 6–20, 6–26, 6–52, 6–53). Nodes encased in cartilage alone are invisible on radiographs of the vertebrae. This explains why Schmorl found such nodes to be three times more common at autopsy than radiographs of living patients would suggest.

VERTEBRAL EDGE DISTURBANCES

The raised bony edges or rims seen around the margins of the vertebral body,

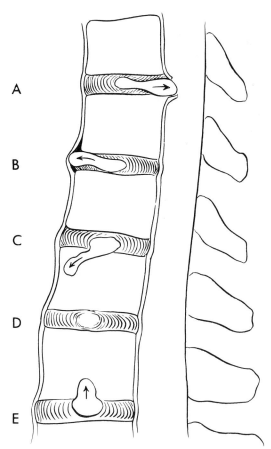

Figure 6–47. Herniations of the nucleus pulposus. *A,* Posterior herniation of the nucleus pulposus may penetrate or circumvent the posterior longitudinal ligament, and exert extradural compression on the spinal cord and nerve roots. *B,* Anterior herniation of the nucleus pulposus may elevate the anterior longitudinal ligament, to produce anterior vertebral osteophyte formation and a diminished intervertebral disk space. *C,* Alternately, nuclear material may herniate anteriorly between the vertebral rim and end-plate to separate a portion of the vertebral body from the remainder. *D,* Normal intervertebral disk and nucleus pulposus, for comparison. *E,* Penetration of the vertebral end-plate by herniating nuclear material results in Schmorl's node formation.

lower corners of the vertebral bodies. These notches are filled by cartilaginous tissue, the precursor of the bony vertebral rims, which appears radiolucent on the radiograph. Ossification within these cartilaginous rims begins in girls between the ages of six and eight, and in boys between the ages of seven and nine. Several areas of ossification may appear simultaneously and may coalesce within the peripheral cartilaginous rim, but fusion of these secondary ossification centers with the main bulk of the vertebral body does not begin until about age 15. Prior to this time, these secondary ossification centers appear on the lateral radiograph as small, radiopaque triangles at the anterior corners of the vertebral bodies but separate from them ("rim

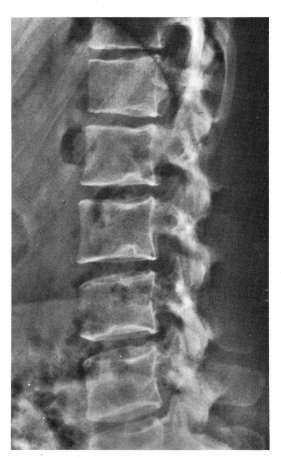

Figure 6–48. Schmorl's nodes. Herniation of nuclear material through the vertebral end-plates into the cancellous bone of the vertebral body elicits a reaction from the surrounding bone, which eventually ossifies to produce the characteristic indentations seen adjacent to the intervertebral disk spaces in this patient. (See also Figs. 6–20, 6–26, 6–52, 6–53A.)

and their separation from the body on the radiograph, have aroused considerable controversy. Are these edge separations normal or abnormal? And if abnormal, do they represent fractures or intervertebral disk injuries?

Schmorl[15] traces the development of the normal vertebral rim or edge ("Randleiste") back to childhood. On the lateral radiograph of a young child's spine, notches or grooves may be noted in the anterior upper and

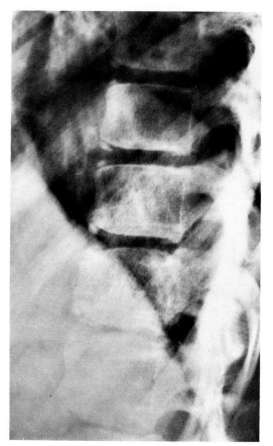

Figure 6–49. Normal vertebral rim apophyses. Small, radiopaque triangles at the anterior vertebral body corners in a child will later fuse with the bodies to produce superior and inferior vertebral rims.

apophyses": Fig. 6–49). These secondary ossification centers radiologically resemble the epiphyseal centers of long bones, but Schmorl and others discourage the use of the term "epiphyses" for these vertebral edge centers. This is because they do not add to the growth of the vertebral body, as one would expect of a true epiphysis. Therefore, these bony rims cannot be considered "epiphyses" in the usual sense of the term.

Fusion of the bony vertebral edge with the body occurs gradually between the 15th and 22nd year. When the vertebral rims have fused with the body, they give insertion to Sharpey's fibers, the strong, outermost containing fibers of the intervertebral disk. The lower lumbar vertebral rims are the last to fuse with their bodies.

Vertebral edge separations have been

noted throughout adult life, most commonly in the anterosuperior corners of the lower lumbar vertebral bodies (Figs. 6–50 to 6–53). Schmorl and Junghanns[15] have shown such vertebral edge separations to represent anterior herniation of nuclear disk material between the vertebral rim and body, extending to the anterior surface of the vertebral body beneath the anterior longitudinal ligament. A diagonal cleavage thus results between the anterosuperior corner and the rest of the vertebral body (Fig. 6–54). Their pathologic sections provide elegant support for this thesis, demonstrating nuclear disk material within the cleft between the vertebral edge and body, and anteriorly beneath the longitudinal ligament.[15] This finding in the adult spine indicates a pathologic process; so the term "limbus vertebra," with its connotation of a normal variant, should be avoided.

Can such findings occur in acute trauma? And how may they be distinguished from the vertebral edge separations described above? Fracture of the anterosuperior corner of a vertebral body during spinal

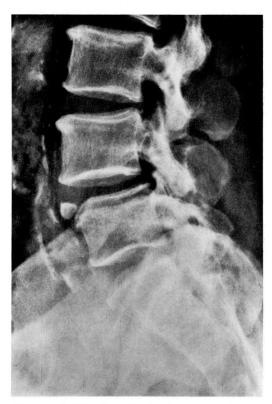

Figure 6–50. Vertebral edge separation at L-5. Note separation involving the anterosuperior corner of L-5 vertebral body.

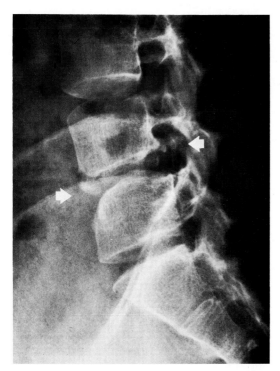

Figure 6–51. Anterior and posterior vertebral edge separations at L-4. Herniation of the nucleus pulposus has occurred both anteriorly and posteriorly at the L-4 disk level, displacing small fragments of the vertebral body (arrows). (Courtesy of Dr. R. H. Freiberger, Hospital for Special Surgery, New York, N.Y.)

flexion injury is a common occurrence, and the distinction between fracture and disk herniation may be difficult to draw. Both may be associated with narrowing of the disk space. In general, however, vertebral edge separations are more frequent in the lower lumbar spine, while compression fractures occur most often near the thoracolumbar junction. Certainly, irregular cleft margins without signs of sclerosis suggest a recent fracture, while smooth, dense, widely separated cleft margins exhibiting proliferative change suggest a more chronic condition, such as might be expected with an old disk injury. Both fracture and vertebral edge separation produce fragments larger than the normal vertebral edge itself, but edge separations often exceed fracture fragments in size. A fracture fragment tends to be displaced downward and anteriorly in compression injury, while edge separations tend to displace the edge fragment upward, with minimal anterior displacement (Fig. 6–55). In recent trauma, other evidence of compression injury is often observed, such

as wedging of the vertebral body or infraction of the end-plates; these changes would not be expected in the edge separations that result from disk degeneration.

SCHEUERMANN'S DISEASE (JUVENILE KYPHOSIS)

This disease of the adolescent spine will be included with traumatic lesions, as trauma is considered to play an important role in its etiology; besides, the wedge-shaped deformities of the vertebral bodies seen in radiographs of Scheuermann's disease may be mistaken for old compression fractures.

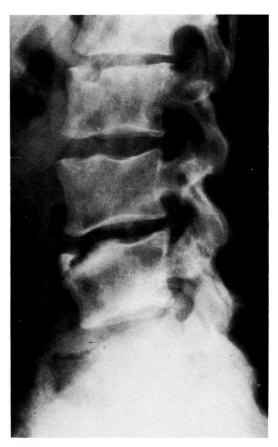

Figure 6–52. L-4 vertebral edge separation, with Schmorl's nodes above. Considerable sclerosis has resulted about the anterior vertebral edge separation at L-4. Schmorl's node formation is especially well marked at L-2. (Both these conditions represent abnormal penetration of the vertebral body by herniated nuclear disk material, reflecting increased permeability of the vertebral end-plates.) (Courtesy of Dr. Robert H. Freiberger, Hospital for Special Surgery, New York, N.Y.)

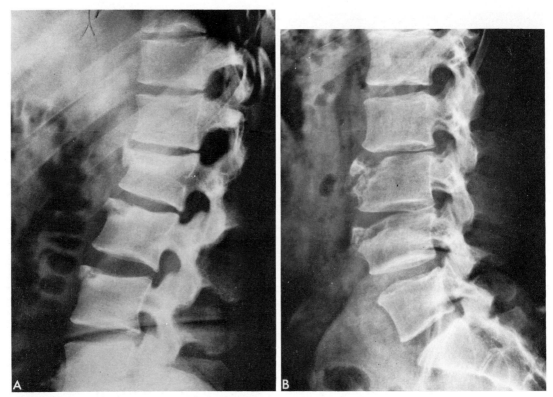

Figure 6–53. Multiple vertebral edge separations. *A*, Edge separations have occurred at vertebrae L-1 through L-3. Note Schmorl's node formation in the lower thoracic spine; both findings indicate vertebral end-plate deficiency, in this case the result of acute axial osteoporosis (Courtesy Dr. R. H. Freiberger, Hospital for Special Surgery, New York, N.Y.). *B*, Vertebral edge separations of L-3 and L-4 show considerable associated reactive change.

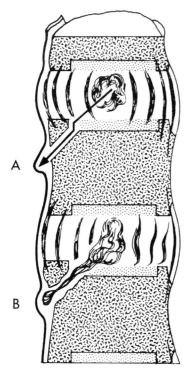

Figure 6–54. Vertebral edge separation. *A*, Anteroinferior herniation of nuclear disk material occurs between the vertebral rim and body, extending to the anterior surface of the vertebral body beneath the anterior longitudinal ligament. *B*, A diagonal cleavage thus results between the anterosuperior corner and the rest of the vertebral body, containing herniated nuclear material on pathologic section. (After Schmorl-Junghanns.)

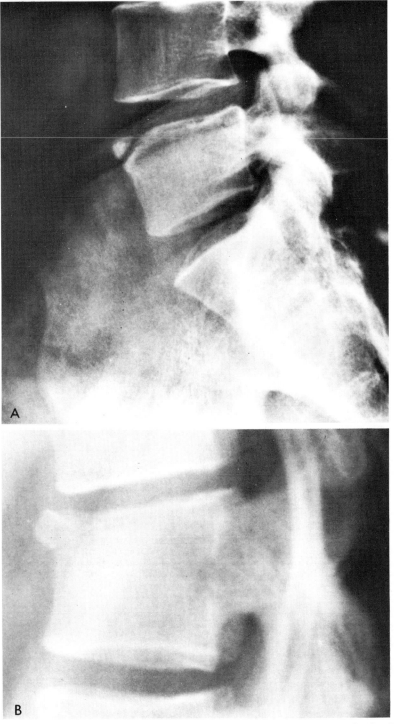

Figure 6-55. Vertebral edge separation vs. compression fracture. *A*, Vertebral edge separation. Note sclerosis about margins of separation, and upward displacement of anterior fragment. *B*, Compression fracture. Note anterior and downward displacement of fracture fragment.

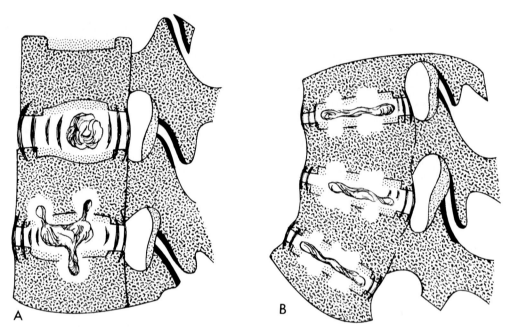

Figure 6–56. Scheuermann's disease. *A*, Nuclear disk material penetrates through defective vertebral end-plates (light stippling) into the vertebral bodies, producing Schmorl's nodes. Collapse of the disk space follows on the escape of the nuclear substance. *B*, Closer approximation of the vertebral bodies results; however, as the intervertebral distance is maintained posteriorly by the apophyseal joints, only the anterior edges of the vertebrae are free to come more closely together. This results in a kyphosis of the spine, putting increased pressure on the growing vertebral bodies anteriorly, eventuating in wedge deformity of the growing vertebrae. (After Schmorl-Junghanns.)

SYNONYMS

Vertebral epiphysitis; juvenile kyphosis; kyphosis dorsalis juvenilis; juvenile diskogenic disorder.

INCIDENCE. Both sexes are about evenly involved. The condition is first noted at puberty, and is rarely encountered before the age of ten.

ETIOLOGY AND PATHOGENESIS. Juvenile kyphosis was first described by Scheuermann in 1921, who regarded the disease as an inflammatory condition affecting the vertebral end-plates — an aseptic necrosis or osteochondritis ("vertebral epiphysitis"). On radiographs of affected patients, he noted progressive irregularities in the vertebral end-plates, narrowing of the intervertebral disk spaces, and gradual anterior wedging of the vertebral bodies, often in the mid- or lower thoracic spine of an older child or an adolescent. Vertebral edge separations appeared in the involved thoracic vertebra, and also in the lower lumbar spine.

Schmorl and Junghanns, in reviewing their vast collection of pathologic material, were subsequently unable to find inflammatory changes or necrosis of bone in cases of Scheuermann's juvenile kyphosis. However, they often found Scheuermann's disease in children with unusually thin, fragile cartilaginous end-plates that were cupped into the vertebral bodies around the disk nuclei, and subject to cracking or fissuring under stress.[15]

The subsequent course of the disease (Fig. 6–56), eloquently documented by their pathologic specimens, was marked by penetration of disk material through the defective end-plates into the vertebral bodies, producing Schmorl's nodes. Collapse of the disk spaces followed the escape of nuclear substance. Closer approximation of the vertebral bodies resulted; however, as the intervertebral distance was maintained posteriorly by the apophyseal joints, only the anterior edges of the vertebrae were free to come more closely together. This produced a mild kyphosis, together with increased pressure upon the anterior aspects of the growing vertebral bodies. The increased pressure suppressed growth in height of the vertebral bodies anteriorly, eventuating in wedge-shaped deformities, with increased kyphosis. Meanwhile, attempted healing of the disrupted intervertebral disks by invasion of capillaries and fibrous tissue from outside the disk produced fibrous and, later, bony ankylosis of the intervertebral disk joint, with rigidity of the kyphotic curve. Associated scoliotic deformity is comparatively mild.[15]

CLINICAL COURSE. Scheuermann's disease is first noted as a round-back deformity of the spine, often by someone other than the patient. Symptoms vary widely. Although considerable back pain may be experienced, young people so affected often have few or no symptoms associated with their gradually progressive deformity. Mild cases may exhibit no physical findings at all, and may come to light only as an incidental finding on radiographs of the spine or chest taken for another purpose. Progression of the disease may be accelerated by vigorous exertion or hard physical labor ("apprentice kyphosis"; "farm boy's back"). The disease has been related in some cases to a single episode of mechanical injury to the back.[15]

RADIOLOGIC FINDINGS. The radiologic findings in Scheuermann's disease are most often found in the mid- and lower thoracic spine, but the cervical and lumbar spine may be affected also. Irregularity of the vertebral end-plates, with extensive Schmorl's node formation and narrowing of the intervertebral disk spaces, typifies the involved segments. A single vertebra may be affected, but more often several are included, and often a segment of six to eight vertebrae shows such changes. Wedging of the vertebral bodies contributes to a kyphotic curve (Fig. 6–57). In later stages, calcifications may appear in the intervertebral disks in affected areas. With age, spondylosis and degenerative change may supervene in the diseased segments of the spine. Avulsion fractures of the spinous processes of the vertebrae involved with juvenile kyphosis sometimes occur.[14, 15] Vertebral edge separations may be seen both in the lower lumbar spine, and in the segments directly involved with Scheuermann's disease.

Associated Conditions

An increased incidence of lumbosacral disk disease has been noted in patients with Scheuermann's disease,[14] with an increase in posterior disk herniations resulting in neurologic compression. Posterior herniations of disk material in the thoracic spine requiring laminectomy for relief of spinal

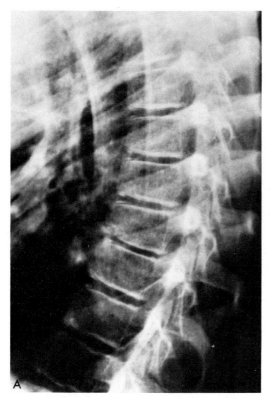

A

Figure 6–57. Scheuermann's disease. *A*, Early Scheuermann's disease: This fifteen-year-old boy presented with painful kyphosis. A lateral view of his thoracic spine demonstrates early narrowing of the anterior intervertebral disk spaces and irregularities of the rim apophyses involving several lower thoracic vertebrae. *B*, More advanced case of Scheuermann's disease. *C*, Severe Scheuermann's disease: Note kyphosis of the spine, with marked vertebral end-plate irregularity in the mid- and lower thoracic region.

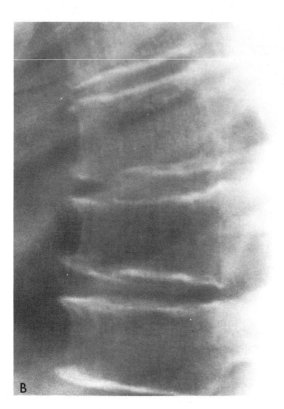

B

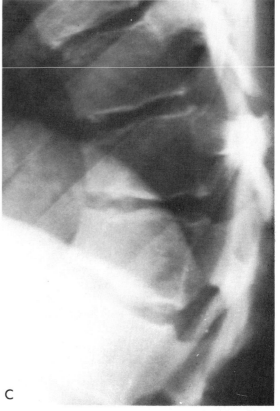

C

cord compression have been noted[3] but are probably infrequent. Thoracic cord compression due to epidural cysts associated with Scheuermann's disease has also been described.[12] Vertebral ischemia due to pressure from the cyst on nutrient vessels supplying the vertebral end-plates has been invoked as the cause of the juvenile kyphosis in such cases.

REFERENCES

1. Böhler, L. The Treatment of Fractures. New York, Grune & Stratton, 1956.
2. Ellis, J. D.: Compression fractures of the vertebral bodies and other changes mistaken for them. J. Bone & Jt. Surg., 26:139, 1944.
3. Epstein, B. S.: The Spine, A Radiological Text and Atlas, 3rd ed. Philadelphia, Lea & Febiger, 1969.
4. Holdsworth, F. W.: Fractures, dislocations, and fracture dislocations of the spine. J. Bone & Jt. Surg., 45-B:6, 1963.
5. Jefferson, G.: Discussion on spinal injuries. Proc. Royal Soc. Med., 21:625, 1928.
6. Kümmell, H.: Über die traumatischen Erkrankungen der Wirbelsäule, Deutsch. med. Wchnschr., 21:180, 1895.
7. Kümmell, H.: Der heutige Standpunkt der posttraumatischen Wirbelkrankung (Kümmellsche Krankheit), Arch orthop. u. Unfall-Chir., 26:491 1928.
8. Lob, A.: Die Wirbelsäulenvertetzungen und ihre Ausheilung, 2nd ed. Stuttgart, George Thieme Verlag, 1954.
9. Morton, S. A.: The differential diagnosis of traumatic lesions of the spine. Radiology, 41:560, 1943.
10. Nicholas, J. A., Wilson, P. D., and Freiberger, R. H.: Pathological fractures of the spine: etiology and diagnosis. J. Bone & Jt. Surg., 42-A:127, 1960.
11. Nicoll, E. A.: Fractures of the dorso-lumbar spine. J. Bone & Jt. Surg., 31-B:376, 1949.
12. Paul, L. W., and Juhl, J. H.: The Essentials of Roentgen Interpretation, 3rd ed., Hagerstown, Harper & Row, 1972, pp. 386–408.
13. Roaf, R.: A study of the mechanics of spinal injuries. J. Bone & Jt. Surg., 42-B:810, 1960.
14. Schinz, H. R., Baensch W. E., Friedl, L., and Uehlinger, E.: Roentgen Diagnostics, Vol. 2. 2nd American edition, by Leo G. Rigler. New York, Grune & Stratton, 1967.
15. Schmorl, G., and Junghanns, H.: The Human Spine in Health and Disease. 2nd American ed., by E. F. Besemann, New York, Grune & Stratton, 1971.

Chapter 7

FRACTURE-DISLOCATION OF THE THORACOLUMBAR SPINE

ANATOMY

The posterior aspect of the vertebral column consists of a column of vertebral arches surrounding the spinal cord, united by a system of interosseous ligaments described by Holdsworth as "the posterior ligament complex."[9] The vertebral arches are themselves composed of laminae and paired pedicles, giving rise to the spinous, articular, and transverse processes.

All these bony structures are known as "posterior elements," an anatomically inexact term widely received in the literature, which we prefer to avoid.

The posterior ligamentous complex uniting these bony structures consists (from back to front) of the supraspinous and interspinous ligaments, the capsular ligaments binding the apophyseal joints together, the ligamenta flava, and the posterior longitudinal ligament (Figs. 7–1, 7–2).

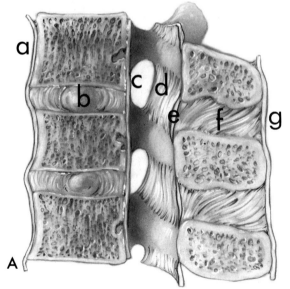 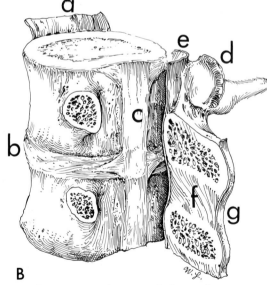

Figure 7–1. Sections of the vertebral column, showing soft-tissue attachments. *A,* Sagittal section. The anterior longitudinal ligament (a), intervertebral disks (b), and posterior longitudinal ligament (c) hold the vertebral bodies together, while the ligamenta flava (d), apophyseal capsular ligaments (e), and interspinous (f) and supraspinous ligaments (g) unite the vertebral arches posteriorly around the canal. Soft-tissue structures (c) through (g), together with the vertebral arches, constitute the *vertebral arch complex. B,* Section exposing the vertebral column from behind and obliquely, with the vertebral arches partially cut away. (a), (b), (c) as in Figure 7–1A; (e) ligamentum flavum; (d) apophyseal capsular ligaments; (f) interspinous ligament, (g) supraspinous ligament.

These ligaments are reinforced by the posterior paraspinal muscles, and are strengthened by the rib cage in the thoracic spine, and by the abdominal muscles in the lumbar spine.

It is this posterior complex of vertebral arches, ligaments, and joint capsules, more than any other structure, that maintains the integrity and continuity of the vertebral column and preserves the spinal cord from injury. We shall refer to it as "the vertebral arch complex" (Figs. 7–1, 7–2). According to Holdsworth, its disruption results in a clinically *unstable* spinal injury, that is, an injury permitting abnormal spinal motion with the threat of producing neurologic injury. Severe damage to the vertebral arch complex must be presumed in any injury sufficient to produce vertebral dislocation. Hyperextension injuries that sever the anterior longitudinal ligament and avulse the intervertebral disk bonds, particularly in the cervical spine, are similarly unstable.

INCIDENCE

The frequency with which vertebral arch complex damage occurs in spinal injuries is difficult to assess, as such damage is not always clinically apparent, and may be difficult to detect on conventional spinal radiographs of less than optimal technique. Böhler,[1] upon reviewing the radiographs of a large series of spinal injuries, was struck by the frequency with which fractures of the vertebral arches and processes accompanied even apparently minor vertebral trauma. Lob[13] found fractures of the vertebral arches and articular processes in 29 per cent of all his cases of spinal injury, and in 69 per cent of all his fracture-dislocation injuries. Kaufer and Hayes[12] noted that dislocation of lumbar segments is seen in 10 to 20 per cent of all thoracolumbar fractures. An increased incidence of anomalies of lumbar segmentation appeared in their series of fracture-dislocations, in comparison with the general population. This led them to suggest that patients with these anomalies showed an increased susceptibility to spinal injury.

MECHANISM OF INJURY

Injury to the vertebral arch complex, which is made up of the vertebral arches

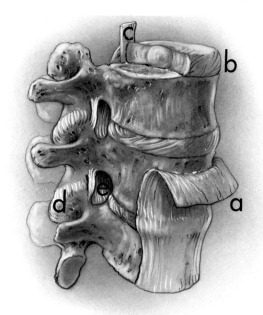

Figure 7–2. Exterior view of vertebral soft tissue attachments. Note the capsular ligaments of the apophyseal joints (d). The anterior longitudinal ligament (a) invests the anterior and lateral aspects of the vertebral bodies, and has been partially reflected. Note the intervertebral disk in cross-section (b), with its central nucleus pulposus, and the narrow posterior longitudinal ligament (c) extending upward behind it.

and the posterior ligament complex, may thus involve bones, ligaments, or both together (Figs. 7–1, 7–2). The vertebral arches may be fractured, resulting in a loss of posterior spinal cohesion. The posterior ligament complex may be avulsed, allowing diastasis of the vertebral arches without fracture. Combinations of both often occur. The apophyseal joints (facets) may be dislocated and may lock to prevent reduction of the injury (Fig. 7–3).

Such injuries involving the posterior vertebral column may result from pure hyperflexion, in which the vertebral arches and processes are distracted from each other on the outside of the curve. More often, however, rotation (axial torsion) or horizontal shearing stresses contribute to the damage. Most posterior spinal injuries are, in fact, the result of a combination of these forces interacting with each other upon the vertebral column, so that the mechanism of injury is rarely pure.[15] For descriptive purposes, however, they will be considered to be the result of pure injury. Indeed, in most spinal injuries, one mechanism of injury is usually

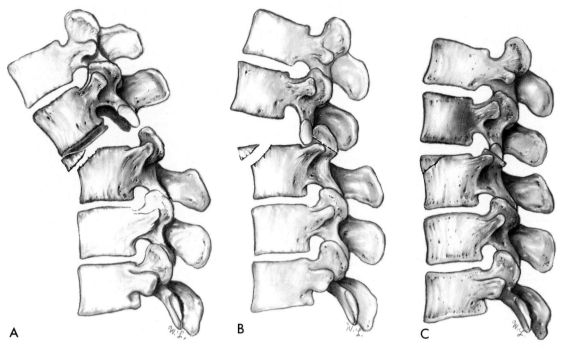

A   B   C

Figure 7–3. Locking of facets (articular processes) in lumbar fracture-dislocation. *A*, Fracture-dislocation of the lumbar spine with distraction of the facets posteriorly. *B*, On attempted reduction of the dislocation by hyperextending the spine, the upper facet cannot slide back, as it is blocked by the lower. The vertebrae are forced apart, and spinal cord injury may be aggravated by the resultant stretching. To reduce the dislocation satisfactorily, osteotomy of the lower facet (dashed line) must be performed at surgery. *C*, Reduction of the dislocation after osteotomy, with normal alignment of the facets restored.

dominant, producing a more or less characteristic deformity by which it can be recognized.

The vast majority of thoracolumbar fracture-dislocations result from flexion violence, in which the vertebral bodies are compressed anteriorly. Vertical loading or compression forces applied in the long axis of the vertebral column may be converted to flexion forces by the mechanisms discussed in Chapter 6. Tension, distraction, or disruption forces are applied posteriorly to the vertebral arch complex on the other side of the fulcrum about which the injury pivots. The distance 2 in Figure 7–4 is usually four times the distance 1. The compression force brought to bear on the vertebral bodies anterior to the fulcrum (distance 1) is therefore four times greater than the distraction force acting on the vertebral arch complex (distance 2). Thus, pure flexion injury exerted on the thoracolumbar spine will produce compression of vertebral bodies long before distraction of the vertebral arch complex

can occur.[19] However, when a force deforming the vertebral column in flexion is too great to be dispelled by collapse of a vertebral body alone, it will produce distraction on the other side of the fulcrum, with damage to the vertebral arch complex; or, if the deforming force persists after compression fractures of the vertebrae have been produced anteriorly, disruption may follow posteriorly.[11] Injuries resulting in posterior vertebral distraction have been described as disruptive hyperflexion,[2] tension injuries,[19] or simply as hyperflexion fractures,[1] in contrast to the anterior compression fractures and disk injuries, which leave the posterior spine intact (flexion injuries).

Roaf,[15] in working with cadaver vertebral columns found it experimentally impossible to tear the posterior ligament complex by applying a pure hyperflexion force, but when he introduced elements of torsion (rotary force about the long axis of the vertebral column) or forward shear (horizontal force) he was readily able to disrupt the posterior ligament complex. Similarly, in hyperextension injuries, application of torsion to the cadaver vertebrae made it much easier to tear the anterior longitudinal ligament.

Pure dislocation injuries are rare in the thoracolumbar spine, because its mobility is less than that of the cervical spine, and the vertebral segments are bound more closely together. The thoracolumbar apophyseal joints do not enjoy as wide a range of motion as do those in the cervical spine. Thoracolumbar vertebral dislocations are thus as likely to be produced by fracturing the articular process as by disengaging them. Indeed, far greater violence is required to dislocate the thoracolumbar vertebrae than the cervical. The resultant injury is likely to be more extensive, entailing multiple vertebral fractures and severe soft tissue injury. Compression fractures of the vertebral bodies associated with dislocation injuries are more likely to show comminution and end-plate infraction of the body than are compression fractures without dislocation (Fig. 7–5).

Fractures involving the pedicles, laminae, or articular processes are of greater significance in terms of spinal function and clinical management than are isolated fractures of the transverse or spinous processes. Evidence of any of these injuries on radiographs, however, suggests disruption of the vertebral arch complex, with the possibility of severe spinal injury.

CLINICAL FINDINGS

The injured patient who has sustained dislocation of the thoracolumbar spine will complain of back pain at the level of injury, and may experience inability to move his legs after the injury. Physical examination of the injured back will reveal a palpable gap between the spinous processes at the level of dislocation. This gap is the most reliable indication of this condition.[12] Swelling, tenderness, and ecchymosis of the skin may be present over the back at the site of injury. Such findings over the shoulder blade or laterally on the upper torso may indicate indirect rotational violence to the spine, and consequently a rotary fracture-dislocation.[9] Gibbus deformity of the spine or neurologic deficit

upon examination of the lower limbs may also be found.

All vertebral injuries with interspinous widening, or other evidence of vertebral arch complex disruption, are clinically *unstable*.[9, 14] This means that improper handling of the patient may damage the spinal cord and nerve roots, if the initial injury has not already done so. It is, therefore, of great importance to recognize injuries of the vertebral arch complex at the earliest possible stage in the patient's management.

Neurologic damage occurs in 53 per cent

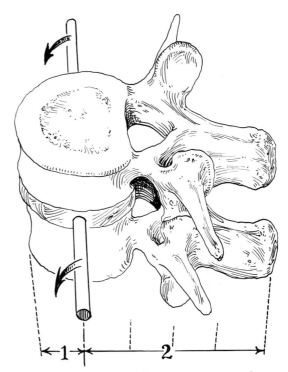

Figure 7–4. Spinal flexion injuries: mechanical considerations. Spinal flexion occurs about a fulcrum passing in the coronal axis through the center of the intervertebral disk, producing compression along *1* and distraction along *2*. Distance *2* is normally four times the length of distance *1*. If distances *1* and *2* are considered to represent lever arms pivoting about a fulcrum, the increased length of arm *2* affords it considerable mechanical advantage over *1*. Compression force brought to bear on the vertebral bodies anterior to the fulcrum (distance *1*) is therefore four times greater than the distraction force acting on the vertebral arch complex (distance *2*). Thus, pure flexion injury will produce compression fractures of the vertebral bodies long before distraction of the vertebral arch complex occurs.

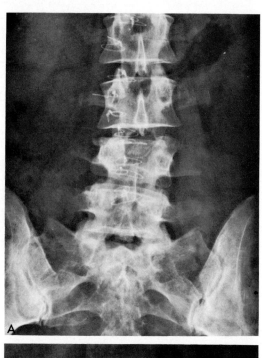

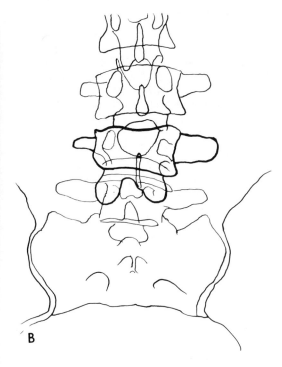

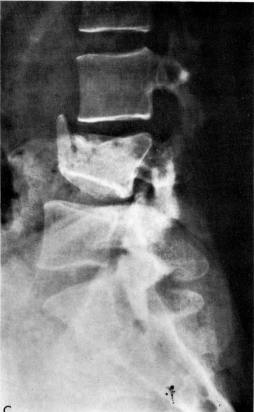

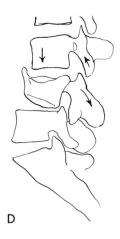

Figure 7–5. Hyperflexion fracture-dislocation at L-3/4 with compression of L-4 vertebral
body. *A, B,* Frontal view: The compressed
vertebral body of L-4 is heavily outlined on the
tracing. Note the interspinous gap at the L-3/4
level. *C, D,* Lateral view: Considerable compression deformity of L-4 vertebral body is readily
apparent. Less apparent but of greater clinical
significance is distraction of L-3/4 apophyseal
joints posteriorly (posterior arrows) and widening of the interspinous distance.

Illustration and legend continued on the following page.

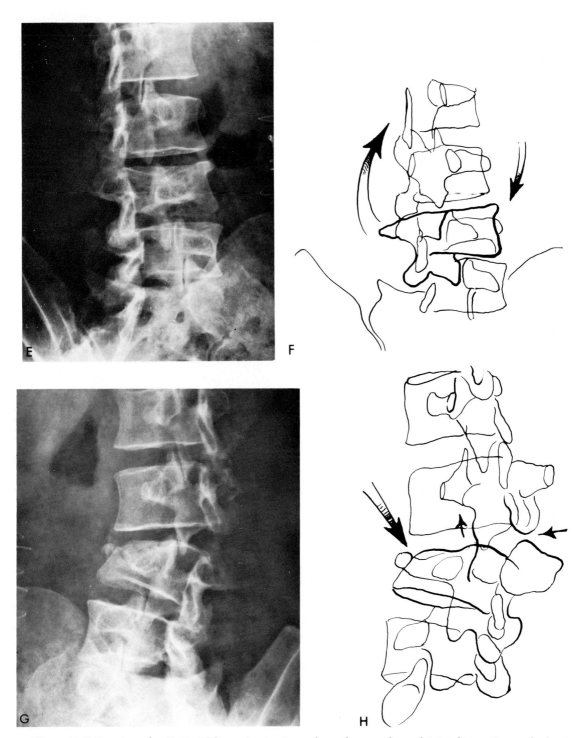

Figure 7–5 *Continued.* *E–H*, Oblique projections show the apophyseal joint distraction to the best advantage (small arrows) and confirm the presence of posterior ligament complex injury. (Large arrows indicate the direction of disruptive forces on the lumbar vertebrae).

Illustration and legend continued on the following page.

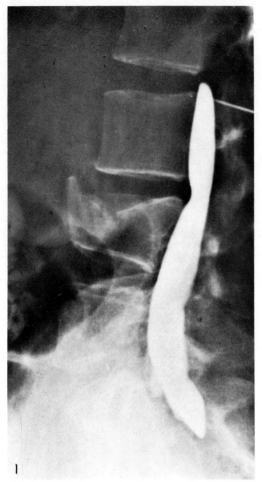

Figure 7–5 Continued. *I*, Myelogram of the same patient, cross-table lateral view: Posterior herniation of the injured intervertebral disk has occurred, compressing the dura at L-3/4.

one moves caudad from the thoracic to the lumbar spine, resulting in an added margin of safety for the nerve roots in traumatic disruption of the lumbar vertebral canal. Unfortunately, however, fracture-dislocations occur most commonly at the thoracolumbar junction where the vertebral canal is relatively less capacious[2] (as is true of thoracolumbar vertebral injuries in general). At this level, the conus medullaris of the spinal cord is vulnerable to injury.

Another cause of neurologic injury in thoracolumbar fracture-dislocations is compression of peripheral nerve roots in the intervertebral foramina between two dislocated vertebral segments.[13] Such injuries may be impossible to detect radiologically, as when soft tissues compress the roots within the intervertebral foramen. These soft tissues may include synovial lining or articular cartilage from the adjacent apophyseal joints. The intervertebral foramina are often difficult to project clearly on conventional radiographic views, especially in the presence of extensive bony and soft tissue injury in the immediate vicinity.

What determines the extent of neurologic damage in a given spinal injury? Several authors have observed that the extent of skeletal damage gives no indication of the degree of neurologic injury. Cord compression in vertebral fractures may result from edema, hematoma, or bone fragments compressing the spinal cord without obvious radiographic compromise of the vertebral canal.[7] A high incidence of paraplegia has been associated with rotary fracture-dislocations of the spine, which notoriously reduce themselves in the supine position to appear almost normal on the radiograph[9, 10] (Fig. 7–6). Jefferson has remarked on the ease with which completed fracture-dislocations of the vertebral column are reduced in patients who have been rendered "hopeless paraplegics," while less severely injured patients often prove much more difficult to reduce.[11] Böhler notes that in spinal fracture-dislocations, vertebral arch fractures may prove the salvation of the spinal cord rather than its destruction, for such fractures allow greater mobility to the cord when it is caught between two dislocated vertebral segments (Fig. 7–7). In Lob's experience, however, spinal fracture-dislocations with vertebral arch fractures are attended by such a severe degree of

to 70 per cent of all thoracolumbar fracture-dislocations, according to various authors.[12, 14, 20] This figure decreases to 15 per cent to 20 per cent when all fractures of the spine are included.[13, 18] Dislocation occurring below the level of L-2 is less likely to produce irreversible neurologic damage, as the spinal cord usually terminates at this level. Neurologic injuries sustained below the level of L-2, therefore, involve the peripheral nerve roots of the cauda equina; these have the capability for regeneration, unlike the spinal cord itself. Peripheral nerve roots possess greater tensile strength than the spinal medulla, and are more resistant to injury.[20] The dimensions of the vertebral canal are another factor in determining neurologic injury. They increase as

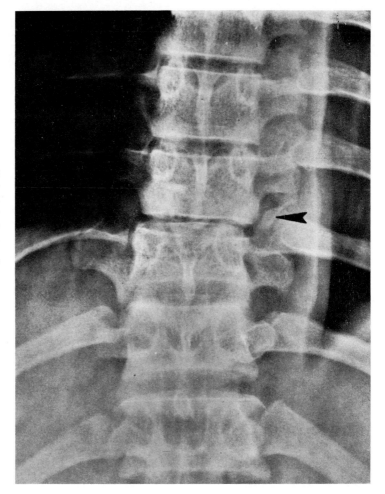

Figure 7–6. Self-reduction in a rotary fracture-dislocation at T-8/9. A severe rotary fracture-dislocation at T-8/9 has rendered this patient paraplegic. The dislocation is reduced in this antero-posterior supine view of the injured spine, so that only a subtle discrepancy in the alignment of the vertebral bodies, pedicles, and spinous processes (arrow) betrays the grave injury sustained.

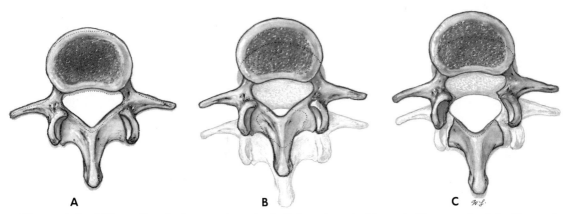

A   **B**   **C**

Figure 7–7. Effect of arch fracture in spinal dislocation. *A*, Normal. The vertebral bodies and arches are superimposed, and the vertebral canal is of normal dimensions. (The contours of the vertebra below are indicated in dotted lines). *B*, Spinal dislocation with intact vertebral arches. The vertebral canal has been severely compromised, with the spinal cord caught between the vertebral arch above the dislocation (in dark shading) and the posterior edge of the vertebral body below the dislocation (dotted lines) (in light shading) in a shearing compression injury. *C*, Spinal dislocation with fracture of the vertebral arch. The integrity of the vertebral canal and its contents has been maintained by "opening" of the fractured vertebral arch.

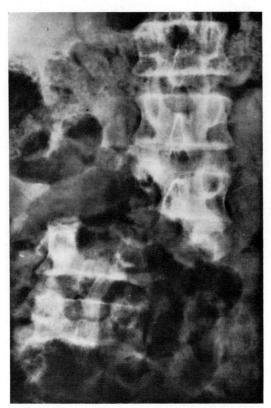

Figure 7–8. Severe lateral shear fracture-dislocation of L-3 on L-4. This lethal injury was sustained by a jeep-driver whose overturned vehicle fell on him. (Courtesy of J. A. Goree, M.D.).

violence that neurologic injury often occurs regardless.[13] Traumatic rupture of the anterior longitudinal ligament is very often associated with neurologic injury. This ligament may be ruptured by forward shearing injuries, markedly displacing vertebral bodies anteriorly or laterally (Fig. 7–8). Less frequently, it may be avulsed in hyperextension injury to the thoracolumbar spine, associated with paraplegia in a high percentage of cases[3] (see p. 347).

RADIOLOGIC DIAGNOSIS OF THORACOLUMBAR SPINE FRACTURE-DISLOCATIONS

Vertebral arches and processes are difficult to see on conventional radiographic views of the spine.[1, 13] In lateral projections only the vertebral bodies are plainly visible; for in the lumbar region four articular and two transverse processes overlap the arches

posteriorly, and in the thoracic spine overlying ribs add further to the confusion. Roentgen rays of sufficient intensity to penetrate the trunk usually blacken the film in the vicinity of the vertebral arches. (Lateral views of the spine should always be inspected over a bright light source to evaluate these structures.)[1]

These difficulties in interpreting conventional radiographs of the vertebral arch complex historically delayed understanding and diagnosis of injuries to this region. (Still today some appear to regard the spine as consisting merely of a column of vertebral bodies!)[1]

Aids to Diagnosis of Vertebral Arch Complex Injuries

1. Close inspection of the anteroposterior and lateral views. When a patient with a potentially unstable spinal injury is brought for radiologic examination, he will usually be immobilized in a supine position on a stretcher or frame. Anteroposterior (frontal) and cross-table lateral radiographs of the injured portion of the spine may then be obtained and studied with minimal disturbance of the patient's position. Depending on the radiographic findings, it may be elected to restrain the injured patient in the supine position for additional views, or to turn the patient for other views in order to complete the study.

In the presence of radiographic signs of injury to the vertebral arch complex on the anteroposterior and cross-table lateral views, *the patient should not be turned, but immobilized in the supine position.* Further views may then be obtained by angling the x-ray tube and film cassettes at 45° to the injured spine. On the other hand, if no signs of vertebral arch complex injury are found, and the back injury does not seem clinically severe, the patient may be moved for additional views at the discretion of the radiologist.

How should the radiographs be interpreted to determine whether or not to move the patient? Systematic inspection of the vetebral arches, processes, and apophyseal joints should be made on the available anteroposterior and lateral

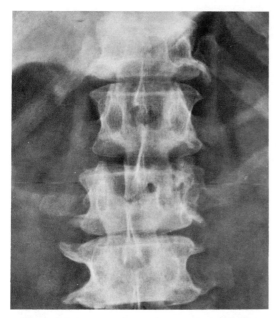

Figure 7–9. Apophyseal joint fracture-dislocation on anteroposterior view. Note spreading of right apophyseal joint and lateral displacement of left apophyseal joint consequent to superior articular process fracture in this patient with a rotary fracture-dislocation of L-1 on L-2.

views. The anteroposterior projection should be viewed as though regarding a transparent spine from behind. In cases of uncertainty, comparison of the radiographs with a skeleton will permit recognition of even minor traumatic changes in the posterior structures.

A. Careful scrutiny of the apophyseal joints is most important, as they are the most sensitive indicators of dislocation or unstable spinal injury. In such cases, they will appear fractured, displaced, or both (Fig. 7–9).

B. The alignment of the pedicles and spinous processes must be studied on the frontal view. Minimal discrepancy in the alignment of these structures at one level may be the only positive radiologic finding in a markedly unstable case of rotary fracture-dislocation of the vertebrae (Fig. 7–10).

C. The intervals between each spinous process must be compared, and, similarly, between each set of laminae. Increased intervals at one level are diagnostic of a tear of the posterior

ligament complex, and consequently of an unstable spinal injury (Fig. 7–11; see also Figs. 7–12, 7–14). Physical examination of the spine will confirm this finding; a gap will be palpable between the spinous processes, corresponding to the increased interval noted on the radiograph.[1]

D. The lateral view should be closely inspected over a bright light source. Compression fractures of the vertebral bodies will be obvious, but separation between spinous processes is often difficult to discern. Again, a gap between two spinous processes is diagnostic of a posterior ligamentous tear (see Fig. 7–12).

E. The distance between the posterior aspects of the vertebral bodies and the spinolaminar line represents the sa-

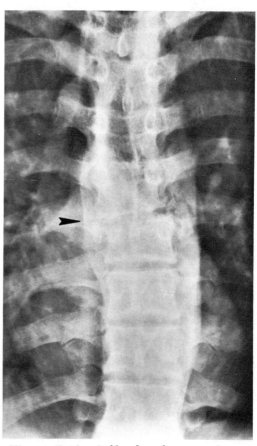

Figure 7–10. Self-reduced rotary fracture-dislocation of T-7 on T-8 on supine anteroposterior view (arrow). A slight discrepancy in alignment is the only clue to this severe spinal injury. (Cf. also Figure 7–6.)

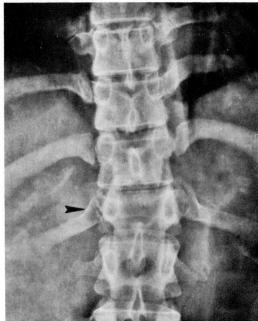

Figure 7–11. Increased interspinous interval in fracture-dislocation of the spine. Note the gap between the spinous processes of T-11 and T-12 (level of arrow) in this patient with rotary fracture-dislocation. The left apophyseal joint at the level of injury is spread. (Also see Figs. 7–12, 7–14.)

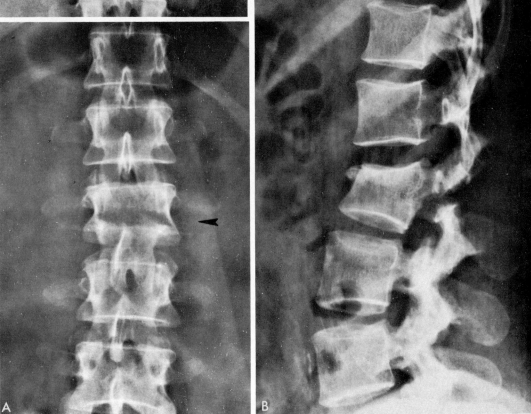

Figure 7–12. Posterior ligamentous tear in seat belt injury. *A,* Frontal view. Note the widening of the L-1/2 interspinous interval and the horizontal fractures of the L-2 pedicles and transverse processes (arrow), producing an "empty vertebra" appearance. These findings on a supine KUB film in an injured patient denote a severe unstable spinal fracture-dislocation which should not be moved. *B,* Lateral view. The anterior compression fracture of L-2 vertebral body is readily seen. Of greater clinical importance, however, is the posterior widening or gap between the L-1 and L-2 spinous processes, diagnostic of a posterior ligamentous tear. (This finding may be seen only when the film is inspected over a bright light source). Both pedicles of L-2 have been split in this seat belt fracture-dislocation of the Smith type. (See also p. 323.)

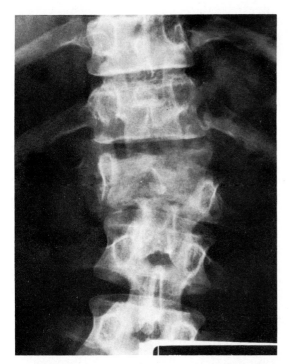

Figure 7–13. Vertebral arch fracture widening vertebral canal. Note increased interpedicular distance at L-1 vertebra in this patient with rotary fracture-dislocation of T-12 on L-1 and disruption of L-1 vertebral arch. Both apophyseal joints are grossly spread as well.

gittal diameter of the vertebral canal on the lateral view, and the interpedicular distance represents its coronal diameter on anteroposterior view. A vertebral arch fracture with separation of the fragments will produce a sudden increase in this diameter, when compared with the vertebral canal above and below the level of injury (Fig. 7–13).

2. Oblique projections of the spine, (first introduced in 1928) are often of considerable assistance in sorting out the confusing overlap of posterior shadows in the spine.[1] These may be obtained by positioning either the patient or the radiographic cassette at an angle to the tabletop. (Some distortion will result when the cassette is angled in this way, but the anatomic relationships remain clear.) Close correlation with a skeleton is of great help. The intervertebral foramina of the thoracic spine are usually best seen on routine lateral views. Occa-

sionally, however, they may be better seen by turning the patient 20° to either side of the true lateral position. The apophyseal joints and articular processes are often seen to best advantage in oblique views.

3. In the cervical spine, *occult views* (including 30° of caudal angulation of the central ray on supine positions) may be the only means of diagnosing some injuries to the vertebral arch.

4. Tomography of the spine is sometimes the best method for distinguishing between superimposed shadows, and should be resorted to promptly if conventional views suggest posterior injury but are not diagnostic (Fig. 7–14). Both anteroposterior and lateral tomographic cuts may be employed. Excellent bony detail may be secured by the use of hypocycloidal tomography if such is available.[4]

5. Myelography is indicated whenever the possibility of neurologic damage arises with spinal injuries. Extradural defects may be produced by edema, hematoma, fracture fragments, disk prolapse, or vertebral dislocation. Less commonly, hematoma formation within the spinal cord will produce an intramedullary mass. A detailed discussion of these topics is beyond the scope of this book.

CLASSIFICATION OF THORACOLUMBAR FRACTURE-DISLOCATIONS

The following classification of fracture-dislocations of the thoracolumbar spine is offered in the hope that it will prove simple but thorough (Table 7–1). Acknowledgment is made to the classifications devised by Böhler,[1] Kaufer and Hayes,[12] Holdsworth,[9, 10] Nicoll,[14] and Rogers.[16]

Hyperflexion fracture-dislocations are characterized as flexion injuries in which anterior compression fractures are associated with distraction injuries of the vertebral arch complex, involving bone (fractures) or the interosseous ligaments (avulsions or dislocations). Seat belt injuries have been excluded from the general category of hyperflexion fracture-dislocations because of their distinctive mechanism of injury (anterior displacement

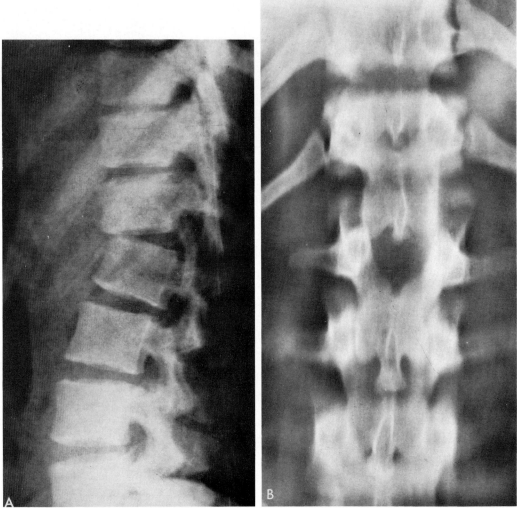

Figure 7–14. Tomographic confirmation of posterior injury. *A,* Posterior ligamentous injury is suggested on the lateral view of this patient with hyperflexion fracture-dislocation, but detail is obscured by technical factors. *B,* Tomographic section through the vertebral arches in the coronal plane readily confirms distraction of the apophyseal joints, with increased space between the laminae and spinous processes at the T-12/L-1 level.

TABLE 7–1. Thoracolumbar Fracture-Dislocations

TYPE OF INJURY	VERTEBRAL BODIES	VERTEBRAL ARCHES
Hyperflexion	A. Compression fracture of body above injury B. Compression fracture of body below injury	A. Separation of arches (with or without avulsion fractures of spinous process) B. Same as "A"
Seat belt injuries	A. Slight compression B. Slight compression, ("avulsion fracture") C. Horizontal body fracture ("fissure fracture")	A. Separation of arches B. Arch fracture (Smith; chance) C. Arch fracture
Rotary fracture-dislocation	A. Slice fracture through cranial end-plate body below injury B. Rupture of intervertebral disk bond	A. Dislocation of apophyseal joints B. Fractures through apophyseal joints C. Fracture of one joint, dislocation of other
Shear fracture-dislocation	Forward shear fracture through vertebral body Shear-induced rupture of disk bond	A. Dislocation of apophyseal joints B. Fractures through apophyseal joints C. Arch fracture (pars, pedicles)
Hyperextension fracture-dislocation	A. Distraction rupture of disk bond B. Fission fracture of body C. Bodies intact	A. Arches intact B. Arches intact C. Compression fracture of arches and articular processes

of the fulcrum) and the high associated incidence of visceral injury. Those spinal fracture-dislocations with strong rotary and forward shear components involved in the mechanism of injury make up further distinctive subgroups within the general category of hyperflexion fracture-dislocations. Hyperextension fracture-dislocations are the result of quite a different mechanism of injury. Although they are relatively rare in the thoracolumbar spine, they too damage the vertebral arch complex and result in vertebral dislocation and neurologic injury.

HYPERFLEXION FRACTURE-DISLOCATION

Hyperflexion fracture-dislocation may be defined as an injury deforming the vertebral column in flexion about a fulcrum through the nucleus pulposus of the intervertebral disk, producing distraction of the vertebral arch complex. Slight axial (rotary) torsion or forward shear forces may play a role in producing the injury,[15] but are not of such magnitude as to significantly alter the characteristic hyperflexion deformity.

Hyperflexion fracture-dislocations described in the earlier literature were frequently the result of falling from a height, or of compression injuries to the vertebral column from above. Many miners trapped beneath rock-falls or in tunnel cave-ins sustained this type of injury (Fig. 7–15). More recently, however, an increasing number of hyperflexion fracture-dislocations are seen in automobile trauma, when the exact mechanism of injury is often difficult to clarify (especially if the patient is thrown from the vehicle).

These injuries compress the vertebral column anteriorly and distract it posteriorly

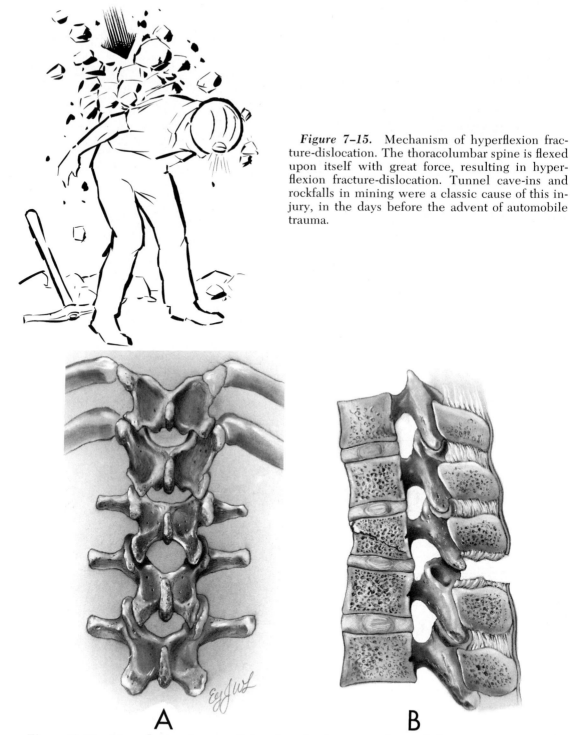

Figure 7–15. Mechanism of hyperflexion fracture-dislocation. The thoracolumbar spine is flexed upon itself with great force, resulting in hyperflexion fracture-dislocation. Tunnel cave-ins and rockfalls in mining were a classic cause of this injury, in the days before the advent of automobile trauma.

A   B

Figure 7–16. Hyperflexion fracture-dislocation. In this type of spinal fracture-dislocation the vertebral column is compressed anteriorly and distracted posteriorly. *A*, Posterior view. Widening of the gap between the laminae and spinous processes is present at the L-2/3 level. *B*, Sagittal section of spine, seen laterally. An anterior compression fracture of the vertebra above the dislocation extends almost, but not quite, to the posterior cortex of the vertebral body. Posteriorly, the apophyseal joints have been avulsed, with their capsules, and the ligamenta flava, interspinous and supraspinous ligaments (posterior ligament complex) have all been torn between the L-2 and L-3 vertebral arches.

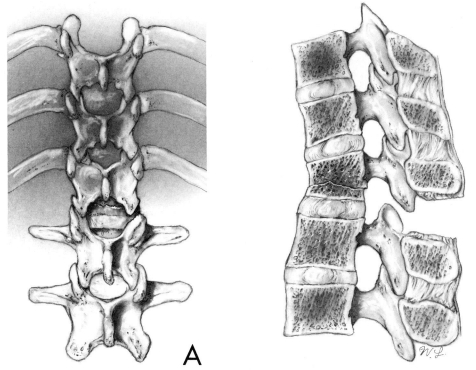

Figure 7–17. Hyperflexion fracture-dislocation. *A*, Posterior section. Similar to Figure 7–16 except that the vertebral body fracture extends through the posterior cortex, where it may be seen under the distracted vertebral arch of T-12. *B*, On lateral section, note the complete vertebral body fracture. The posterior injury is one of pure distractive dislocation, as in Figure 7–16.

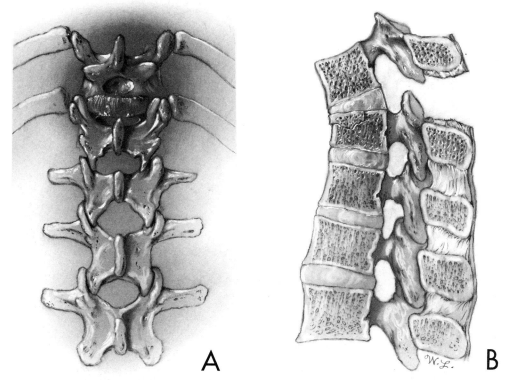

Figure 7–18. Hyperflexion fracture-dislocation. *A*, Posterior view. The posterior aspect of the T-11 intervertebral disk has been exposed by distraction of the vertebral arches. *B*, Lateral section. In this case it is the vertebral body below the level of dislocation that has sustained a compression fracture.

(Figs. 7–16, 7–17, 7–18). The anterior compression fractures of the vertebral bodies that result are no different from the compression fractures discussed in the previous chapter. They tend to be more severe, with fractures of the vertebral end-plates and penetration of disk material vertically into the body, often with comminution of the body on the radiograph. Posteriorly, distraction of the posterior ligament complex produces radiographic diastasis or separation of the vertebral arches and their spinous processes. In some cases, fragments of the spinous process may be avulsed along with tearing of the ligaments. Rupture of the posterior ligaments is often complete, so that at surgery, when the skin and subcutaneous tissues of the back have been incised, the next intact layer of tissues to be encountered is the dura mater of the spinal cord.[12]

On physical examination of the back, a palpable gap between the spinous processes at the level of injury is the most reliable sign of distraction of the vertebral arch complex. Localized tenderness, soft tissue swelling and ecchymosis, and a gibbus deformity of the spine may be noted as well. When the injury is indirect, the blow producing the spinal fracture-dislocation has landed at a distance from the fracture site. In such cases, a bruise may be found over the upper part of the back or neck, where force was applied to the vertebral column.[9] It must always be remembered that disruption of the vertebral arch complex implies a clinically unstable spinal injury, and these patients must be immobilized or managed in such a way that further trauma to the vertebral column is prevented.

The radiologic diagnosis of hyperflexion fracture-dislocation depends on identification of the posterior injury, for compression fractures of the vertebral bodies anteriorly are usually easy to see. The spinous processes and pedicles should be closely inspected on the frontal view. Normally, the pedicles cast paired, smooth, oval shadows aligned vertically to either side of the midline, while the spinous processes appear like a row of teardrops in the midline.[16] Fractures through the vertebral arch will appear as clefts through these structures, and their smooth outer contours will be disrupted. These changes are made clear by comparing the fractured spinous processes and pedicles with intact ones above and below the level of injury.

On the other hand, when a posterior ligamentous tear has spared the bony structures, the interspinous distance will be increased at the level of injury when compared with normal intervals above and below. The space between the laminae of the vertebral arches is also enlarged on the frontal view, when compared with normal spaces above and below the injury (Figs. 7–5A, 7–14, 7–19, 7–20).

On the lateral view, the existence of a fracture-dislocation may be confirmed by careful inspection of the spinous processes and vertebral arches (Figs. 7–5C, 7–19, 7–20). Examination of the film over a bright light source is usually required to do this effectively. Fractures involving the spinous processes, or an increased interspinous distance at the level of injury, may then be confirmed. Further evaluation by means of oblique views and tomograms may be obtained if desired.

SEAT BELT INJURIES

Seat belt injuries differ from the more usual hyperflexion fracture-dislocations of the vertebral column. While hyperflexion injuries pivot about a fulcrum through the intervertebral disk, seat belt injuries pivot about a fulcrum situated at the anterior abdominal wall, where the lap seat belt makes contact with the body in vehicular deceleration (Fig. 7–21), if a cross-body belt is not worn simultaneously. The fulcrum of injury is thus displaced ventrally (Fig. 7–22). This injury usually selects the upper to mid-lumbar spine (L-2, 3, or 4), owing to the position in which lap seat belts are usually worn, being fastened about the lower abdomen over the thighs. A similar injury may result without a seat belt in rapid vehicular deceleration, if a passenger riding in the hind seat is thrown violently forward over the back of the front seat, forcing the body into acute flexion. Any injury in which the body is hurled forward against a horizontal object, such as a railing, fence, or the limb of a tree, may produce the same result.[16]

The spinal injury produced in this way differs from all other spinal injuries in that it is a pure distraction or tension injury—the vertebral column is literally "pulled apart."[19] Compression fractures of the vertebral bodies anteriorly are minimal or absent, as the axis of flexion is completely anterior

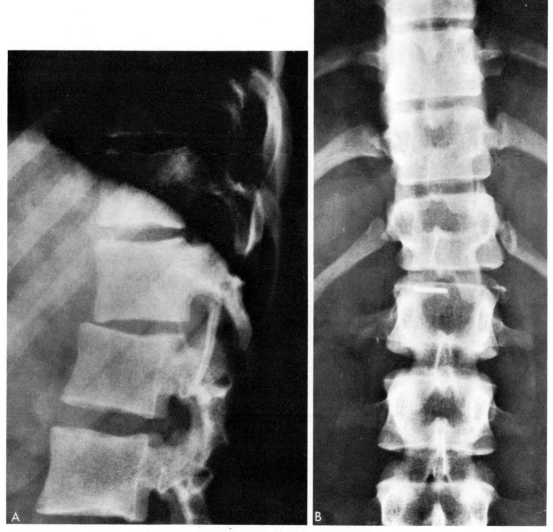

Figure 7-19. Hyperflexion fracture-dislocation. *A*, On lateral view, slight vertebral malalignment may be noted, with a reduced intervertebral disk space, at T-12/L-1 level. *B*, On frontal view, widening of the space between the laminae and spinous processes of T-12 and L-1 (at metallic clip) confirms the presence of posterior ligamentous injury. (Courtesy of Dr. Robert H. Freiberger, Hospital for Special Surgery, New York, N.Y.)

to the vertebral column. These fracture-dislocations fall into two categories:

1. Posterior ligament avulsions, in which the posterior ligament complex is avulsed. This may occur as a pure dislocation, in which the apophyseal joints, posterior longitudinal ligament, and intervertebral disk are disrupted without any bony injury (Fig. 7-23, 7-24) or may be associated with avulsion fractures of the articular processes and posterior fragments of the vertebral bodies at the

level of injury (Fig. 7-25). As noted earlier, disruption of the posterior ligamentous complex is more likely to occur when an element of rotational force is introduced in the injury; such injuries tend to be clinically unstable, and may require internal fixation for satisfactory immobilization.[19] Posterior ligament avulsions are more apt to occur in younger patients, as the bones are more resilient in youth, and the vertebral arch is therefore less subject to distraction or

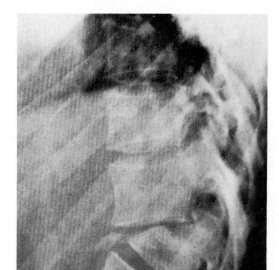

Figure 7–20. Hyperflexion fracture-dislocation. A, Lateral view indicates a more severe vertebral body fracture than Figure 7–19, with wedge deformity resulting from hyperflexion and considerable posterior displacement of the injured vertebral body into the vertebral canal. B, Frontal view demonstrates interspinous widening indicative of posterior distraction injury, and a widened interpedicular distance resulting from vertebral arch fracture.

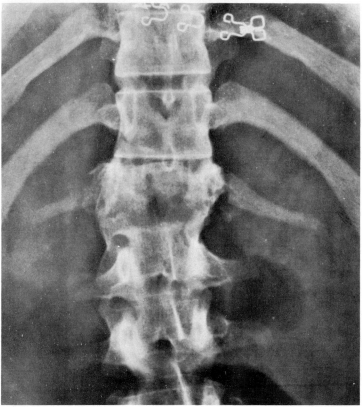

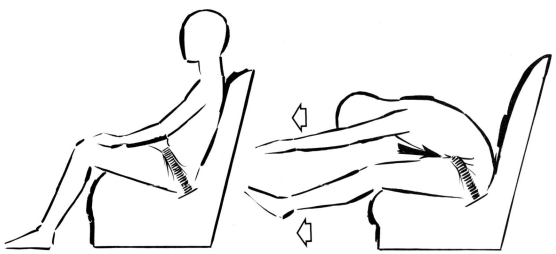

Figure 7–21. Mechanism of seat belt injury. The body is thrown forward against the restraining lap seat belt in rapid vehicular deceleration when a cross-body belt is not worn, producing fracture dislocation of the lumbar spine. Any injury in which the body is hurled forward against a horizontal object may produce the same result.

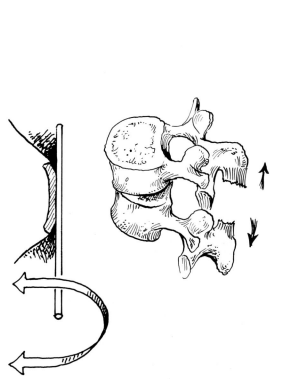

Figure 7–22. Fulcrum displacement in seat belt injury. Normally, the axis of spinal flexion is centered through the interval disk (compare Fig. 7–4). In seat belt injury, however, this fulcrum of flexion is displaced ventrally to the anterior abdominal wall, where the lap seat belt restrains the torso in rapid deceleration. The force of injury on the spine is thus converted from a combination of compression and distraction to one more nearly representing pure distraction (arrows) (After Smith and Kaufer).

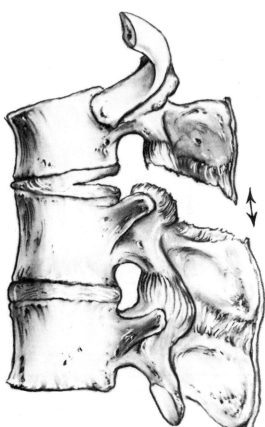

Figure 7–23. Seat belt injury: pure dislocation. The posterior ligament complex has been disrupted, producing a distraction injury between two vertebral arches (arrows). The apophyseal joint capsules have been avulsed, and the posterior longitudinal ligament and intervertebral disk disrupted as well. These injuries are more likely to occur in younger individuals.

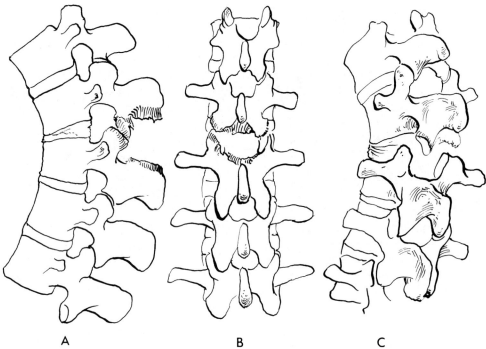

Figure 7-24. Seat belt injury: pure dislocation. Posterior distraction of the vertebral arches in seat belt injury is diagrammed in (A) lateral view, (B) posterior view, (C) posterior oblique view, resulting from disruption of the posterior ligament complex. This injury is more apt to occur in younger patients, and is often associated with rotary force to the spine. (After Smith and Kaufer).

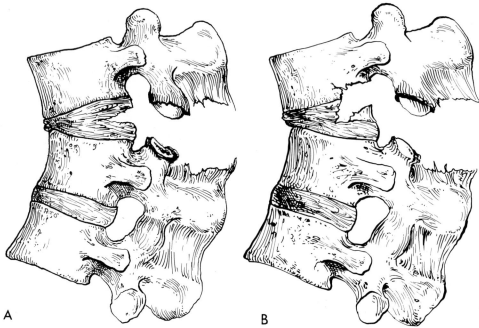

Figure 7-25. Posterior ligamentous disruption. The distraction force exerted on the spine in seat belt injury may dislocate the vertebrae posteriorly by rending the posterior ligament complex, avulsing an articular process (A) or a small posteroinferior corner of the vertebral body (B) in the process.

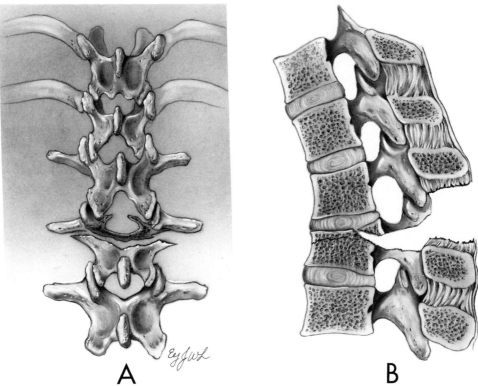

A   **B**

Figure 7–26. Posterior dislocation with avulsion fractures ("Smith fracture"). *A*, Posterior view. A widened interspinous interval indicates tearing of the posterior ligament complex. Note the horizontal fracture through the transverse processes, pedicles, and superior aspect of the vertebral arch. *B*, Lateral section. The supraspinous and interspinous ligaments have been avulsed posteriorly. More anteriorly, the superior articular process and a posterior vertebral body fragment have been separated by avulsion fracture.

"fissure" fracture than it would be in the older patient.

2. Posterior distraction fracture of the vertebral arch, in which avulsion forces acting on the vertebral arch produce a more or less horizontal fracture of the vertebral arch. Three variants of this injury may occur: (1) the Smith fracture, in which a small posterior fragment of the vertebral body and the superior articular processes are included with the arch fracture. The spinous process remains intact, and rupture of the interspinous and supraspinous ligaments occurs instead (Fig. 7–26). (2) When the fracture line extends posteriorly through the spinous process, this injury becomes the Chance fracture, consisting of a "horizontal splitting of the spine and neural arch, ending in an upward curve which usually reaches the upper surface of the body just in front of the neural foramen," described by G. Q. Chance in 1948. Horizontal fissuring of

the laminae, pedicles, and transverse processes is associated. Chance's original injury exhibited a slight anterior compression fracture of the vertebral body as well (Fig. 7–27).[5] (3) The most extensive fracture of these three variants is the horizontal fissure fracture (sometimes mistakenly described as a Chance fracture), in which the horizontal arch fracture, is extended anteriorly through the vertebral body to produce a complete transverse fissuring or splitting of the vertebra, opening posteriorly (Figs. 7–28, 7–29). Increased bony brittleness of the vertebral arch in older patients makes them more subject to this type of fracture.

As the abdomen and its contents are interposed between the fulcrum of injury and the spine, the possibility of coexisting abdominal trauma in these patients must always be borne in mind. Significant abdominal soft tissue injuries oc-

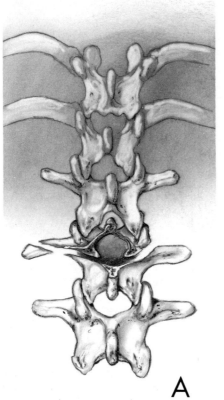
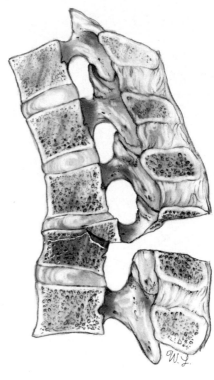

A

B

Figure 7–27. Chance fracture. G.Q. Chance's original fracture, as described in 1948, consisted of "a horizontal splitting of the spine and neural arch, ending in an upward curve which usually reaches the upper surface of the body just in front of the neural foramen."[4] *A*, Posterior view. The fissure involves the superior portion of the spinous process, laminae, pedicles, and transverse processes (here showing unilateral transverse process involvement.) *B*, Lateral section. A slight anterior compression fracture of the vertebral body is associated.

curred with 15 per cent of these spinal fracture-dislocations in one series.[16] Such injuries have included ruptures or tears of the duodenum, distal small bowel, colon, spleen, pancreas, gravid uterus, and the musculature of the anterior abdominal wall. These injuries may pose a more immediate hazard to the patient than the spinal fracture-dislocation itself.[6]

On clinical examination of patients with this type of spinal injury, the findings are those of hyperflexion fracture-dislocation discussed previously. In addition, however (and especially when a clear history of the injury is not forthcoming), the finding of bruising or ecchymosis over the anterior abdominal wall should suggest the possibility of a seat-belt injury, and a careful investigation for possible blunt abdominal trauma should follow. Spinal neurologic injury has been noted in 15 per cent of patients injured in this manner.[16] This is considerably less than the incidence of neurologic injury noted with spinal fracture-dislocations in general (53 to 70 per cent), and may result from the greater distance between the vertebral canal and the point of impact of the injury.

The radiographic findings in seat-belt injuries involve the vertebral arch complex, as discussed with hyperflexion fracture-dislocations. The subtypes described previously may be recognized, the posterior ligamentous complex avulsions, or the posterior distraction fractures involving the vertebral arch. As the

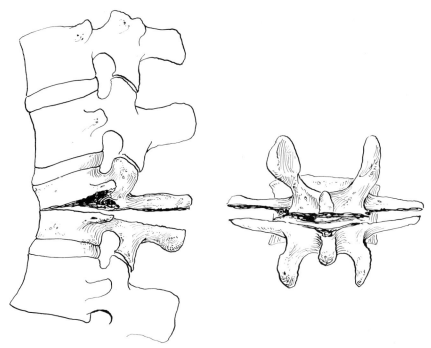

Figure 7–28. Seat belt injury: horizontal "fissure" fracture. A pure distraction injury, this fracture splits the vertebra horizontally, opening it posteriorly as one would open the covers of a book. The posterior ligament complex remains essentially intact. (After Smith and Kaufer.)

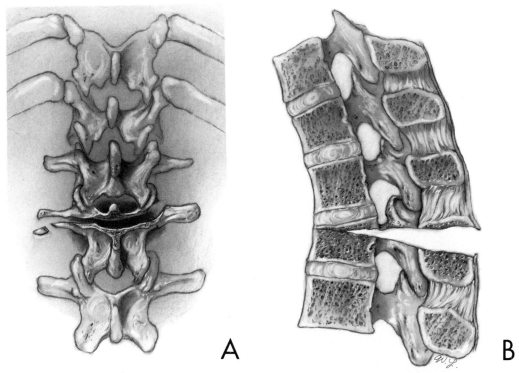

Figure 7–29. Seat belt injury: horizontal "fissure" fracture. *A*, Posterior view. The vertebral arch is horizontally split, including spinous process, superior laminae, pedicles, and both transverse processes. *B*, Lateral section: As the injury is primarily one of distraction, no anterior compression of the vertebral bodies is associated. Note intact ligaments.

vertebral column injury is essentially distractive, anterior compression fractures of the vertebral bodies are minimal or absent.

On the frontal view, the pedicles and spinous processes must be scrutinized for fractures, dislocations, or malalignment. Separation and elevation of a vertebral arch may give an empty or vacant appearance to an involved vertebral body[16] when compared with others above and below (Fig. 7–12). Fracture lines passing obliquely or transversely through the transverse processes should always alert the observer to the possibility of a fractured vertebral arch. Confirmation of the distraction injury may be made on the lateral view (Figs. 7–30, 7–31). In the event of abdominal trauma, a full-sized KUB film of the abdomen should be included with the spine study. This should be carefully inspected for free air or fluid in the peritoneal cavity, abnormalities of the bowel gas pattern, or other evidence of significant abdominal soft tissue injury. Contrast studies of the gastrointestinal or genitourinary tracts may be required for further evaluation if necessary.[6]

ROTARY FRACTURE-DISLOCATIONS

Rotary fracture-dislocations result from a rotary or torsion force applied about the long axis of the vertebral column. They are usually associated with a hyperflexion injury resulting from vertical loading or compression of the thoracolumbar spine from above. A blow falling on the shoulder blade

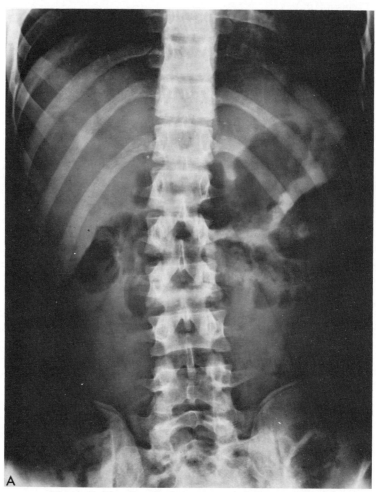

Figure 7–30. Seat belt injury. *A*, Abdominal film.
Illustration and legend continued on the opposite page.

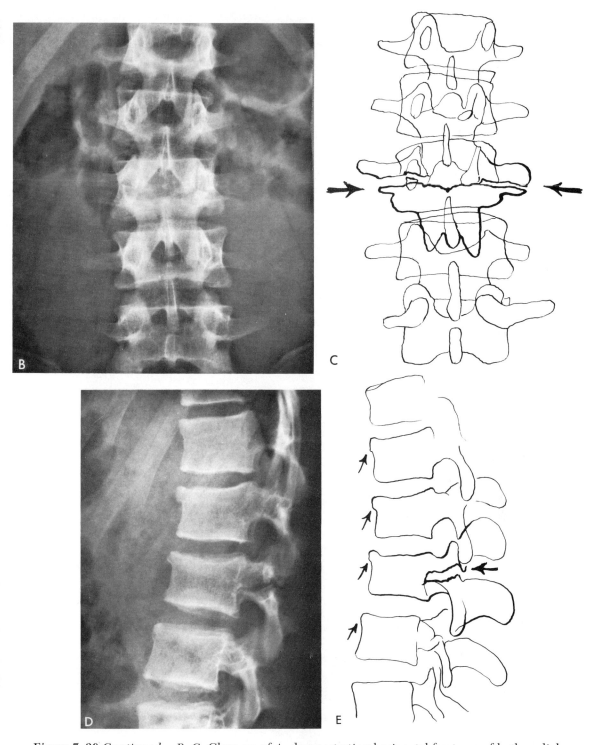

Figure 7–30 Continued. B, C, Close-up of A, demonstrating horizontal fractures of both pedicles and transverse processes of L-3 vertebra (arrows). Minimal widening of the L-2/3 interspinous gap may be appreciated when compared with similar intervals above and below; this finding denotes posterior ligament complex rupture and a potentially unstable spinal injury. D, E, Lateral view, with horizontal fracture of pedicles and vertebral arch of L-3 (large arrow), and minimal anterior compression fractures of several lumbar vertebral bodies (small arrows).

Illustration and legend continued on the following page.

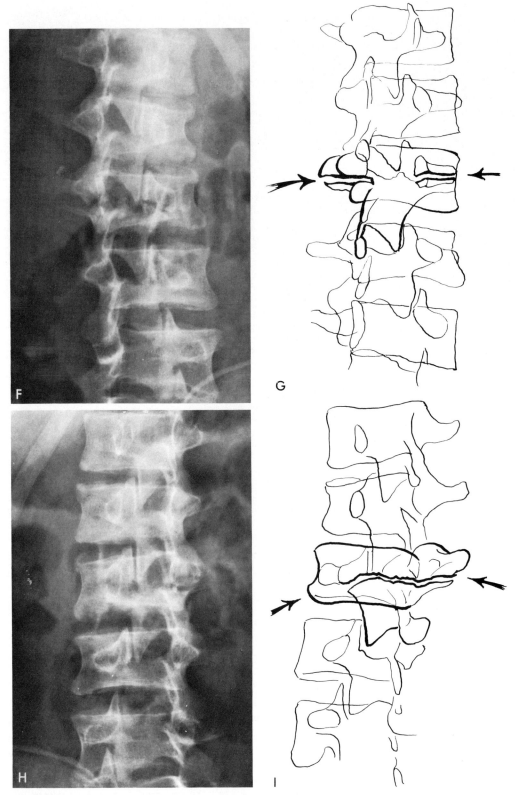

Figure 7–30 *Continued.* *F–I,* Oblique views demonstrating the vertebral arch fractures (arrows) to better advantage.

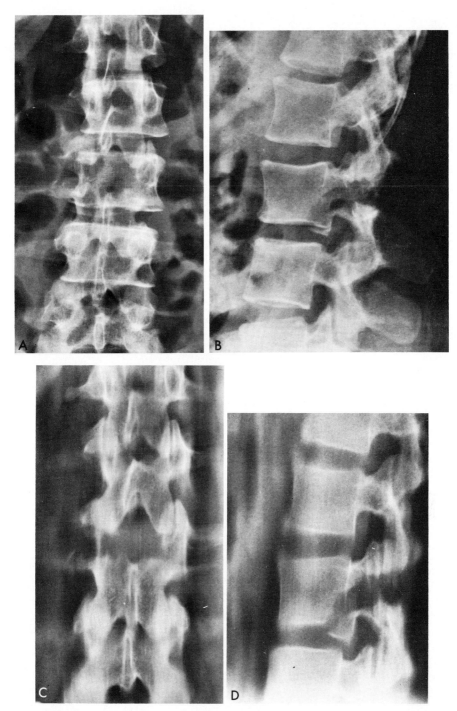

Figure 7–31. Seat belt injury. *A,* Frontal view: The right pedicle of L-3 vertebra has been fractured transversely, and the left pars interarticularis of L-3 has been fractured as well. A gap between the spinous processes at this level indicates that rupture of the posterior ligament complex has occurred. ("Smith fracture"). *B,* Lateral view: The fracture line passes through the pedicles and pars interarticularis region, with avulsion of a posterior fragment of the vertebral body. The injury continues posterior to the fracture as a tear of the posterior ligament complex, with separation of the spinous processes. *C,* Tomographic cut of *A.* Note the interlaminar gap at the level of injury, with separation of the spinous processes. The fracture extends horizontally through the transverse process. *D,* Tomographic cut of *B,* showing the fracture line more clearly. Note the absence of vertebral body compression in comparison with Figure 7–30*D,* indicating this injury to be more purely distractive in origin. (Courtesy of Dr. Robert H. Freiberger, Hospital for Special Surgery, New York, N.Y.).

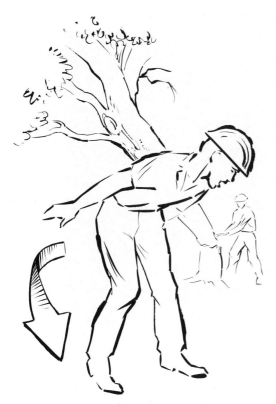

Figure 7–32. Mechanism of rotary fracture-dislocation. The torso is deflected laterally at the same time that the spine is compressed from above, bending and simultaneously rotating the thoracolumbar spine about its long axis.

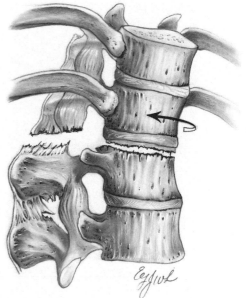

Figure 7–33. Rotary fracture-dislocation, anterolateral view. The direction of the rotary force of injury is indicated by the curved arrow, about the long axis of the vertebral column. A "slice" fracture involves the cranial end-plate of L-1 vertebral body anteriorly, and the posterior ligament complex has been torn by the rotary injury.

may compress the vertebral column while deflecting the torso laterally to produce such an injury (Fig. 7–32).[9, 10] Roaf[15] has demonstrated that the posterior ligament complex is readily ruptured in this manner, with dislocation or fracture of the apophyseal joints (Figs. 7–33 to 7–36). Rotary fracture-dislocations are among the most clinically unstable of all the thoracolumbar spinal injuries, and they are attended by a very high incidence of neurologic damage.[9, 10] Clinically, a bruise or skin injury over the scapular region may alert the examiner to the possibility of an indirect rotary injury to the spine.[11]

Radiologically, rotary fracture-dislocations may be deceptive, as they show a sinister tendency to self-reduction when the patient is immobilized in the supine position, often making the correct diagnosis extremely difficult.[8, 9] The vertebral arches essentially return to their normal positions. A small discrepancy in the alignment of the pedicles and spinous processes on the fron-

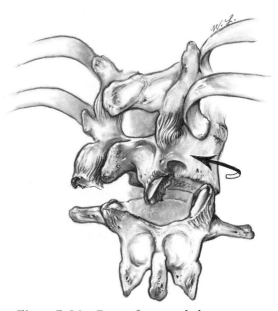

Figure 7–34. Rotary fracture-dislocation, posterior view. The direction of the rotary force of injury is indicated by the curved arrow. The posterior ligament complex has been avulsed at the T-12/L-1 level, and normal alignment of the spinous processes has been disrupted. The apophyseal joints have also been disrupted with distraction on the right, and fracture-dislocation on the left (not clearly seen in this drawing).

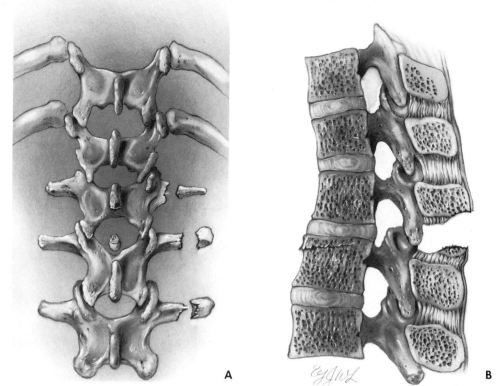

Figure 7–35. Rotary fracture-dislocation. *A*, Posterior view: Rotational deformity has been reduced, so that the spinous processes are in normal alignment. Unilateral fracture of several transverse processes attests to the rotary mechanism of injury, however. A small avulsion of the spinous process on L-1 has resulted from hyperflexion. *B*, Lateral section: Note the characteristic "slice fracture" through the cranial end-plate of the injured vertebral body. Posteriorly, rotation and distraction have disrupted the apophyseal joints and avulsed the posterior ligament complex, with a small fragment of the spinous process above.

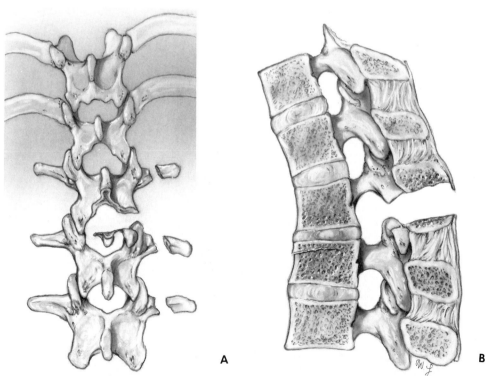

Figure 7–36. Rotary fracture-dislocation. This fracture-dislocation is similar to Figure 7–35, except that one inferior articular process has been fractured and a larger segment of the spinous process above has been avulsed. Again, multiple transverse process fractures limited to one side indicate a rotary mechanism of injury.

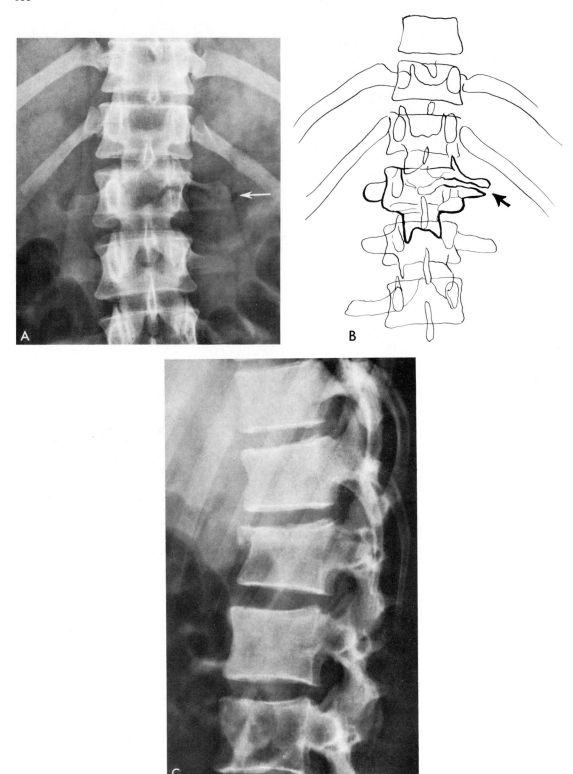

Figure 7–37. Rotary fracture-dislocation. *A, B,* Frontal view: Unilateral fracture of the transverse process and pedicle of L-1 vertebra (arrow) suggests a rotary mechanism of injury, as does the distraction of the opposite apophyseal joint at T-12/L-1. *C,* Lateral view: Anterior "slice" fracture of the cranial end-plate L-1 vertebral body, often seen with rotary fracture-dislocations.

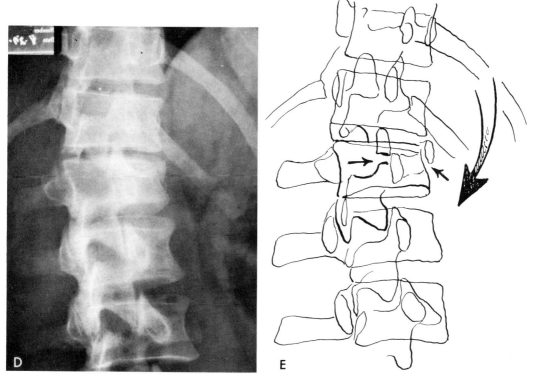

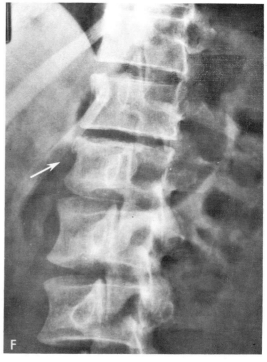

Figure 7–37 Continued. D, E, Right anterior oblique view confirms pedicle and transverse process fracture of L-1 on the left (small arrows). Large arrow indicates the direction of disruptive force on the vertebral column. *F,* Left anterior oblique view confirms distraction of apophyseal joints between T-12 and L-1 on the right. Arrow indicates "slice" fracture fragment of L-1 vertebral body.

tal view may provide the only clue to the existence of this severe injury. Great care must, therefore, be taken to confirm the normal radiographic alignment of these struc-

tures before allowing the patient to be moved for additional views! (Figs. 7–6, 7–10). Oblique or horizontal fractures of the transverse processes may also suggest rotary injury to the vertebral arch complex, especially if they are confined to one side.[1] (Fig. 7–37).

Posterior changes may also be difficult to appreciate on the lateral view if the injury has reduced itself. The apophyseal joints should be closely inspected for dislocation, fracture of the articular processes, or both together (Fig. 7–38). An anterior "slice" fracture through the cranial end-plate of the vertebral body at or just below the level of injury is a characteristic finding in rotary fracture-dislocations. The cranial portion of the injured body is often displaced slightly forward or laterally with respect to the remainder (Figs. 7–37, 7–39, 7–40, 7–41). Alternatively, rupture of the intervertebral disk bond may occur, as in shear fracture-dislocations (Fig. 7–38).

SHEAR FRACTURE-DISLOCATIONS

Shear fracture-dislocations occur with subjection of the thoracolumbar vertebral column to a forward shearing force, displacing the upper vertebrae anteriorly on the lower at the level of injury. Such a force is transmitted horizontally, usually as a blow from behind (Fig. 7–42). This type of dislocation is more common in the thoracic than in the lumbar spine.[9, 10] As with rotary or torsional injuries, the posterior ligament complex is more easily disrupted by forward shearing force than by pure hyperflexion.[15]

Shear fracture-dislocations are of two types: those in which the vertebral arch remains intact, and those in which the arch is fractured (*traumatic spondylolisthesis*).

SHEAR FRACTURE-DISLOCATIONS WITH INTACT VERTEBRAL ARCH. This injury occurs with overriding of the apophyseal joints, with either dislocation or fractures of the articular processes. The anterior longitudinal ligament is torn or severely stretched, and vertebral body fracture or shearing of the intervertebral disk bond completes the injury, allowing anterior displacement of the vertebral column (Fig. 7–43). In cases in which the articular processes remain intact, locking of the articular processes at the level of injury may result

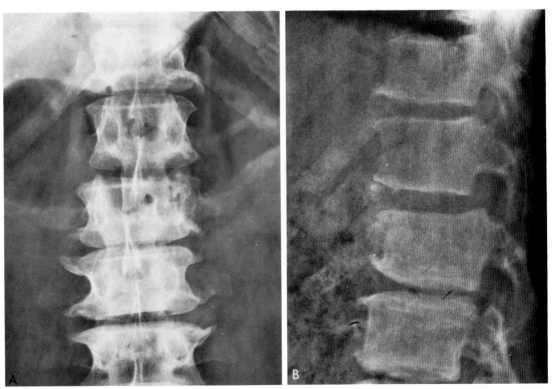

Figure 7–38. Rotary fracture-dislocation. *A*, Frontal view. The right apophyseal joint at L-1/2 is dislocated; the left apophyseal joint has been fractured through the superior articular process of L-2 vertebra. (Same case as Fig. 7–11.) *B*, Lateral view. L-1 vertebra has been rotated and displaced anteriorly on L-2.

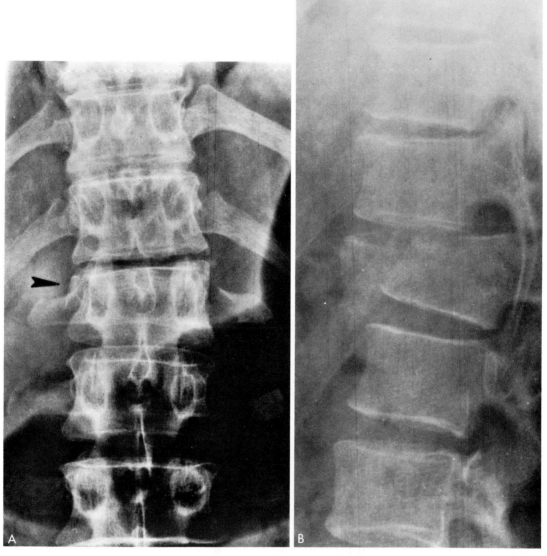

Figure 7–39. Rotary fracture-dislocation. *A*, Frontal view. Minimal changes are present to suggest the severity of spinal injury. A fragment of the L-1 vertebral body has been avulsed (arrow) and the T-12 intervertebral disk space is narrowed. Transverse process fractures of L-1 and L-2 are present on the left only, suggesting rotary injury. *B*, Lateral view: Severe dislocation is revealed at the T-12 L-1 level, with a "slice" fracture through L-1 vertebral body.

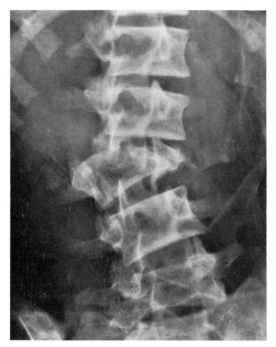

Figure 7–40. Rotary fracture-dislocation. The radiologic findings in rotary fracture-dislocation are not always subtle. Note gross dislocation, vertebral arch fracture at L-3, and transverse process avulsions.

from the displacement. These dislocations may require open surgery for successful reduction. A shearing stress is applied to the spinal cord at the level of injury when the vertebral arch remains intact (Fig. 7–44). The cord is pinched between the arch of the anteriorly displaced vertebra above and the body of the stationary vertebra below, resulting in a high incidence of neurologic injury.[1]

TRAUMATIC SPONDYLOLISTHESIS. In these fracture-dislocations, fractures of the vertebral arch accompany forward shear displacement of the vertebral column. The arch fractures widen the vertebral canal at the level of injury, allowing greater mobility to the spinal cord or cauda equina when they are caught between the two dislocated vertebral segments (Figs. 7–44, 7–45). Böhler writes: "Fractures of the arch . . . signify not a destruction but a salvation of

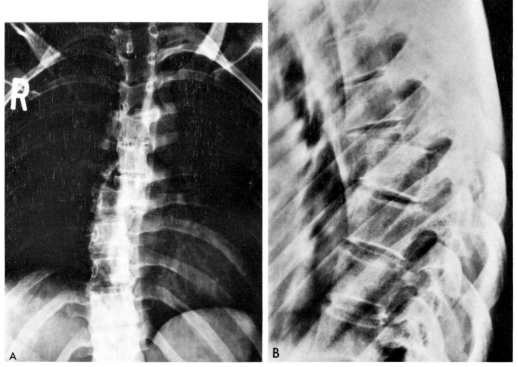

Figure 7–41. Rotary fracture-dislocation involving the thoracic spine. *A,* Frontal view: A severe automobile accident has dislocated the thoracic spine. Such dislocations occur more frequently in the cervical or lumbar spine than in the thoracic, where the ribs and intercostal muscles act to stabilize the vertebral column against injury. *B,* Lateral view: A rotary mechanism of injury has disrupted the thoracic vertebral column.

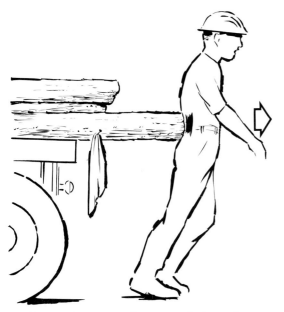

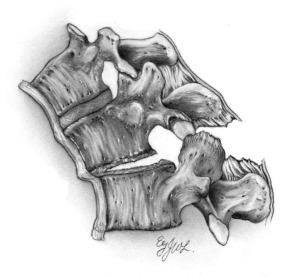

Figure 7–42. Mechanism of shear fracture dislocation. A shearing force displaces the upper spine anteriorly upon the lower, usually transmitted as a horizontal blow from behind.

Figure 7–43. Shear fracture-dislocation with intact vertebral arch. Dislocation of the apophyseal joints has occurred, with overriding of the articular processes and avulsion of the posterior ligament complex. Anteriorly, shearing of the intervertebral disk bond between the vertebral bodies may be noted, with severe stretching of the anterior longitudinal ligament.

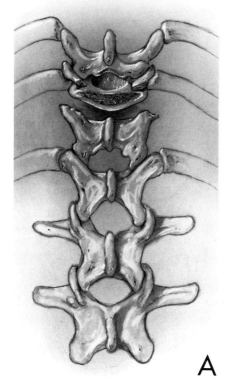

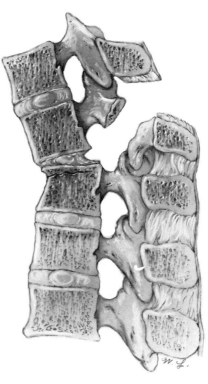

A

B

Figure 7–44. Shear fracture-dislocation with vertebral arch fracture. A, Posterior view: Widening of the interspinous distance has occurred at the T-11/12 level, associated with fracture of the vertebral arch. B, Lateral section: The arch fracture is again shown with avulsion of the posterior ligament complex. This arch fracture may "release" the spinal cord to save the patient from neurologic injury. Anteriorly, shearing of the intervertebral disk and fracture of the vertebral body below have occurred.

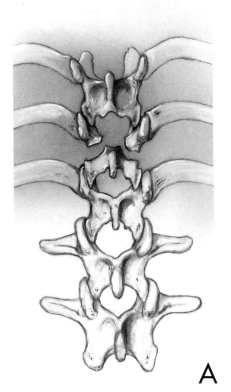
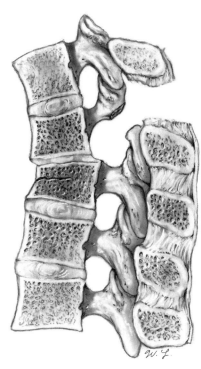

A

B

Figure 7–45. Shear fracture-dislocation with traumatic spondylolisthesis. Similar to Figure 7–44 but with vertebral arch fracture involving each pars interarticularis. Again note disruption of the posterior ligament complex and anterior disk injury with vertebral body fracture. The extent of this fracture-dislocation injury readily distinguishes it from the more common spondylolysis or spondylolisthesis with an associated history of back injury.

the spinal cord." Lob,[13] however, has noted that the vertebral arches are quite stout and strong in the lumbar region, and a spinal injury of sufficient violence to fracture them often causes neurologic injury in any case, associated with a severely comminuted fracture-dislocation.

Shear fracture-dislocations are best appreciated radiographically on the lateral view, where the displacement of the vertebral column resulting from the forward shear injury becomes obvious (Figs. 7–46, 7–47). When the vertebral arches remain intact, the apophyseal joints should be closely inspected on the lateral view for fracture, dislocation, or possible locking. In such cases, the vertebrae are displaced but remain essentially intact (Fig. 7–48). When the vertebral arch is fractured, however, the posterior portion of the arch and the spinous process remain behind, while the anterior parts of the arch shift forward with the displaced portion of the vertebral column. The

actual fracture lines in the vertebral arch may become clearly visible only upon oblique projections or tomography. A widened sagittal diameter of the vertebral canal at the level of the injured vertebra readily confirms the existence of vertebral arch fracture on lateral view, however.

Shear fracture-dislocations with vertebral arch fractures occurring in the lower lumbar region are usually quite severe injuries, as considerable force is required to fracture the stout lower lumbar vertebral arches. Comminuted fractures often result, with severe displacement and extensive soft tissue injury. These can usually be distinguished on radiographic appearances from cases of preexisting lumbar spondylolisthesis with a recent history of back trauma, which show only isolated pars defects with a greater or lesser degree of forward slipping of the vertebral bodies, often accompanied by chronic changes of intervertebral disk degeneration.[13]

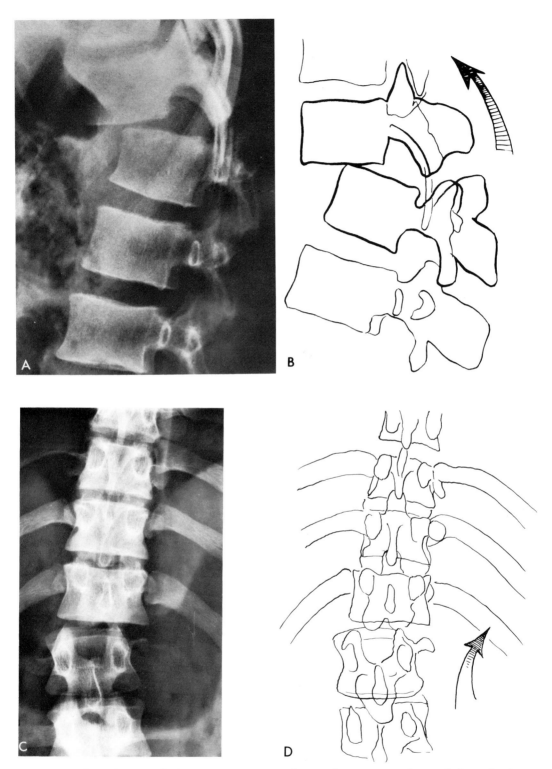

Figure 7–46. Shear fracture-dislocation. *A, B,* Lateral view demonstrates forward shear displacement (arrow) of T-12 vertebra on L-1, which has torn the intervertebral disk between them. *C, D,* Frontal view exhibits a gap between the laminae and spinous processes of T-12 and L-1 vertebrae. The transverse processes of L-1 are fractured as well. (Arrow indicates direction of vertebral disruption.)

Illustration and legend continued on the following page.

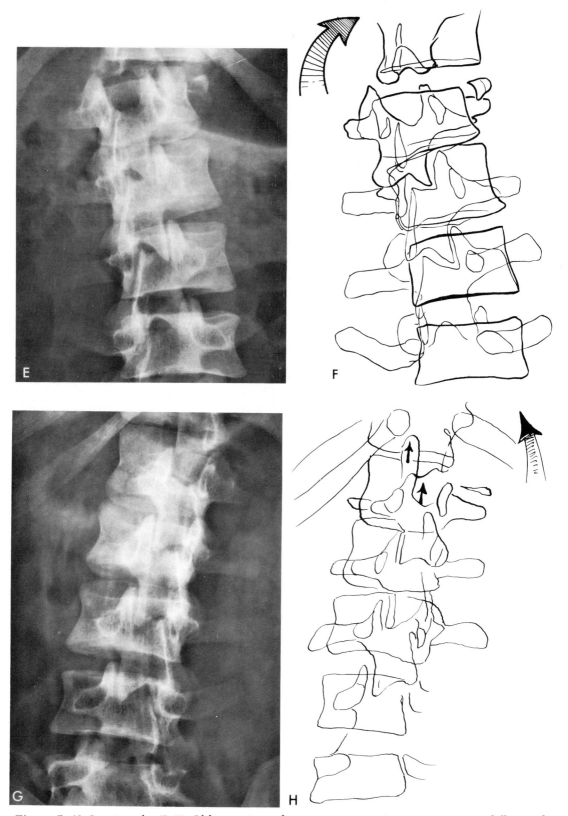

Figure 7–46 Continued. E–H, Oblique views demonstrate posterior structures in a different dimension (near top of illustrations). Large arrows reflect vertebral disruption. Small arrows on left anterior oblique view indicate distraction of apophyseal joint at T-12/L-1.

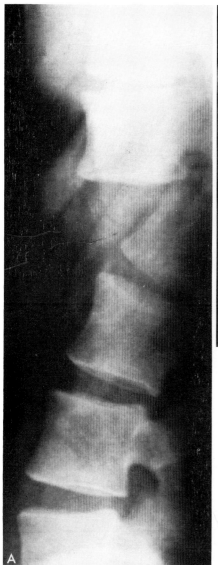

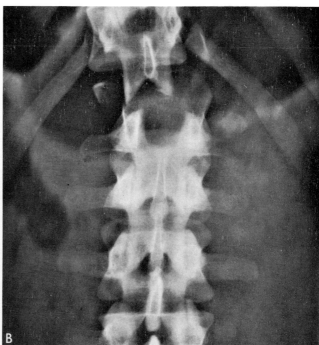

Figure 7–47. Shear fracture-dislocation. *A*, Lateral view. Extreme forward dislocation of T-12 on L-1 vertebrae may be noted. *B*, Frontal view. Marked distraction of the apophyseal joints is apparent at this level. A corner of L-1 vertebral body has been avulsed as well (beneath T-12 body).

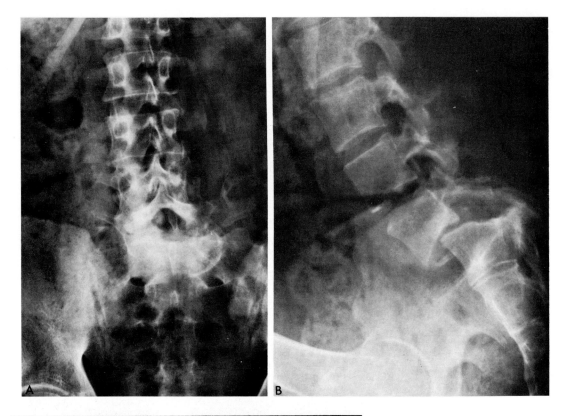

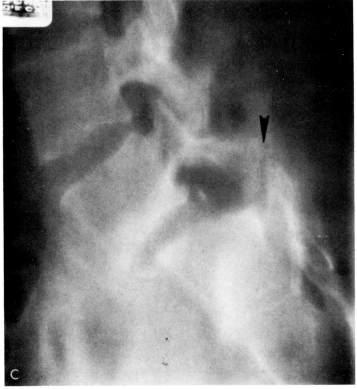

Figure 7–48. A, B Shear dislocation with articular process locking. This patient sustained a "sprung back" injury (see p. 388) in the form of a pure lumbosacral dislocation. Locking of the facets is shown to advantage on the tomographic cut (*C*) (arrow). This complication may block attempts at closed reduction, and require surgery for repositioning of the vertebrae. (See also Fig. 7–3.)

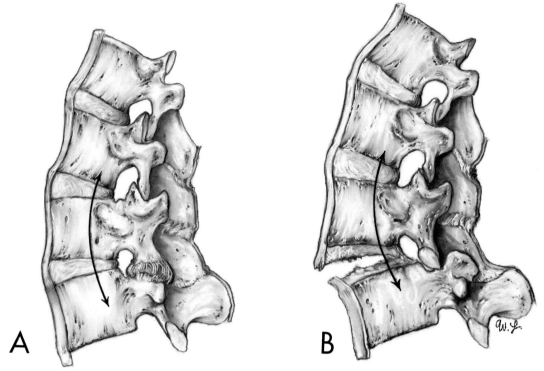

Figure 7–49. Two types of hyperextension fracture-dislocation. *A*, In this type of hyperextension fracture-dislocation, posterior compression fractures of the apophyseal joints (note bulging joint capsule) and spinous processes may result. Distraction forces anteriorly (curved arrow) are resisted by the intact anterior longitudinal ligament and intervertebral disk bonds. *B*, Disruption of the anterior longitudinal ligament and intervertebral disk has been produced, and the vertebral column is distracted anteriorly. Dislocation of the apophyseal joints has resulted posteriorly, but no compression fractures have occurred in this region.

HYPEREXTENSION FRACTURE-DISLOCATIONS

The mechanism of injury in hyperextension fracture-dislocations is completely opposite to that seen in the injuries discussed up to this point, all of which involve spinal flexion. In hyperextension, the vertebral column pivots in the opposite direction about the fulcrum through the nucleus pulposus of the intervertebral disk, being distracted anteriorly and compressed posteriorly. Roaf,[15] in his work with cadaver spines, was unable to disrupt the anterior longitudinal ligament by application of a pure hyperextension force; he succeeded only in producing posterior compression fractures of the vertebral arches and processes (Figs. 7–49, 7–50). As with flexion injuries, however, he found he could readily disrupt the anterior longitudinal ligament if he added components of rotation or forward shear to

the hyperextension force. The intervertebral disk bond would then be pulled apart, and the vertebral column could be dislocated (Figs. 7–49, 7–51, 7–52).

Hyperextension fracture-dislocations, although common in the cervical region, are relatively infrequent in the thoracolumbar spine. Only four cases were observed in one series of 154 thoracolumbar injuries, representing 2.5 per cent of the total. These hyperextension fracture-dislocations all occurred in the thoracic spine, from T-3 to T-11 vertebrae. All four patients sustained severe neurologic injuries, two by transection of the cord at the site of injury, and two by massive spinal cord necrosis resulting from traction on the cord. The prognosis for hyperextension injuries of the thoracolumbar spine in this series was noted to be poor.[3]

Radiographically, hyperextension fracture-dislocations are best demonstrated

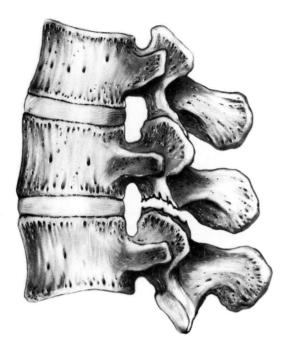

Figure 7–50. Hyperextension fracture-dislocation with posterior compression fractures. The inferior articular processes have been compressed posteriorly. Anteriorly, the anterior longitudinal ligament and intervertebral disk bonds remain intact.

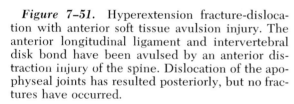

Figure 7–51. Hyperextension fracture-dislocation with anterior soft tissue avulsion injury. The anterior longitudinal ligament and intervertebral disk bond have been avulsed by an anterior distraction injury of the spine. Dislocation of the apophyseal joints has resulted posteriorly, but no fractures have occurred.

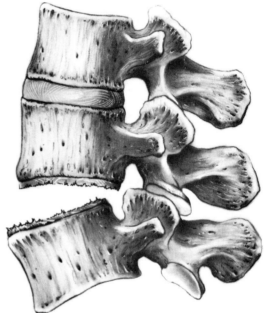

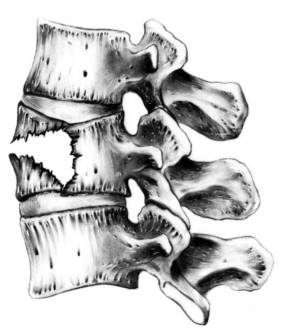

Figure 7–52. Hyperextension fracture-dislocation with anterior "fissure" fracture. A variant of the injury illustrated in Figure 7–51, the anterior longitudinal ligament has been avulsed, but the intervertebral disk bonds have remained intact, while a "fissure" or distraction fracture of the vertebral body has resulted instead.

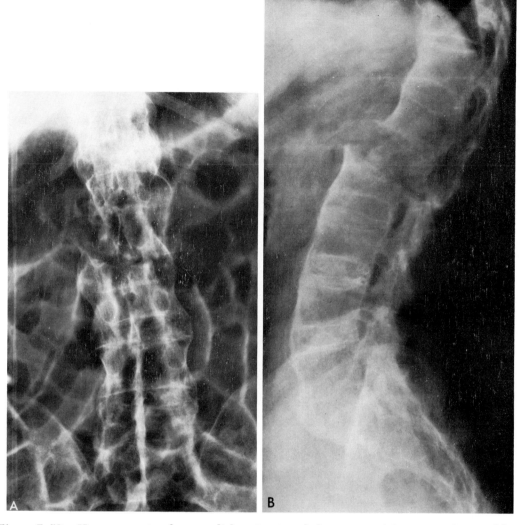

Figure 7–53. Hyperextension fracture-dislocation in ankylosing spondylitis. *A, B,* 50 year old male with ankylosing spondylitis who fell backward across a table while drinking with a friend, and was subsequently unable to move his legs. He was sustained on alcohol for five days thereafter by his friend, who dragged him to the roadside and left him there when he began to smell offensive. He was then found by the police and brought to the regional hospital, where he was diagnosed as having a hysterical conversion reaction and admitted to the psychiatric service. There he informed his physician that he was now able to lie flat on his back in bed, which he had not been able to accomplish for years. Radiologic evaluation of the spine was subsequently obtained, and the correct diagnosis made.

on the lateral view. Posterior compression fractures of the vertebral arch complex may result (Fig. 7–50) in cases in which the anterior longitudinal ligament remains intact.[1] Anterior distraction injuries may arise from tearing of the anterior longitudinal ligament and avulsion of the disk bond (Fig. 7–51), or by a distraction or "fissure" fracture of the vertebral body (Fig. 7–52). Small diagonal fractures involving the posteroinferior corner of a lumbar vertebral body have also been described in lumbar hyperextension injury,[17] presumably on the basis of vertebral compression. These fragments may be displaced posteriorly to produce cord compression. Fracture-dislocations in vertebral columns solidified by ankylosing spondylitis are alleged to result only from hyperextension injury, never from hyperflexion (Fig. 7–53).[8]

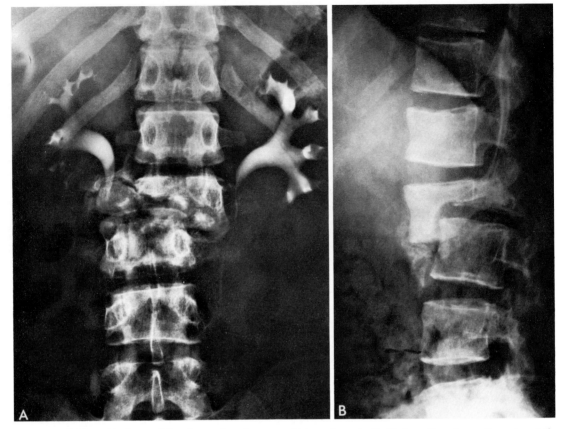

Figure 7–54. Healing of lumbar spine fracture-dislocation. *A, B,* Note callus formation about the fracture fragments in this shear fracture-dislocation of L-2 on L-3 vertebrae. (Courtesy of Dr. Robert H. Freiberger, Hospital for Special Surgery, New York, N.Y.)

HEALING OF VERTEBRAL ARCH COMPLEX INJURIES

Fractured vertebral arches unite as do fractured long bones, with callus deposition between the fracture fragments. The callus appears as a dense cloud of calcium density on the radiograph, at first indistinct, and later becoming denser and more clearly defined (Fig. 7–54). Healing of the associated soft tissue injuries (ligamentous and muscular tears, hematoma formation) is frequently accompanied by extensive soft tissue ossification ("myositis ossificans"), which may fuse with the fracture callus to produce large, irregular, asymmetric accretions of bone at the site of injury. Such masses of bone may produce synostoses of adjacent vertebrae; this may usually be distinguished from congenital synostosis or block vertebra formation by its irregularity and asymmetric appearance on the radiograph. Severe degenerative arthritis of the injured intervertebral disk and apophyseal joints frequently occurs rapidly after fracture-dislocation, radiographically similar to that seen with intervertebral disk degeneration, but chronologically more acute in its onset. The costovertebral articulations may be similarly involved.[13]

REFERENCES

1. Böhler, L.: The Treatment of Fractures. New York, Grune & Stratton, 1956.
2. Braakman, R., and Penning, L.: Injuries of the Cervical Spine. Amsterdam, Excerpta Medica, 1971.
3. Burke, D. C.: Hyperextension injuries of the spine. J. Bone & Jt. Surg., 53-B:3, 1971.
4. Casey, B. M., Eaton, S. B., Jr., et al.: Thoracolumbar neural arch fractures: evaluation by hypocycloidal tomography. J.A.M.A., 224:1263, 1973.

5. Chance, G. Q.: Note on a type of flexion fracture of the spine. Brit. J. Radiol., *21*:452, 1948.

6. Dehner, J. R.: Seatbelt injuries of the spine and abdomen. Amer. J. Roentgenol., *111*:833, 1971.

7. Epstein, B. S.: The Spine, A Radiological Text and Atlas, 3rd. ed., Philadelphia, Lea & Febiger, 1969.

8. Guttmann, L.: Traumatic paraplegia and tetraplegia in ankylosing spondylitis. Paraplegia, *4*:188, 1966.

9. Holdsworth, F. W.: Fractures, dislocations, and fracture-dislocations of the spine. J. Bone & Jt. Surg., *45-B*:6, 1963.

10. Holdsworth, F. W.: Fractures, dislocations, and fracture-dislocations of the spine. J. Bone & Jt. Surg., *52-A*:1534, 1970.

11. Jefferson, G.: Discussion on spinal injuries. Proc. R. Soc. Med., *21*:625, 1928.

12. Kaufer, H., and Hayes, J. T.: Lumbar fracture-dislocation. J. Bone & Jt. Surg., *48-A*:712, 1966.

13. Lob, A.: Die Wirbelsäulenverletzungen und ihre Ausheilung, 2nd ed. Stuttgart, George Thieme Verlag, 1954.

14. Nicoll, E. A.: Fractures of the dorso-lumbar spine. J. Bone & Jt. Surg., *31-B*:376, 1949.

15. Roaf, R.: A study of the mechanics of spinal injuries. J. Bone & Jt. Surg., *42-B*:810, 1960.

16. Rogers, L. F.: The roentgenographic appearance of transverse or Chance fractures of the spine: the seat belt fracture. Amer. J. Roentgenol., *111*:844, 1971.

17. Schinz, H. R., Baensch, W. E., Friedl, L., and Uehlinger, E.: Roentgen Diagnostics. Vol. 2., 2nd American edition by L. G. Rigler, New York, Grune & Stratton, 1967.

18. Schmorl, G., and Junghanns, H.: The Human Spine in Health and Disease. 2nd American ed. by E. F. Besemann. New York, Grune & Stratton, 1971.

19. Smith, W. S.,and Kaufer, H.: Patterns and mechanisms of lumbar injuries associated with lap seat belts. J. Bone & Jt. Surg., *51-A*:239, 1969.

20. Stanger, J. K.: Fracture-dislocation of the thoracolumbar spine. J. Bone & Jt. Surg., *29*:107, 1947.

Chapter 8

ISOLATED POSTERIOR FRACTURES OF THE THORACOLUMBAR SPINE

ISOLATED VERTEBRAL ARCH FRACTURES

Incidence

Isolated fractures of the vertebral arch resulting from acute trauma are quite rare injuries.[2, 9] No fractures fitting this description were found in a series of over 700 cases of vertebral injury.[6] Most such fractures occur in conjunction with fracture-dislocations of the spine, as discussed in Chapter 7.

Mechanism of Injury

Isolated vertebral arch fractures are alleged to result from a direct blow to the spinous process, collapsing the arch.[9] Böhler[2] claims that he has never seen such an injury resulting from direct violence. The vertebral arches in the lower thoracic and lumbar spine are composed of stout, dense cortical bone. Indirect violence to the vertebral column sufficient to produce vertebral arch fractures nearly always results in a more extensive injury, usually a fracture-dislocation.

Radiologic Findings and Differential Diagnosis

Most cases of posttraumatic vertebral arch fracture in fact represent *preexisting spondylolysis or spondylolisthesis* with a history of acute back injury.[9, 11] The interarticular isthmus, or pars interarticularis of the lamina, has undergone stress fracture or resorption in these patients (see Chapter 10). Absolute confirmation of the chronic nature of the defect may be made only by comparison with radiographs of the patient's spine obtained prior to the injury, if this is possible. However, radiographic findings of elongation of the injured pars interarticularis, inconsistencies in bony density about the margins of the defect (either an increase or a decrease in radiodensity), or absence of a segment of the vertebral arch (congenital aplasia) strongly suggest a preexisting stress fracture or defect of the bone in this region. Reactive sclerosis of the opposite pedicle (the result of altered weight transmission) indicates that the lesion is of long standing.[7]

An *acute fracture* of the vertebral arch, by comparison, would be expected to exhibit sharp edges and irregularity of the fractured bone, without radiologic evidence of prior changes in bone texture (Fig. 7–33). No sclerosis of the opposite pedicle or pars interarticularis would be expected. Neither would absence of a substantial segment of the vertebral arch be anticipated (congenital aplasia).

Congenital clefts may occur in many parts of the vertebral arch (Fig. 8–1). It is not always possible to distinguish them from fractures in the acutely injured patient. Retroisthmic clefts (Fig. 8–2), although rela-

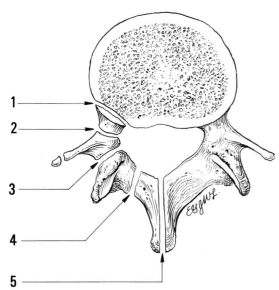

1
2
3
4
5

Figure 8–1. Composite diagram of congenital vertebral arch clefts. Congenital clefts may occur in many parts of the vertebral arch. (1) At the root of the pedicle, splitting off a small portion of the vertebral body posteriorly (retrosomatic cleft). (2) In the pedicle. (3) In the interarticular isthmus (although bony defects in this region usually represent spondylolysis). (4) In the lamina (retroisthmic cleft). (5) In the spinous process (spina bifida).

tively infrequent, may cause confusion in this region. Smooth edges and dense cortical margins about a cleft suggest a congenital, rather than a traumatic, origin. Reactive sclerosis of the contralateral pedicle adds support for a congenital lesion, as opposed to an acute injury. Oblique projections of the spine and tomography may be required to show congenital arch clefts to advantage.

Hypoplasia or aplasia of the pedicle is presumed to result from a congenital disturbance in the cartilage model of the vertebral arch in utero, leading to abnormal subsequent ossification.[9] The affected pedicle may be thinner than its fellow on the normal side (hypoplasia), or absent altogether (aplasia); the pars interarticularis and superior articular process on the same side may be deficient also (Fig. 8–3). Vertical clefts of the pedicle, presumably congenital, have been reported but are apparently quite rare.[7, 9]

The normal distribution of weight-bearing stress through the vertebral arches of the spine is disturbed by the deficient pedicle; stress is shunted to the opposite side, and reactive sclerosis of the contralateral pedicle results, which may involve the adjacent pars interarticularis and superior articular process also. Such reactive sclerosis bespeaks a long-standing lesion. (It is not always apparent with milder degrees of pedicle hypoplasia, however.)[7]

Radiologically, the ring shadow of the deficient pedicle appears faint or absent on the anteroposterior view of the spine, while its fellow appears more dense than normal. Malalignment of the spinous processes may be noted at the level of the defect, similar to that seen in rotary fracture-dislocation (Chap. 7): the spinous process above the affected vertebra is deflected toward the side of the deficient pedicle, when compared with the spinous process of the involved vertebra. This deflection may be spontaneously corrected by positioning the patient supine for filming (as is also the case with rotary fracture-dislocations) and may be brought out only when the patient is erect.

Oblique views of the spine exhibit the defect to best advantage. When extensive, such pedicle defects are less likely to be confused with fracture than with primary or metastatic tumor. In such cases, sclerosis of the contralateral pedicle again affords a clue to the congenital nature of the lesion.[7]

Healing

Healing of the vertebral arch clefts may occur both in fractures and in spondylolysis, and in itself does not distinguish between them.[9, 11] Massive callus formation about the divided vertebral arch, however, suggests healing of an acute fracture. Vertebral arch fractures require three to seven months of complete immobilization for solid union to occur, if no complications are present.[6] Acute injuries of a dysplastic pars interarticularis in a patient predisposed to spondylolysis characteristically show little or no evidence of callus formation.[11]

ISOLATED ARTICULAR PROCESS FRACTURES

Incidence

Isolated fractures of the articular processes, in the absence of other spinal injuries,

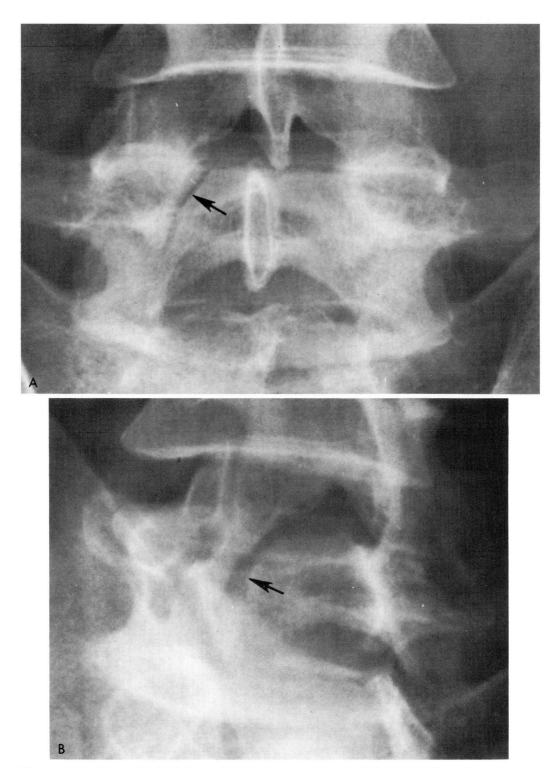

Figure 8–2. Retroisthmic cleft. *A,* Anteroposterior view: A cleft divides the right lamina of L-5 vertebra (arrow). *B,* Left anterior oblique view of the right retroisthmic cleft (arrow).

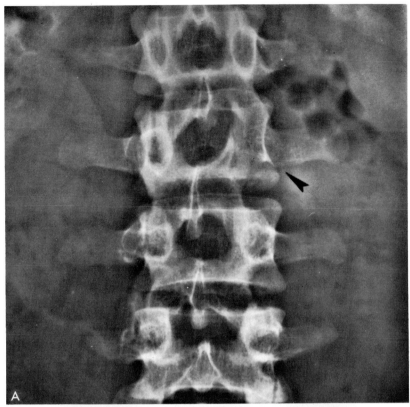

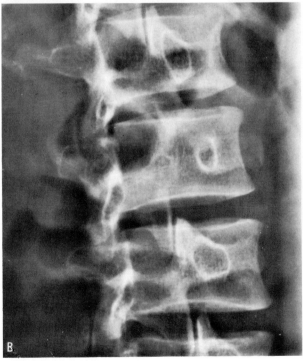

Figure 8–3. Congenital aplasia of the pedicle. *A,* Anteroposterior view. The left pedicle of L-2 vertebra is absent (arrow); the opposite pedicle is sclerotic. The spinous process of L-2 is deflected away from the side of the absent pedicle. Although absence of a pedicle usually suggests metastatic malignancy, the finding of sclerosis in the opposite pedicle indicates the process to be of long standing, making metastatic disease considerably less likely. *B,* Right anterior oblique view. A substantial defect in the left pars interarticularis of L-2 vertebra is present as well. (Compare this with the vertebral arches above and below.) *(Illustration continued next page.)*

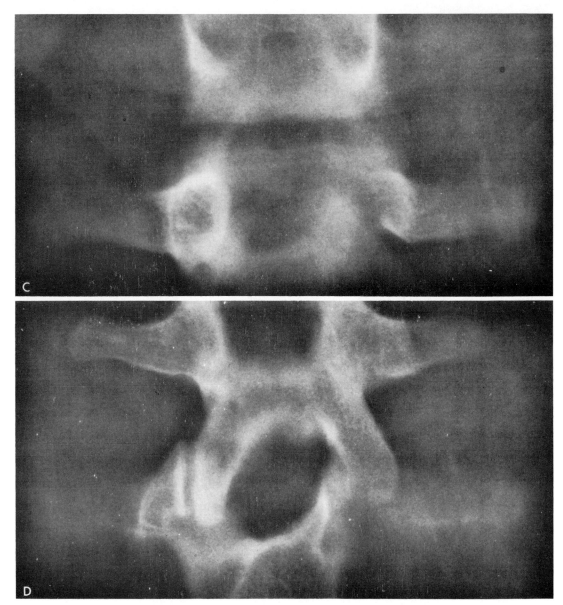

Figure 8–3 Continued. *C*, Tomographic cut through the pedicles of L-2 vertebra confirms the absence of the left pedicle, with sclerosis of the right. *D*, A tomographic cut taken several millimeters posterior to *C* demonstrates absence of the left superior articular process of L-2. The inferior articular process of L-1 is free on the affected side, not articulating with L-2 vertebra at all. The bony defect of L-2 vertebral arch extends to involve the left pars interarticularis as well.

are relatively infrequent.[1] They occur quite commonly in association with fracture-dislocations, however (see Chapter 7).

Mechanism of Injury

Isolated articular process fractures are usually the result of a sideways twist injury, with rotation about the long axis of the spine. Leverage is thereby exerted against the articular processes, and they may fracture. Avulsion of the fracture fragments may result from ligamentous pull.

Clinical Presentation

Patients injured in this way complain of persistent severe, disabling back pain oc-

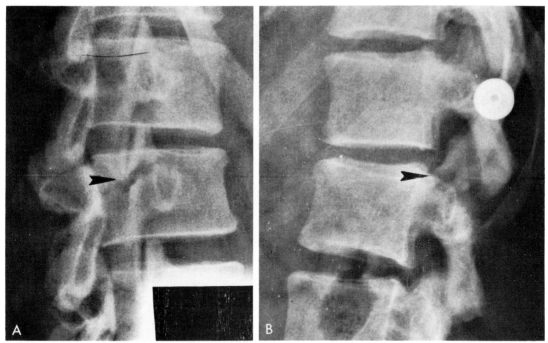

Figure 8–4. Fracture of the superior articular process. *A,* Right anterior oblique view. The left superior articular process of L-1 has been fractured (arrow). Distraction of the fracture fragments has resulted from ligamentous pull. Note the jagged edges of the fracture line (best demonstrated on oblique view) without marginal sclerosis. *B,* Lateral view. The fractured superior articular process has been elevated and displaced slightly forward (arrow).

curring promptly after a twisting injury. Such a history is an important factor in differentiating articular process fractures from unfused apophyses (see below).[1]

Radiologic Findings

Fractures of the articular processes may be most clearly demonstrated on oblique views of the injured spine (Figs. 8–4, 8–5, 8–6). The fracture line shows some irregularity on close inspection, and comminution of the fragments may occur. The free fragment may be retracted by ligamentous pull, thus widening the fracture line.[1]

Differential Diagnosis

Unfused apophyses of the articular processes are considerably more common than isolated fractures (Fig. 8–7). Ten cases were observed in one series of 2000 spinal radiographs, an incidence of 0.5 per cent.[1] They are believed to represent accessory os-

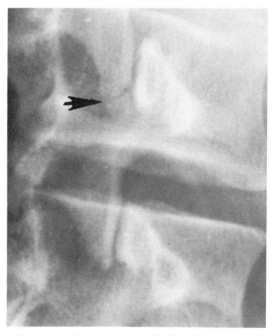

Figure 8–5. Fracture of left inferior articular process of L-2 vertebra (right anterior oblique view). Note the jagged edges of the fracture line, without marginal sclerosis.

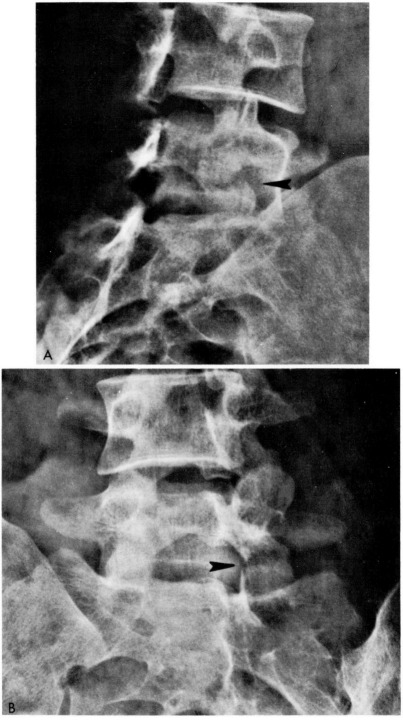

Figure 8–6. Fracture of the inferior articular process. *A,* Right anterior oblique view. The left inferior articular process of L-5 vertebra has been fractured (arrow). This patient noted immediate pain in the left lower back region after twisting her back, and manifested local tenderness over the left lumbosacral area. *B,* Left anterior oblique view. Note irregular fragment edges (arrow).

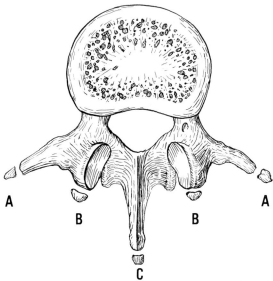

Figure 8–7. Composite diagram of unfused vertebral arch apophyses. Unfused apophyses may involve many of the vertebral arch appendages, where they may be confused with fractures. A,A: In the transverse process. B,B: In the articular processes. C: In the spinous process.

sification centers that have failed to unite normally with the remainder of the articular process. Similar unfused apophyses occur

in the transverse and spinous processes of the vertebral arch. They may be differentiated from fractures in several ways.

1. Unfused apophyses of the articular processes show predilection for the inferior articular processes rather than the superior, and are noted most commonly in the lumbar region at the levels of L-2 and L-3 (Figs. 8–8, 8–9). They are more likely to be bilateral and symmetric than are fractures.

2. A history of trauma is often equivocal or absent with unfused apophyses of the articular processes. The classic history of disabling back pain coincident with a rotary injury is usually not forthcoming.

3. Unfused apophyses exhibit smooth margins with rounding of corners, circumscribed by well-defined cortical bone. This is not seen in acute fractures. At times partial fusion of apophyses with the articular process is noted. This usually extends along the lateral aspect of the articular process, leaving a partial cleft or notch in the medial aspect of the process dividing the apophysis from the remainder (Fig. 8–10). When unilateral apophyses are considered as part of the articular process, the process thus

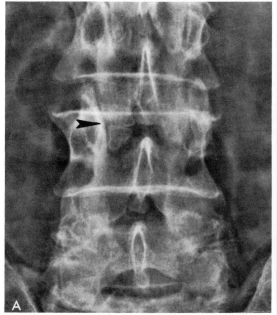

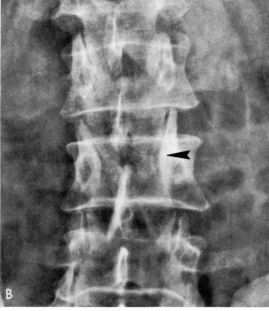

Figure 8–8. Unfused articular process apophyses. *A,* The inferior articular process of L-3 vertebra exhibit an unfused apophysis on the right (arrow). Note the well-defined cortical bone about the margins of the apophysis. When considered as a part of the articular process, the apophysis appears larger and bulkier than its fellow on the opposite side. *B,* The left inferior articular process of L-3 vertebra demonstrates an unfused apophysis in this patient (arrow). Note rounding of the corners of the apophysis, circumscribed by well-defined cortical bone.

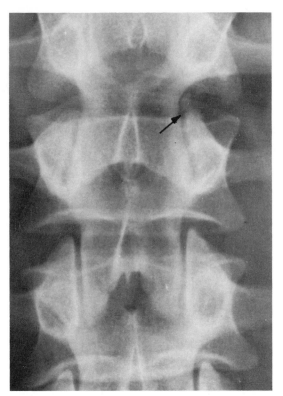

Figure 8–9. Unfused superior articular process apophysis. The left superior articular process of L-2 vertebra exhibits an unfused apophysis (arrow).

formed is larger and bulkier than the uninvolved articular process on the opposite side.

Healing

Immobilization of acutely fractured articular processes is advised both to facilitate firm union of the fractures and to relieve the patient's pain. Fractures involving the base of an articular process are more likely to heal completely than those occurring near the tip.[1] Considerable callus formation and soft tissue ossification often result about fractures of the articular processes and of the vertebral arch. This may become extensive enough to produce a bony synostosis of adjacent vertebral arches at the site of injury. Such changes may usually be distinguished from congenital block vertebra formation by their irregular and asymmetric appearance on the radiograph.

FRACTURES OF THE TRANSVERSE PROCESSES

Incidence

Transverse process fractures occur most frequently in the lumbar spine, although they may involve any vertebral level. L-3 is most commonly fractured, followed by L-1.

Mechanism of Injury

The transverse processes may be fractured by direct injury, such as a blow to the back or flank, or indirectly, as a consequence of violent overpull by the psoas and quadratus lumborum muscles. The psoas muscle arises in part from the anterior surfaces of the transverse processes, whereas the quadratus lumborum originates from their lateral tips. Violent contractions of

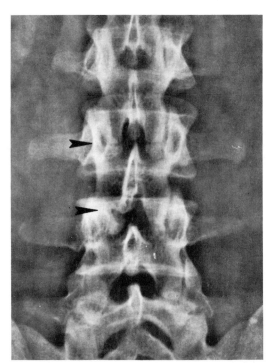

Figure 8–10. Unfused articular process apophyses. The inferior articular processes of L-2 vertebra exhibit bilateral unfused apophyses (upper arrow). An apophysis of the right inferior articular process of L-3 vertebra is partially fused with the process along its lateral aspect, leaving a partial cleft or notch in the medial aspect of the process dividing the apophysis from the remainder (lower arrow).

these muscles, especially of the quadratus lumborum, may break the tips off the transverse processes (Fig. 8–11).

Böhler[2] believes that direct injury is a more frequent cause of these fractures. They have been described in forcefully tackled football players.[3] Transverse process fractures frequently accompany rotary fracture-dislocations and seat-belt injuries of the spine (see Chapter 7).

Associated Injuries

Fractures of the transverse processes most often represent isolated skeletal injuries, although 27 per cent of cases are associated with other fractures of the ribs or spine.[9] Associated soft tissue injuries include hematoma formation in the abdominal muscles retroperitoneally or subcutaneously, and abdominal visceral injuries, especially of the kidneys and ureters. Lumbar nerve injury associated with transverse process fractures occur infrequently.[2]

Radiologic Findings

Transverse process fractures typically appear on the radiograph as vertical fracture lines through the transverse process at a variable distance from the spine (Figs. 8–12, 8–13). Several transverse processes may be fractured on one side, but bilateral fractures are infrequent. Muscular pull on the free fragment of the transverse process may displace it caudally and widen the fracture line. In acute injuries, irregularity or comminution of the fracture line may be appreciated on close inspection.

Horizontal or oblique fractures of the transverse processes may be associated with horizontal fractures of the vertebral body or arch, and consequently with a spinal fracture-dislocation. When horizontal or oblique fractures of the transverse processes are noted, therefore, the vertebrae should be carefully inspected for evidence of fracture-dislocation (see Chapter 7) (Fig. 8–14). This possibility must be excluded before allowing the injured patient to be moved.

Hematuria, when associated with transverse process fractures in the acutely injured patient, is an indication for intravenous urography to exclude tears of the kidneys or ureters.

Differential Diagnosis

Conditions mimicking transverse process fractures on the radiograph include the following.

Lumbar ribs. These represent a thoracolumbar transition anomaly occurring in 7.75 per cent of all autopsied spines.[6] They usually involve L-1, and are of two types: the *thoracic type*, which represents an extra set of ribs similar in all respects to thoracic ribs (Fig. 8–15); and the *lumbar type*, small, irregular stubs of bone articulating with the transverse processes of L-1 (Figs. 8–16, 8–17). It is the latter that may be confused with fractures of the first lumbar transverse processes. Their smooth edges lined with dense cortical bone at their articulations with the transverse processes, however, distinguish them from recent fractures. Moreover, bilateral vertical transverse process fractures restricted to a single lumbar level would be unusual. In cases of doubt, no evidence of healing would be expected on later radiographs of the spine taken one to two months subsequently.[6]

Rudimentary twelfth ribs are occasionally observed. To differentiate these from lumbar ribs with accuracy, it is necessary to radiograph the entire vertebral column and count the segments.

Unfused apophyses at the tips of transverse processes similarly exhibit smooth edges with dense cortical margination, allowing them to be differentiated from recent fractures (Fig. 8–17).

Urinary tract stones may cast shadows over the transverse processes on frontal views of the abdomen resembling transverse process fractures. Oblique views of the abdomen usually succeed in "throwing them off" the spine by confirming their anterior relationship to it. *Calcified abdominal lymph nodes* may be dealt with similarly.

Radiolucent soft tissue lines may be cast across the transverse processes by bowel gas shadows (Fig. 8–18) or the psoas margins of properitoneal fat (Fig. 8–19) to simulate fractures. Close inspection of the radiograph will usually reveal these shadows to extend beyond the margins of the transverse

Text continued on page 367.

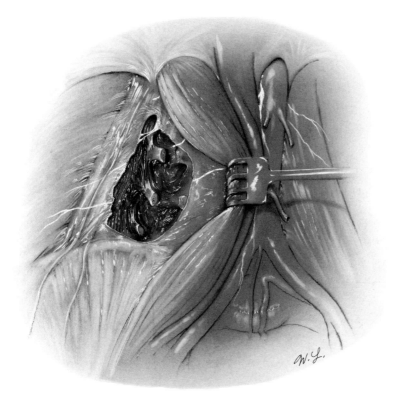

Figure 8–11. ·Soft tissue injuries associated with transverse process fractures. Transverse process fractures are often associated with avulsions of the quadratus lumborum muscle, shown here on the right by retraction of the psoas muscle. Along with this muscle avulsion, extensive injury to fascia, blood vessels, nerves, and ligaments in the retroperitoneal region frequently occurs, together with considerable bleeding.

Figure 8–12. Transverse process fractures. On the right, vertical transverse process fractures are noted at L-3 and L-4 levels (arrows). On the left, an oblique fracture of L-3 transverse process is present (arrow).

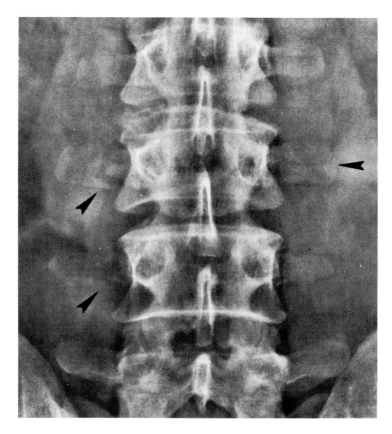

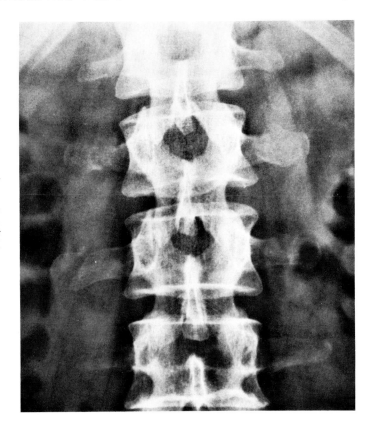

Figure 8–13. Transverse process fractures. Bilateral fractures of L-2 and L-3 transverse processes are present. Muscular pull on the right transverse process of L-3 has widened the fracture line. (Courtesy of Dr. R. H. Freiberger, Hospital for Special Surgery, New York, N.Y.)

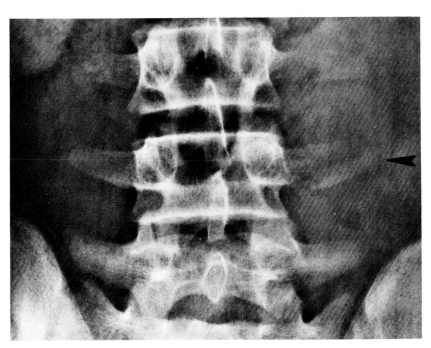

Figure 8–14. Horizontal transverse process fracture. The left transverse process of L-4 vertebra has been fractured in a horizontal manner (arrow). The possible coexistence of vertebral column fracture-dislocations must always be suspected in patients with this type of transverse process fracture.

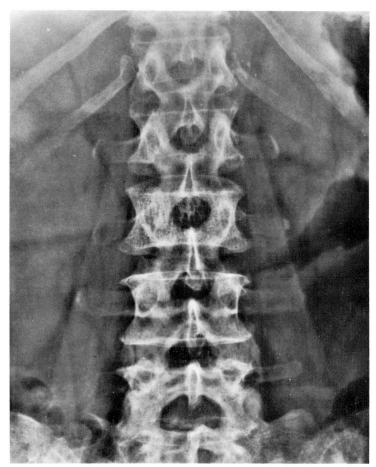

Figure 8–15. Lumbar ribs, thoracic type. An extra set of ribs is present at L-1 level, similar in all respects to lower thoracic ribs. (A hemangioma of L-3 vertebral body represents an incidental finding in this patient.)

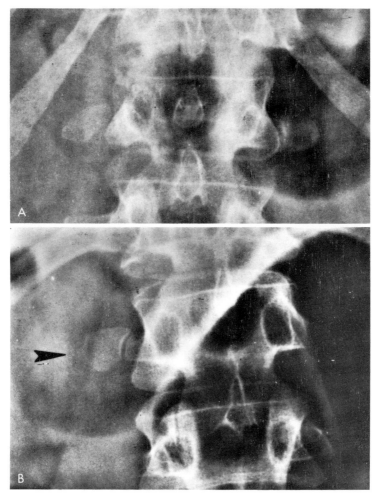

Figure 8–16. Lumbar ribs, lumbar type. *A,* Small, irregular stubs of bone articulate with the transverse processes of L-1 vertebra bilaterally. Their smooth edges and dense cortical margins distinguish them from recent transverse process fractures. *B,* Unilateral lumbar rib, lumbar type (arrow).

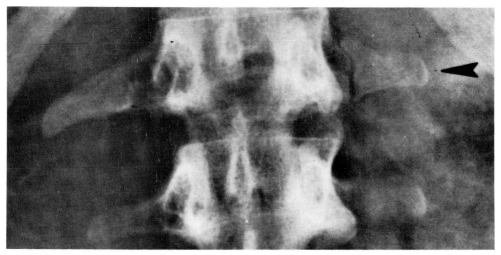

Figure 8–17. Lumbar ribs, mixed types. A thoracic type lumbar rib is present on the right, and a lumbar type lumbar rib on the left (arrow).

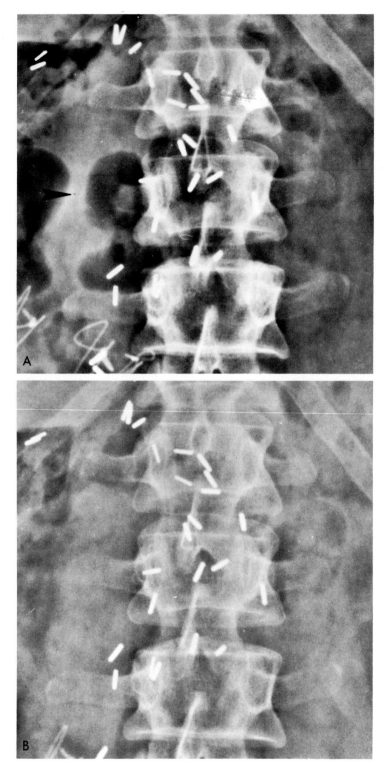

Figure 8–18. Bowel gas shadows simulating transverse process abnormality. *A,* Colonic gas overlying the right transverse process of L-2 vertebra partially obliterates its outlines, suggesting fracture or metastatic destruction (arrow). *B,* A later film of the same patient reveals the transverse process in question to be normal, after the bowel gas has disappeared.

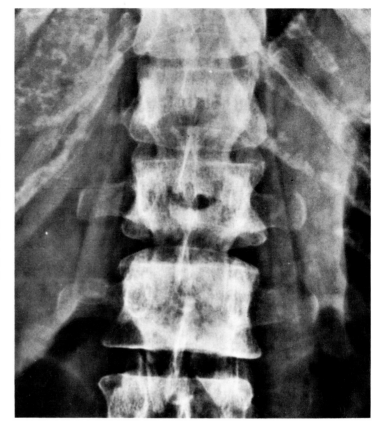

Figure 8–19. Psoas shadows simulating transverse process fractures. Properitoneal fat silhouetting the psoas margins may be projected across the lumbar transverse processes to simulate fracture lines. If fractures are suspected, oblique abdominal views may "throw" the psoas margins off the transverse processes to resolve confusion. (Abnormal bone density in this patient is the result of metastatic disease.)

processes, thus confirming them to be unrelated. If necessary, oblique views or even abdominal compression may shift these lines away from the transverse processes in question.

In the thoracic spine, *osteoarthritis of the costotransverse articulations* may be confused on the radiograph with fractures of the transverse processes (Fig. 8–20), especially since they may be associated with back pain. Similar osteoarthritic changes may involve the *costovertebral joints* as well (Fig. 8–21).

Healing

Isolated fractures of the transverse processes, although painful at first, usually heal soundly with little or no treatment in two to three months after the injury.[6] When the fracture fragments are widely distracted by muscular pull, however, extensive callus formation or pseudoarthroses may result at the fracture sites[5, 6] (Fig. 8–22). Massive

new bone formation may arise within injured muscle, bridging several lumbar transverse processes. Previously described as a congenital malformation, such new bone deposition has been documented to occur following transverse process fractures.[5, 6] It may represent "posttraumatic myositis ossificans" arising in retroperitoneal hematoma associated with the fractures (Fig. 8–23). Painful pseudarthroses may occur in these bony masses, requiring surgical excision for relief.[5]

Similar findings involving the lumbar transverse processes may arise in patients who deny previous significant injury to the back or abdomen, however.[8, 12] We have seen such a case. Bony bridging of the lumbar transverse process ends is noted, sometimes with anomalous joints between them, as described above. Such cases may in fact represent congenital malformations; their differentiation from cases of previous back injury will depend upon an adequate clinical history.

Spinal injury may alter the relationship of

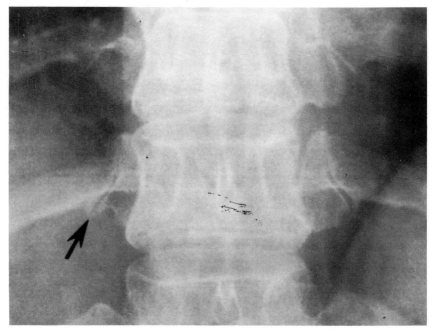

Figure 8–20. Osteoarthritis of costotransverse articulations. Marginal osteophytes have formed at the edges of the synovially lined costotransverse articulations of T-10 vertebra (arrow). The appearance may be confused with fracture.

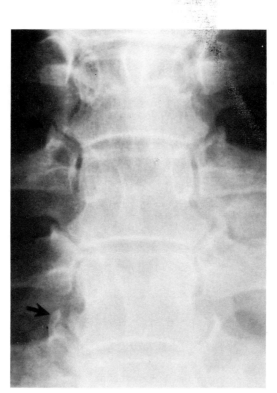

Figure 8–21. Osteoarthritis of costovertebral articulations, lower thoracic spine. Marginal osteophytes (arrows) may be confused with fracture fragments.

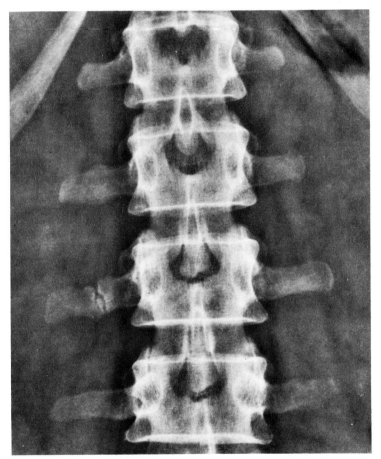

Figure 8–22. Healing in transverse process fractures. Slight enlargement of the right transverse process of L-2 vertebra indicates callus about a healed fracture. At the L-3 level, however, a pseudarthrosis has resulted, with sclerotic margins and rounding off of the fragment corners.

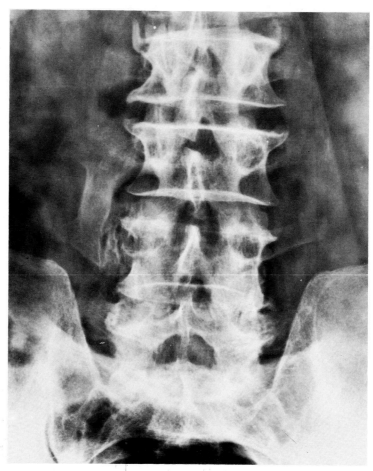

Figure 8–23. Healing in transverse process fractures. Bony bridging has occurred between the right transverse processes of L-3 and L-4 vertebrae, following fracture of the right transverse process of L-4, which has eventuated in a pseudarthrosis at the fracture site and ossification of the associated retroperitoneal hematoma.

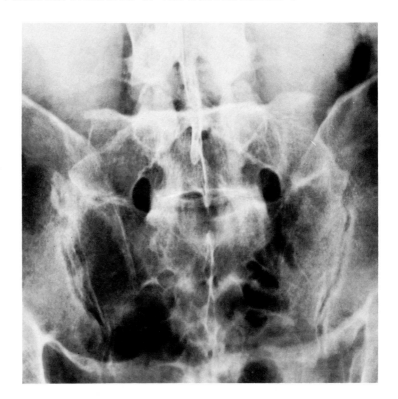

Figure 8–24. Bilateral lumbosacral assimilation joints. "Assimilation joints" are present between the transverse processes of L-5 vertebra and the top of the sacrum, shown to advantage on this "tilt" view of the sacrum with the central ray angled 30° toward the head, patient supine. These joints are believed to arise most commonly as a result of transitional anomalies at the lumbosacral junction, that is, partial sacralization of the last lumbar vertebra, or partial lumbarization of the first sacral element.

the lowest free pair of lumbar transverse processes to the iliac crests to produce pseudarthroses between them.[6] These may give rise to symptoms of back pain on an acquired, rather than a congenital, basis. Similarly, "assimilation joints" between the lowest lumbar vertebra and the sacrum may sometimes be acquired on a posttraumatic or degenerative basis (Figs. 8–24, 8–25).[6]

FRACTURES OF THE SPINOUS PROCESSES

Incidence

Fractures of the spinous processes most commonly occur near the cervicothoracic junction, being considerably less frequent elsewhere. The first thoracic vertebra is the most commonly injured, followed by the seventh cervical and the second thoracic in that order.[2, 9]

Mechanism of Injury

Several types of injury may produce fractures of the spinous processes.

"Clay-shoveler's fracture" usually involves the cervicothoracic junction. In attempting to lift shovelfuls of wet clay or snow adherent to the shovel, musculoligamentous overstrain results in this region, which may avulse fragments from the spinous processes posteriorly (Fig. 8–26). Forceful pulling may have the same effect ("root-puller's fracture").[4] Similar injuries have been reported in cricket players and in those engaging in heavy manual labor who have been previously idle.[2]

Cervical hyperextension injuries may produce compression fractures of the spinous processes posteriorly.

Thoracic hyperflexion and seat-belt injuries may include ligamentous avulsion of the spinous processes posteriorly, especially when the spinous process fractures are horizontally or obliquely disposed. This finding signifies damage to the vertebral arch complex, and therefore an unstable spinal fracture-dislocation (see Chapter 7).

Direct violence to the neck or back may fracture the spinous processes on impact (Fig. 8–27). This is a less common cause of spinous process fracture, especially in the

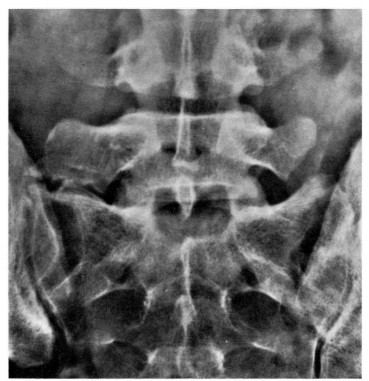

Figure 8–25. Degenerative change in a unilateral assimilation joint. When unilateral, assimilation joints may "tether" the lumbosacral junction and interfere with normal movement of the lumbosacral joint. This may result in degenerative changes in the assimilation joint itself, or elsewhere in the lumbosacral region.

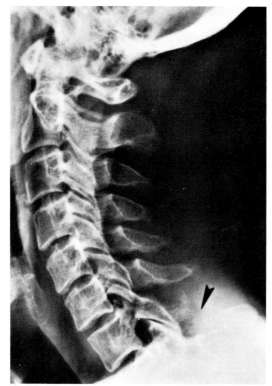

Figure 8–26. Clay-shoveler's fracture. The spinous process of C-7 vertebra has been avulsed (arrow). This injury usually involves the cervicothoracic junction, and results from musculoligamentous overpull.

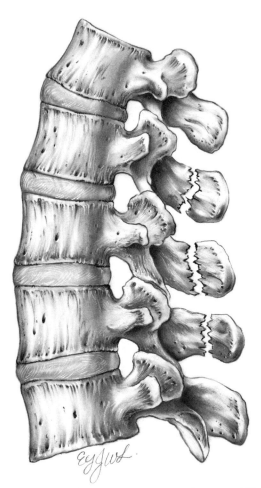

Figure 8–27. Spinous process fractures. The vertical orientation of these fractures is in keeping with a direct blow to the back as the mechanism of injury. When the fracture lines are horizontally or obliquely disposed, a potentially unstable fracture-dislocation injury of the vertebral column should be suspected.

lumbar region, where the spinous processes are comparatively stout and strong.

Radiologic Findings

Inspection of the frontal view radiograph in spinous process fracture reveals a characteristic double shadow to the spinous process silhouette, owing to juxtaposition of the fracture fragments. On the lateral view, a vertical fracture line may be seen at a variable distance from the tip of the spinous process, with downward displacement of the free posterior fragment. A horizontal spinous process fracture should arouse suspicion of further damage to the spine resulting from a hyperflexion injury, such as a Chance fracture.

Differential Diagnosis

The differential diagnosis of spinous process fractures includes the following:

Unfused apophyses of the spinous processes are analogous to those encountered in the articular and transverse processes, and differentiation from fractures involves the same criteria (Fig. 8–7).

Soft tissue ossification occurring posteriorly in the neck, giving rise to the so-called *"fabella nuchae,"* may mimic avulsion fractures of the spinous processes (Fig. 8–28). Examination of all the adjacent spinous processes will reveal them to be intact.

Congenital malformations of the spinous processes, including bifid and sagittally cleft spinous processes (spina bifida occulta), may produce irregularity and distortion of their radiologic outlines (Figs. 8–1, 8–29, 8–30, 8–31). Close inspection of both frontal and lateral views, however, will usually suffice to differentiate them from fractures.

Healing

Union of isolated spinous process fractures is almost invariable, and most authors agree that minimal or no immobilization is required to treat them.[2, 9]

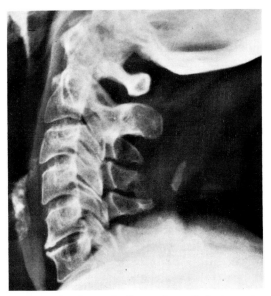

Figure 8–28. Fabella nuchae. Soft tissue ossification in the nape of the neck, the so-called "fabella nuchae," may mimic avulsion fractures of the spinous processes radiologically. Close inspection of the adjacent spinous processes reveals them to be intact.

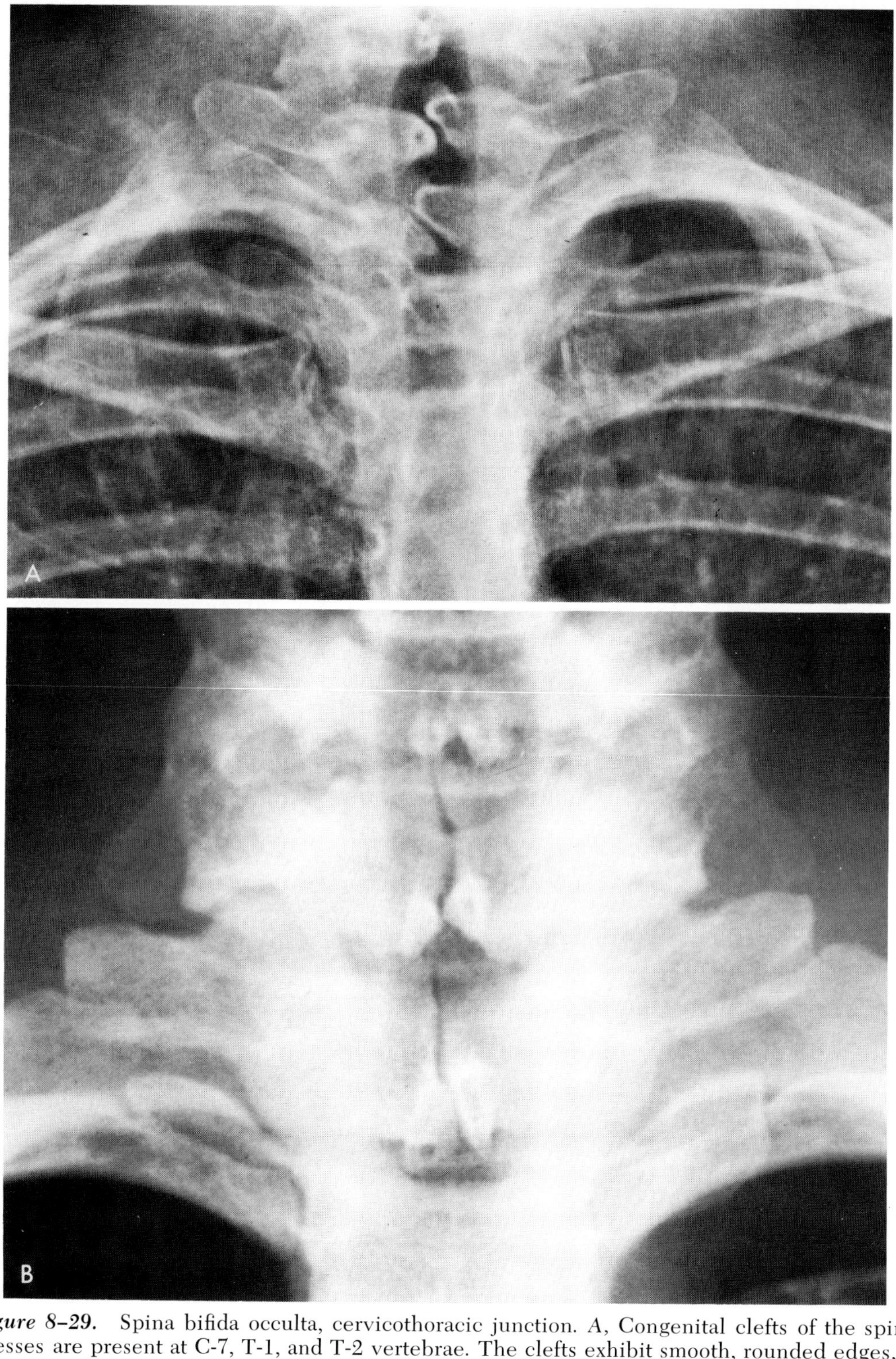

Figure 8–29. Spina bifida occulta, cervicothoracic junction. *A,* Congenital clefts of the spinous processes are present at C-7, T-1, and T-2 vertebrae. The clefts exhibit smooth, rounded edges, and their sagittal orientation is characteristic: a fracture line in this direction would be most unusual. *B,* Another case of cervicothoracic spina bifida involving C-7, and T-1 vertebrae.

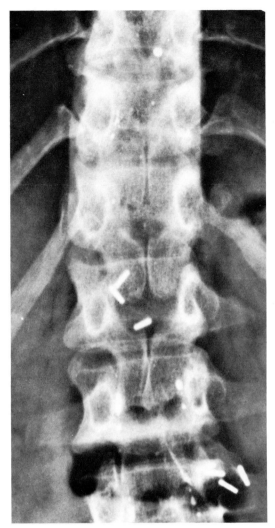

Figure 8–30. Spina bifida occulta, thoracolumbar junction. Congenital clefts of the vertebral arches posteriorly are present at T-11, T-12, and L-1 levels. (Spinous processes have failed to form altogether at the T-11 and T-12 levels.)

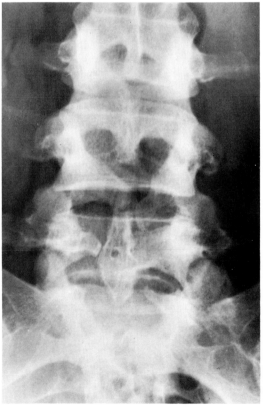

Figure 8–31. Spina bifida occulta, lumbosacral junction. Spina bifida occulta of L-4, L-5, and S-1 levels is noted, with a centralized agglutination of the spinous processes at these three levels.

REFERENCES

1. Bailey, W.: Anomalies and fractures of the vertebral articular processes. JAMA, *108*:266, 1937.
2. Böhler, L.: The Treatment of Fractures. New York, Grune & Stratton, 1956.
3. Bowerman, J. W., and McDonnell, E. J.: Radiology of athletic injuries: Football. Radiology, *117*:33, 1975.
4. Cancelmo, J. J.: Clay-shoveler's fracture. Amer. J. Roentgenol., *115*:540, 1972.
5. Hyman, G.: A case of pseudarthrosis following fractures of the lumbar transverse processes. Brit. J. Surg., *32*:503, 1945.
6. Lob, A.: Die Wirbelsäulenverletzungen und ihre Ausheilung. 2nd. ed. Stuttgart, Georg Thieme Verlag, 1954.
7. Maldague, B. E., and Malghem, J. J.: Unilateral arch hypertrophy with spinous tilt: a sign of arch deficiency. Radiology, *121*:567, (1976).
8. Neumann, R.: Eine linksseitige Brückenbildung zwischen den Querfortsätzen des 3. u. 4. Lendenwirbelkörpers. Arch. Orthop. Unfall-Chirg., *45*:548, 1953.
9. Schmorl, G., and Junghanns, H.: The Human Spine in Health and Disease. 2nd Amer. ed. by E. F. Besemann. New York, Grune & Stratton, 1971.
10. Seegelken, K., and Keller, H.: Retroisthmische Spalte der Lendenwirbelsäule. Fortschr. Röntgenstr., *121*:659, 1974.
11. Wiltse, L. L.: Spondylolisthesis, *In* The A.A.O.S. Symposium on the Spine. St. Louis, C. V. Mosby Co. 1967.
12. Zimmer, E. A.: Fragekasten. Fortschr. Röntgenstr., *104*:735, 1966.

Part IV

INJURIES OF THE SACRUM AND COCCYX

Chapter 9

INJURIES OF THE SACRUM AND COCCYX

SACRAL INJURIES

The sacrum arises from the coalition of five vertebrae below the lumbar spine. It forms a part of the bony pelvic ring, contributing its posterior wall. The sacrum is firmly bonded within the pelvic ring by the sacroiliac joints, and functions as an integral part of the pelvis. It is therefore no surprise that fractures of the sacrum usually accompany other fractures of the pelvic ring.

Incidence

Sacral fractures may be detected in 44 per cent of all fractures of the pelvic ring.[1, 5]

Anterior pelvic fractures of the pubic and ischial rami are frequently associated, as the anterior portions of the pelvic ring are structurally weaker than the posterior parts, and are the first to break in compression injuries of the pelvis. The sacral fracture lines are usually aligned vertically, or sometimes obliquely (Figs. 9–1, 9–2, 9–3); horizontal sacral fractures are relatively infrequent. Although reported as rare by several authors,[3, 4] vertically oriented fractures of the sacrum predominate over horizontal or oblique types in several large series.[1, 5] Most sacral fractures are unilateral. Isolated fractures of the sacrum are rare, accounting for but 1 per cent of all fractures involving the sacrum.[5, 7] These are usually the horizontal ones, crossing the sacrum above or below the sacroiliac articulations (Fig. 9–4).

Mechanisms of Injury

Sacral fractures are more commonly produced by violence transmitted through one leg or through one side of the body to the pelvis.[1] The sacroiliac joint resists rupture or separation, owing to its oblique orientation and to the great tensile strength of the fibers that hold it together (Figs. 9–5, 9–6). Violence directed at the sacroiliac joint is thus as likely to fracture the bone to either side of the joint (iliac wing laterally, sacral ala medially) as to disrupt the sacroiliac joint itself. Adjacent fractures may lead into the sacroiliac joint to produce a combined fracture-dislocation (Fig. 9–7).

The foramina for the first and second sacral nerve roots, perforating the sacral wing, or ala, medial to the sacroiliac joint, structurally weaken the bone in this vicinity. A compressive force applied to the pelvis is thus more likely to break the pelvic ring along this "dotted line" of weakness than elsewhere, producing a vertical fracture through the sacral foramina along one side (Figs. 9–1, 9–2). Such a compressive force may be applied to the pelvis in one of three ways:[1]

1. By *rotation*, in which one leg is hyperextended, thereby rotating the hip bone backward about a horizontal axis and stressing the sacroiliac articulation (Figs. 9–8, 9–9).
2. By *leverage*, in which the pelvis is flattened from front to back by a compressing force (often with multiple pelvic fractures) and buckling of the sacroiliac

Text continued on page 386.

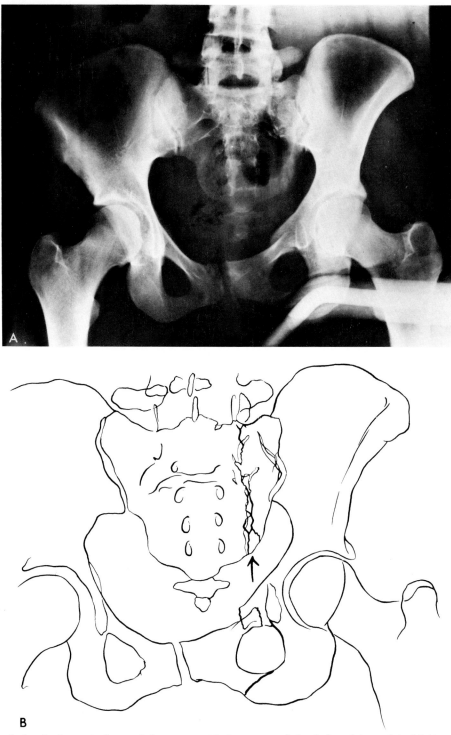

Figure 9–1. Left vertical sacral fracture, with fractures of the left pubic and ischial rami. *A,B,* A vertical fracture through the left sacral wing has disrupted the superior foraminal lines on the left, avulsed the superior articular process on that side, and extended through the lower aspect of the sacrum (arrow). Fractures of the rami anteriorly have completed the fracture through the left pelvic ring.

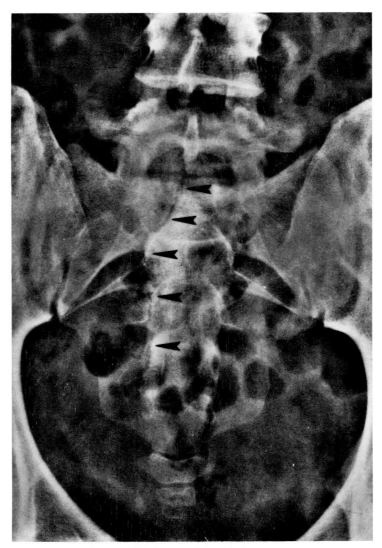

Figure 9-2. Vertical sacral fracture. Note the vertical fracture line (arrows) passing through the lower right sacral foramina but deviating obliquely towards the midline superiorly.

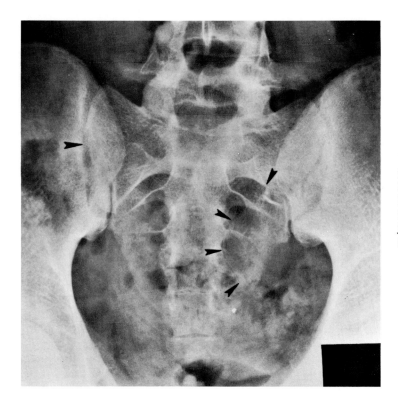

Figure 9–3. Oblique sacral fracture, left. The sacral fracture line on the left pursues an oblique course (arrows). Diastatic injury to the right sacroiliac joint was sustained as well (single arrow).

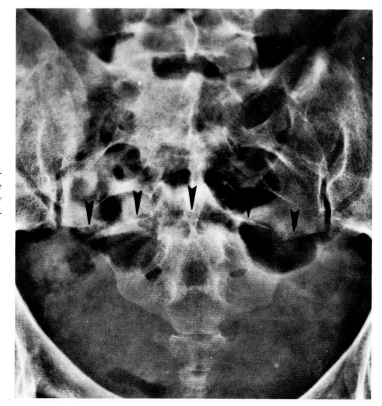

Figure 9–4. Transverse sacral fracture. The fracture line crosses the sacrum transversely just below the sacroiliac articulations (arrows).

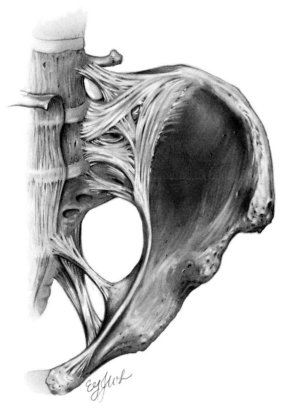

Figure 9-5. Pelvic ligaments: anterior view. The sacroiliac joint is secured by ligaments of great tensile strength, binding the bones together. More inferiorly, the sacrospinous and sacrotuberous ligaments cross the pelvis, arising from the free edge of the lower sacrum.

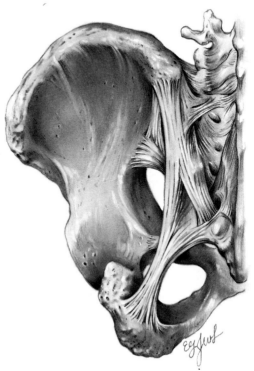

Figure 9-6. Pelvic ligaments: posterior view. The sacroiliac ligaments are oriented obliquely along the course of the joint.

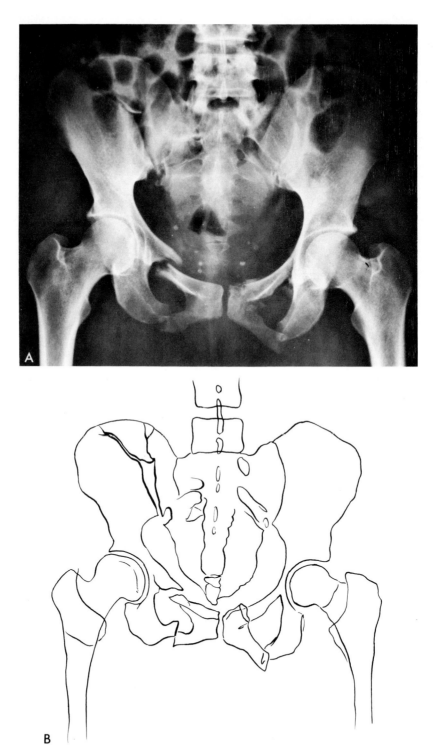

Figure 9–7. Fracture-dislocation of the right sacroiliac joint, with fractures of the pubic and ischial rami. *A,B,* A fracture-dislocation has disrupted the right sacroiliac joint, with fracture of the iliac wing lateral to the joint and the sacral ala medial to it, shown by discontinuity of the superior foraminal lines. All four pubic and ischial rami have been fractured as well.

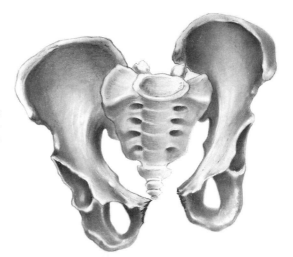

Figure 9–8. Pelvic rotation fracture. The left hip bone has been rotated backward about a horizontal axis, disrupting the symphysis pubis and the left sacroiliac joint.

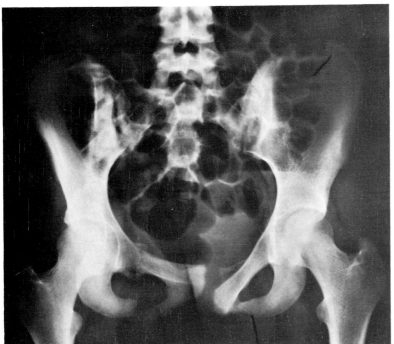

Figure 9–9. Pelvic rotation fracture. The right hip bone has been rotated backward about a horizontal axis, disrupting the symphysis pubis and right sacroiliac joint, and fracturing the right pubic and ischial rami. (Courtesy of R. H. Freiberger, M.D., Hospital for Special Surgery, New York, N.Y.)

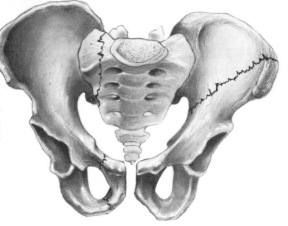

Figure 9–10. Pelvic leverage fracture. Anteriorly, the right pubic rami are fractured; posteriorly, the right sacral ala and left iliac wing are fractured, the result of a compressing force exerted on the pelvis from front to back.

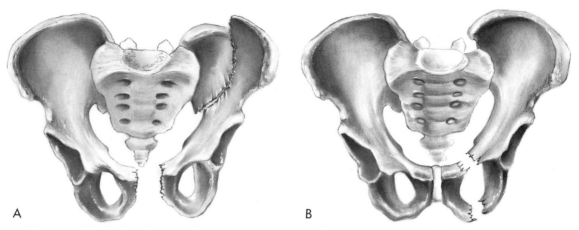

A   **B**

Figure 9–11. Pelvic leverage fractures. *A*, The pelvis has been compressed from front and behind, breaking the pelvic ring anteriorly and posteriorly. The symphysis pubis and left iliac wing have been disrupted. *B*, Another example of a pelvic leverage or compression injury in which the left pubic rami and sacroiliac joint have been disrupted.

articulations or sacral fractures results (Figs. 9–10, 9–11, 9–12).

3. By *shear.* The patient sustains a blow against the knee while sitting erect, in the typical dashboard injury of vehicular trauma. This force is transmitted through the long axis of the femur to the hip bone, which is driven backward and upward. The usual result is posterior fracture-dislocation of the hip, but the sacrum may fracture if the leg is moderately abducted at the moment of impact, thus directing the force medially (Figs. 9–13, 9–14).

A direct blow to the sacrum from behind may produce a transverse sacral fracture, usually below the sacroiliac joints, often with anterior displacement of the distal fragment. Isolated fractures of the sacrum are usually of this nature.

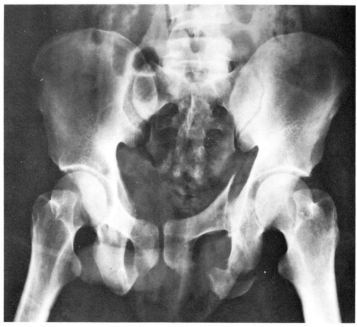

Figure 9–12. Pelvic leverage fracture. The pelvis has been flattened from front to back by a compressing force, producing multiple fractures of the pubic and ischial rami, and buckling of the right sacroiliac articulation.

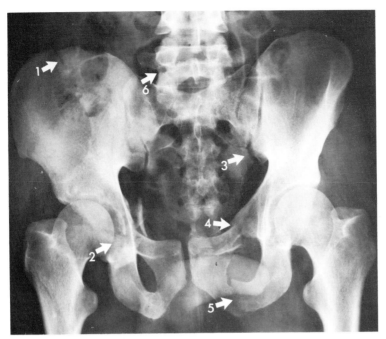

Figure 9–13. Pelvic shear fracture. Force transmitted through the long axis of the right femur has produced a central fracture-dislocation of the right hip joint (arrow 2), after which the pelvis has been fractured at the right iliac wing and sacroiliac joint (arrow 3), left pubic and ischial rami (arrows 4 and 5). Bilateral spondylolysis at L-5 level is incidentally present (arrow 6). (Courtesy of R. H. Freiberger, M.D., Hospital for Special Surgery, New York, N.Y.)

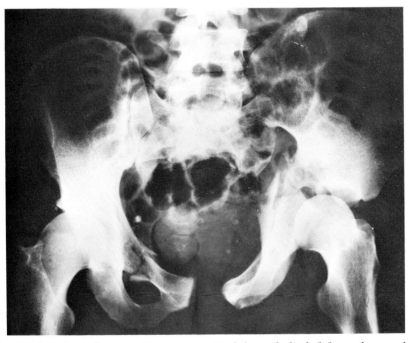

Figure 9–14. Pelvic shear fracture. Force transmitted through the left femur has produced a central fracture-dislocation of the left hip joint, and dislocated the entire left hip bone upwards and backwards. The right pubic and ischial rami have been fractured as well. (Courtesy of R. H. Freiberger, M.D., Hospital for Special Surgery, New York, N.Y.)

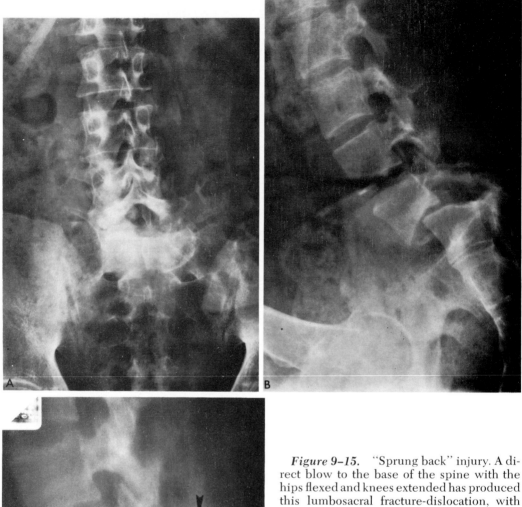

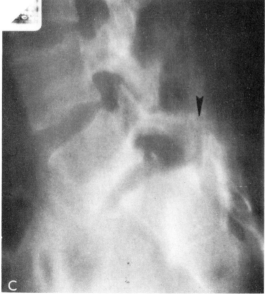

Figure 9–15. "Sprung back" injury. A direct blow to the base of the spine with the hips flexed and knees extended has produced this lumbosacral fracture-dislocation, with the lumbar spine displaced forwards on the sacrum. *A,* Frontal view: Note disruption of the vertebral arch alignment and fractures of the left lower lumbar transverse processes, from avulsion of the quadratus lumborum muscle. *B,* The lumbosacral fracture-dislocation is clearly shown on lateral view. *C,* Lateral tomographic cut showing locking of the lumbosacral articular processes (arrow) preventing closed reduction of the dislocation.

A direct blow to the upper sacrum or lower lumbar spine, with the lumbar spine and hips flexed but with the knees extended, may produce an unstable dislocation at the lumbosacral joint (Fig. 9–15) or a fracture-dislocation at the S-1/S-2 level, the so-called "sprung back." This injury may fracture the upper sacrum transversely just above the level of bonding to the pelvis through the sacroiliac joints, forcing the entire vertebral column forward on the pelvis. Associated fractures of the lower lumbar transverse processes may result from avulsive injury to both quadratus lumborum muscles.[2]

Compressive injuries to the pelvis resulting in abnormal traction on the sacrospinous and sacrotuberous ligaments may produce avulsion fractures of the inferior margins of the sacrum, where the ligaments insert (Fig. 9–18 C). These fragments may be further avulsed by the pulling effect of the external rotator muscles of the hip, which originate along their margins.

Radiologic Findings

Sacral fractures are often extremely difficult to detect radiologically, especially if they are undisplaced. The sacral ridges and foraminal margins cast an intricate network of linear densities on the frontal view of the sacrum, in which a thin, undisplaced fracture line may easily lie concealed. Overlying gas and soft tissue shadows add to the complexity, and may obscure bony detail. Small wonder, then, that a sacral fracture may occasionally go undetected until hematoma spreads the fracture line or callus appears to announce its presence!

When injury to the sacrum is suspected, the standard frontal and lateral sacral views may be supplemented by oblique projections to cast off confusing shadows. With the patient supine, the central x-ray beam may be angled 30° toward the head, projecting the full length of the sacrum onto the film. This allows a thorough evaluation of sacral bony detail (Fig. 9–16). If the central ray is angled toward the feet, an obstetric view of

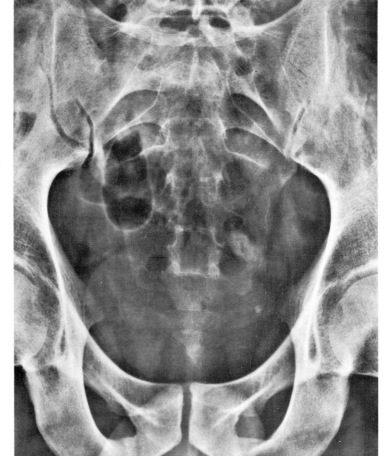

Figure 9–16. 30° tilt view of sacrum. With the patient supine, the central x-ray beam is angled 30° toward the head, projecting the full length of the sacrum onto the film. Thorough evaluation of bony sacral detail may then be obtained. Note the normal sacrococcygeal articulation.

the pelvis is obtained, readily revealing bony displacement in compression fractures of the pelvis.[1] Tomographic cuts of the sacrum in both anteroposterior and lateral planes may provide additional information in difficult cases, and may be especially useful with subtle, undisplaced fractures through the sacral foramina.[6]

The following points should be noted when inspecting sacral radiographs for suspected injury (Fig. 9–17):

1. The left and right halves of the sacrum should be examined for symmetry on frontal views. A vertical fracture through the sacral ala may cause it to appear foreshortened when compared with the ala on the unaffected side. On a true anteroposterior view, the sacroiliac joint on the injured side may thus appear displaced toward the midline (Figs. 9–1; 9–18 A-A; B-B).[1]

2. The lumbosacral intervals between the transverse processes of L-5 and the superior surfaces of the sacroiliac joints will also reveal asymmetry in true anteroposterior projections of the sacrum with vertical fractures (Fig. 9–19).

3. The free borders of the lower sacrum (below the sacroiliac joints) should be closely inspected for avulsion fractures (Fig. 9–18C), or for cracks extending into the bone (Fig. 9–1; 9–3; Fig. 9–18 E-E). Rarely, unfused apophyses of the articular surface and lateral margin of the sacrum may be confused with fracture (Fig. 9–20).

4. The bony ridges extending laterally between the sacral nerve foramina are projected obliquely on the standard frontal view of the sacrum and give the appearance of a series of curved lines arching over each foramen like eyebrows over the eyes (anterior superior sacral foraminal lines) (Fig. 9—16). These superior foraminal lines should appear precisely symmetric on a true anteroposterior view and will amply repay close scrutiny when injury is suspected. In many sacral fractures, the only positive radiologic finding consists of a minimal disturbance or inconsistency in the superior foraminal lines, best established by comparing them with their fellows on the opposite side (Fig. 9–18 D, Fig. 9–21).

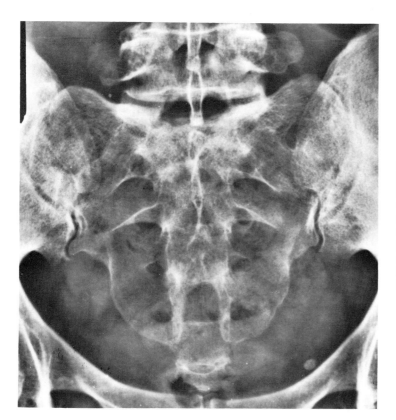

Figure 9–17. Normal sacrum. Note: (1) symmetry of both sacral alae, (2) symmetry of intervals between the transverse processes of L-5 vertebra and the sacrum, (3) intact lower sacral borders, (4) symmetric, paired anterior superior foraminal lines arching over the sacral foramina, like eyebrows over the eyes.

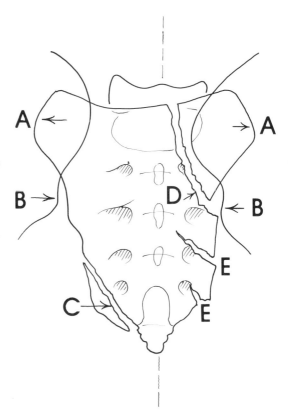

Figure 9–18. Composite drawing of sacral fractures. This drawing outlines some characteristics of sacral fractures. *A-A* and *B-B*: The affected sacroiliac joint has been displaced toward the midline (dotted lines) when compared with its fellow on the opposite side. *C*: Avulsion fracture, resulting from pull on the sacrospinous and sacrotuberous ligaments. *D*: Disruption of superior foraminal lines. *E-E*: Cracks in the free borders of the lower sacrum extending into the bone. (After Bonnin.)

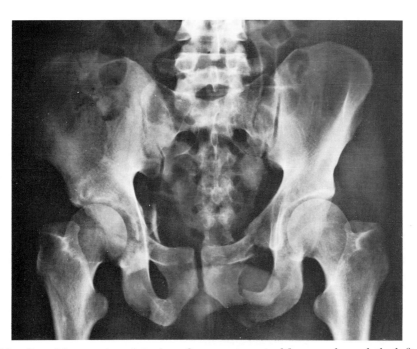

Figure 9–19. Sacral fracture in pelvic shear fracture. A vertical fracture through the left sacral ala has resulted in a discrepancy in the lumbosacral intervals between the transverse processes of L-5 vertebra and the superior surfaces of the sacrum. (Same case as Fig. 9–13.)

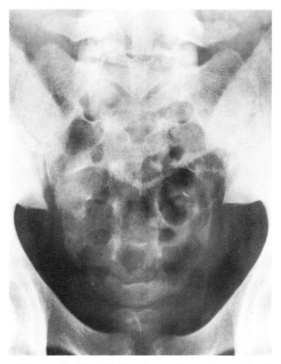

Figure 9–20. Unfused sacral apophyses. Both the articular surfaces and the lower free borders of the sacrum exhibit lucent lines parallel to the margins, becoming scalloped in the lower portion. These should not be confused with fractures.

This is especially true for incomplete, undisplaced sacral fractures, which occur not infrequently.[1, 5, 6]

5. On the lateral projection, displacement or angulation in transverse sacral fractures or dislocations may best be demonstrated, either above the sacroiliac joint level in the "sprung back" injury (Fig. 9–15 B), or below in distal sacral fractures (Figs. 9–22 to 9–26).[2]

Associated Injuries

Pelvic and sacral fractures are often associated with other conditions that pose a greater threat to the patient than the fractures themselves. These include the following:

SHOCK. When sufficient violence has been directed to the body to fracture the pelvis, massive internal bleeding often results, leading to surgical shock. Correction of this condition takes priority over other considerations.

VISCERAL INJURY. Tears of the bladder and urethra constitute the most frequently encountered visceral injury in pelvic frac-

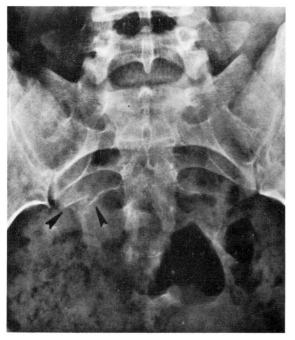

Figure 9–21. Undisplaced transverse sacral fracture. This patient sustained a fall onto the buttocks, resulting in a transverse sacral fracture below the level of the sacroiliac articulations, essentially undisplaced on lateral view. The only clue to the presence of the fracture on the films lies in the asymmetry of the superior foraminal lines on the right (arrows).

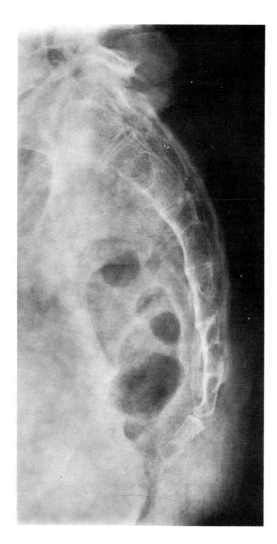

Figure 9–22. Normal sacrum and coccyx, lateral view. An additional sacral segment is present. Note the normal sacrococcygeal joint. (Same case as Fig. 9–16.)

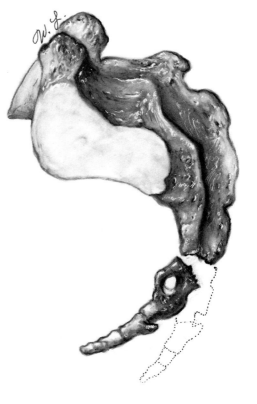

Figure 9–23. Transverse sacral fracture (lateral view). Angulation of the sacral fracture fragments may be noted following transverse fracture of the distal sacrum. (Normal position of the distal fragment indicated by dotted lines.)

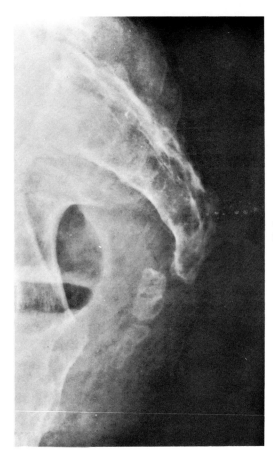

Figure 9–24. Transverse sacral fracture (lateral view). Note the anterior displacement of the distal fracture fragment.

Figure 9–25. Transverse sacral fracture (lateral view). In this sacral fracture, the distal fracture fragment is displaced posteriorly. (Courtesy of Henry M. Selby, M.D., New York, N.Y.)

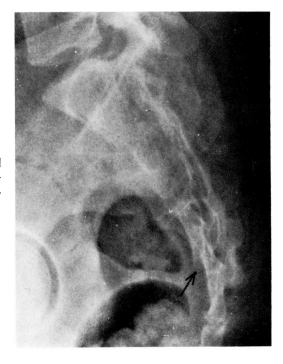

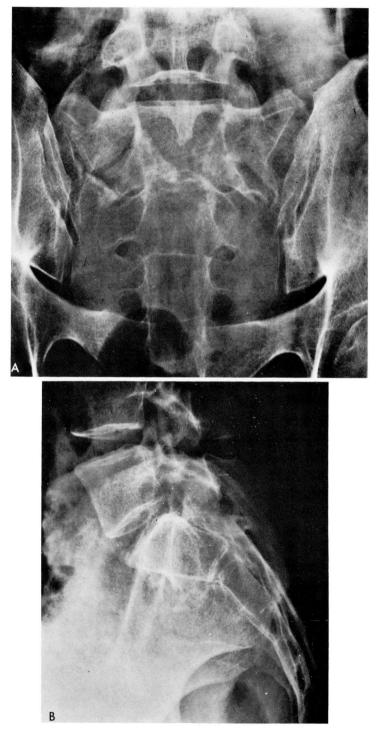

Figure 9–26. Transverse sacral fracture. *A,* Frontal view. This sacral fracture passes through a residual sacral intervertebral joint, associated with a posterior defect at the first sacral level, and is unusual in that it passes between the sacroiliac articulations, rather than above or below them. *B,* Lateral view. Angulation of the sacral fracture fragments is demonstrated. (Courtesy of R. H. Freiberger, M.D., Hospital for Special Surgery, New York, N.Y.)

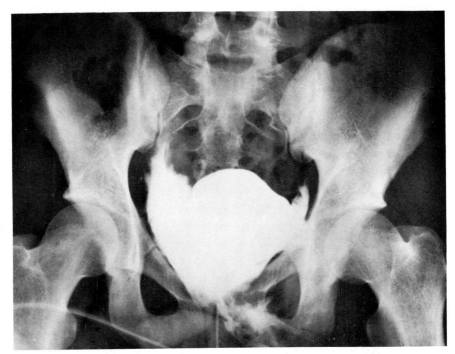

Figure 9–27. Bladder tears with pelvic injury. Cystography demonstrates both intraperitoneal and extraperitoneal bladder tears in this patient with pelvic fracture-dislocation. (Same case as Fig. 9–3.)

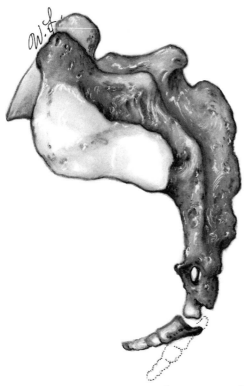

Figure 9–28. Sacrococcygeal joint injury, lateral view. Anterior displacement of the coccyx on the sacrum is demonstrated as a result of injury to the sacrococcygeal joint. (Normal position of the coccyx is indicated by dotted lines.)

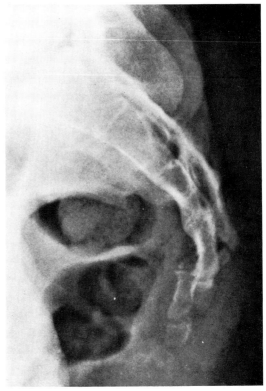

Figure 9–29. Sacrococcygeal joint injury, lateral view. The coccyx has been displaced anteriorly on the distal sacrum on lateral view, the result of a direct blow to the sacrococcygeal joint.

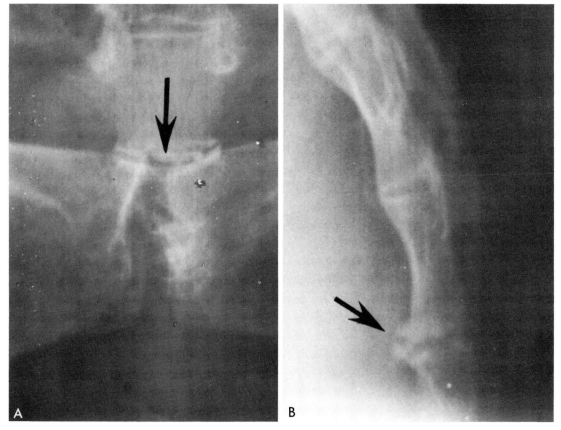

Figure 9–30. Ossification of the sacrococcygeal disk. *A*, Frontal view (arrow). (Disk superimposed on symphysis pubis.) *B*, Lateral view (arrow).

tures. This complication usually manifests itself clinically by hematuria. Urethral catheterization in such cases, if successful, should be followed by radiologic contrast examinations of the lower urinary tract as indicated (Fig. 9–27). Other pelvic viscera may also be injured, including the rectum, small bowel, and vagina.[4]

NEUROLOGIC INJURY. The first and second sacral nerve roots are the most frequently injured in sacral fractures, often owing to inclusion of the nerve foramina in the fracture line. This may give rise to a characteristic syndrome consisting of sensory loss involving the outer aspect of the foot, muscular weakness in the hamstrings and glutei, pronounced weakness of the calf muscles, and impairment of the ankle jerk reflex. Initially, these findings may be overlooked; diagnosis of a sacral fracture may then prompt their detection on further neurologic evaluation.[1, 2]

COCCYGEAL INJURIES

Injuries to the coccyx or to the sacrococcygeal joint most often result from a direct blow to the coccygeal region, such as would be sustained by a fall onto the buttocks. These injuries more commonly occur in women. Although fractures of the coccyx or displacement of the sacrococcygeal joint may be noted on the radiograph (Figs. 9–28, 9–29), the examination is often negative. Sacrococcygeal pain is often disproportionately severe in the light of unremarkable clinical and radiologic findings. Although most patients will respond to conservative therapy, in some cases satisfactory treatment may require excision of the offending sacrococcygeal joint.[4]

Differential Diagnosis of Coccygeal Injuries

Ossification of the sacrococcygeal disk is shown in Figure 9–30 *A, B*. This small, bony fleck could be mistaken for a fracture.

Lateral deviation of the coccyx from the midline, an unusual variant, may be impossible to distinguish from an acute fracture-dislocation, especially in cases of injury. Clinical correlation is required in such cases to arrive at the correct diagnosis.

REFERENCES

1. Bonnin, J. G.: Sacral fractures and injuries to the cauda equina. J. Bone & Jt. Surg., 27·113, 1945.
2. Bucknill, T. M., and Blackburne, J. S.: Fracture-dislocations of the sacrum. J. Bone & Jt. Surg., 58-B:467, 1976.
3. Epstein, B. S.: The Spine, A Radiological Text and Atlas. 3rd ed. Philadelphia, Lea and Febiger, 1969.
4. Key, J. A., and Conwell, H. E.: The Management of Fractures, Dislocations, and Sprains. 5th ed. St. Louis, C. V. Mosby Co., 1951.
5. Medelman, J. P.: Fractures of the sacrum. Amer. J. Roentgenol., 42:100, 1939.
6. Northrop, C. H., Eto, R. T., and Loop J. W.: Vertical fractures of the sacral ala. Amer. J. Roentgenol., 124:102, 1975.
7. Schmorl, G., and Junghanns, H.: The Human Spine in Health and Disease. 2nd American ed. by E. F. Besemann. New York, Grune & Stratton, 1971.

Part V

SPONDYLOLISTHESIS

Chapter 10

SPONDYLOLISTHESIS WITH SPONDYLOLYSIS

DEFINITIONS

The term *spondylolysis* is derived from two Greek roots, *spondylos*, meaning a vertebra, and *lysis* meaning a splitting; thus we have "splitting of a vertebra." This term specifically refers to defects in the pars interarticularis (interarticular isthmus) of the vertebral arch, either on one or on both sides (Figs. 10–1, 10–2). *Spondyloschisis* has been used as a synonym for spondylolysis (*schisis* in Greek meaning a break or cleavage) but might perhaps be more accurately restricted to acute fracture of the pars interarticularis.

Spondylolisthesis (*listhesis,* a slipping) means displacement of one vertebra upon another. Spondylolisthesis may be associated with defects in the vertebral arch (*spondylolisthesis with spondylolysis, spondylolytic spondylolisthesis*) or may occur without them. Spondylolytic spondylolisthesis (Fig. 10–3) has also been described as *isthmic spondylolisthesis, Newman Type II spondylolisthesis*, or simply as *spondylolisthesis* without qualification, although this may lead to confusion with nonspondylolytic varieties, which will be considered in Chapter 11.[5, 9, 15, 26]

INCIDENCE OF SPONDYLOLYSIS

A voluminous literature on spondylolysis and spondylolisthesis has accumulated with the years. Wiltse,[25, 26] in his overall reviews of the subject, reckons the average incidence of pars interarticularis defects (spondylolysis) in the general population to be about 5 per cent. Moreton,[14] in reviewing 32,600 lumbar spine radiographs of asymptomatic individuals, found the incidence of

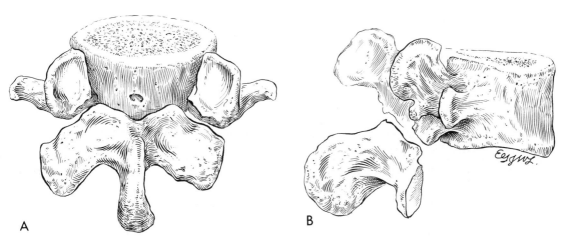

Figure 10–1. Bilateral spondylolysis. *A*, Posterior view. The vertebral arch is divided bilaterally by defects through each pars interarticularis. *B*, Lateral view, slightly oblique. Note the relationship of the pars defect to the (paired) superior articular and transverse processes above, and to the inferior articular and spinous processes below.

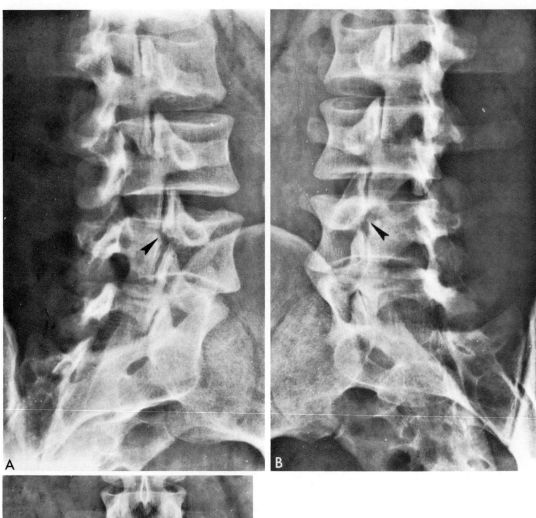

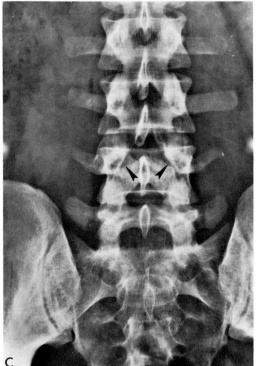

Figure 10–2. Bilateral spondylolysis of L-4 vertebra. *A,B,* Oblique views demonstrating the defects in each pars interarticularis, or spondylolysis (arrows) on L-4 level. These defects are usually best demonstrated on oblique views. (Compare these defects with the normal vertebral arches above and below.) *C,* Frontal view, also demonstrating the bilateral L-4 defects (arrows).

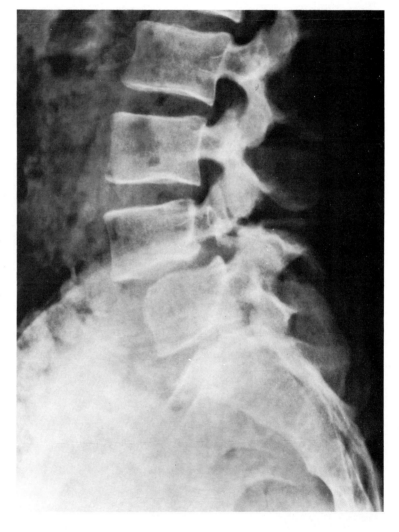

Figure 10–3. Spondylolytic spondylolisthesis. The anterior portion of L-4 vertebra has slipped forward on L-5 vertebra, as a consequence of bilateral spondylolysis dividing the L-4 vertebral arch. The inferior articular processes, laminae, and spinous process of L-4 vertebra have remained behind.

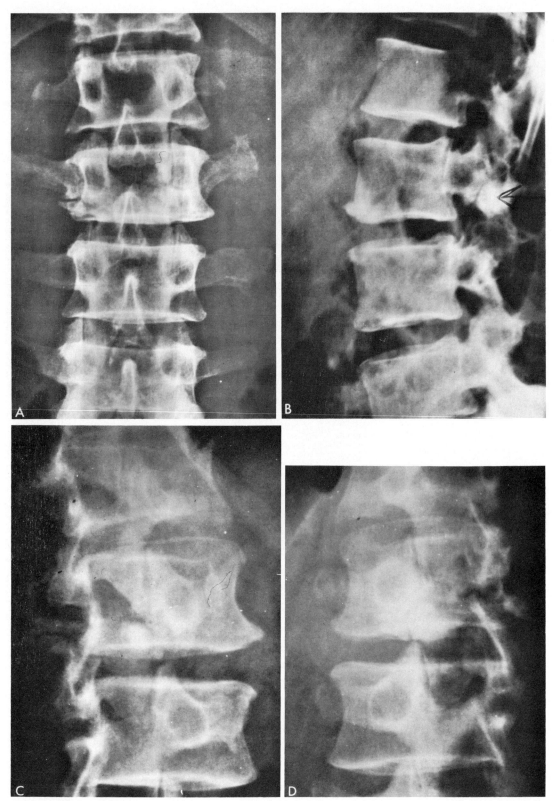

Figure 10–4. Bilateral spondylolysis at L-2 vertebra, *A,B,C,D,* Anteroposterior, lateral, and both oblique views reveal bilateral spondylolysis of L-2 vertebral arch. (The arrow on the lateral view points to the defect and adjacent reactive sclerosis.)

pars defects to average 7.2 per cent, of which 74 per cent were bilateral. In series of patients complaining of low back pain, the incidence of spondylolysis rises to about 10 per cent.[7] A clear-cut relationship between spondylolysis and low back pain does not exist, however; many individuals with spondylolysis remain asymptomatic, and the defects are only incidentally discovered. The highest reported incidences of spondylolysis have been noted by Stewart in Alaskan Eskimos, 26.3 per cent of whom demonstrated vertebral arch defects, this figure rising to over 50 per cent in isolated Eskimo communities north of the Yukon.[6, 23]

Wiltse[26] stated that about half of his cases of spondylolysis were associated with some degree of slipping of the vertebral bodies (spondylolytic spondylolisthesis.) In Lerner and Gazin's series, 36 per cent of their cases of spondylolysis exhibited spondylolisthesis as well.[7] Defects of the pars interarticularis (interarticular isthmus) demonstrate a strong predilection for the fifth lumbar level; 67 per cent to 91.2 per cent of all such defects occur at L-5 in multiple series.[13, 14, 18, 23] Defects at the L-4 level account for about 10 per cent of the remainder, and involvement of higher levels occurs relatively infrequently (Fig. 10–4). More than one level may be involved (Fig. 10–5). Alaskan Eskimos, in addition to a much higher overall incidence of spondylolysis compared with other groups, demonstrate a proportionately higher percentage

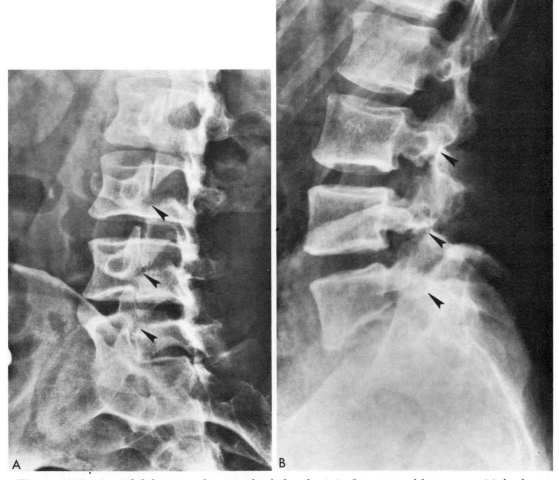

Figure 10–5. Spondylolysis involving multiple levels. *A*, Left anterior oblique view. Multiple pars interarticularis defects are demonstrated on the right, involving L-3, L-4, and L-5 vertebrae (arrows). All were bilateral. *B*, Lateral view. Arrows again demonstrate multiple-level spondylolysis.

of upper lumbar involvement than has been observed in other series.[23]

With respect to race, comparatively higher incidences of spondylolysis have been reported in Mongolian Lapps and in Japanese, as well as in the Eskimos mentioned. United States Blacks, on the other hand, show a decreased incidence of spondylolysis (2.4 per cent) when contrasted with their Caucasian counterparts (5.8 per cent).[18] A strong familial incidence has been reportedly noted. Male predominance has been reported in all series, perhaps reflecting increased physical activity as an etiologic factor. An increased incidence of spondylolysis has been noted in some athletes, including weight lifters and football linemen, compared to the general population.[2]

Spondylolysis increases with advancing age in all series, but only to a point. Stewart initially noted a gradual increase of spondylolysis in his Alaskan Eskimo population to the age of 40 years.[23] Newman and Stone[15] noted a peak age incidence of 35 years at the time of diagnosis of "stress fracture" spondylolisthesis. Rowe and Roche[18] found pars defects rare before the age of ten, but by the age of 20 they had risen to a constant level, with no significant increase in incidence thereafter. More recently, Wiltse[27] has stated that whereas pars defects are quite rare in five year old Caucasian children in the United States, by first grade school level (age six to seven years) the incidence increases to 5 per cent (Fig. 10–6). Beyond this age, an additional increase of only 0.8 per cent occurs by adulthood.

Congenital defects involving the spinous processes are reported to be five to ten times more common in patients with spondylolysis than in the general population.[3] A thirteenfold increase in spina bifida is noted in patients with pars defects in comparison with the general population (Fig. 10–7) and a fourfold increase in the incidence of significant scoliosis associated with pars defects.[26] Spondylolysis in a transitional lumbosacral vertebra has recently been reported,[4] although Wiltse has noted that "transitional vertebrae, being rather stable, are virtually immune to the defect."[26] More commonly, spondylolysis will involve the vertebra just above a transitional vertebra (Fig. 10–8; same case as Fig. 10–3).

Other, less frequently encountered types of vertebral arch defects that may result in spondylolisthesis include clefts or fractures

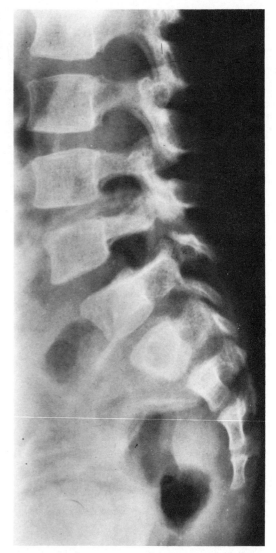

Figure 10–6. Spondylolytic spondylolisthesis in early childhood. Spondylolysis of L-5 vertebra has resulted in a Grade I spondylolisthesis in this three-year-old girl. Pars defects are unusual before the age of six. (Courtesy of R. H. Freiberger, M.D., Hospital for Special Surgery, New York, N.Y.)

of the pedicle (often encountered unilaterally in Alaskan Eskimos with a conventional pars defect on the other side of the vertebral arch)[23, 26] and retroisthmic clefts involving the laminae.[21] Spondylolisthesis resulting from spinal fusions or laminectomies will be discussed later in the chapter. Those types of spondylolisthesis in which the vertebral arch remains intact will be discussed in Chapter 11. Of all the types of spondylolisthesis, that associated with spondylolysis is the most common.[15]

ETIOLOGY OF SPONDYLOLISTHESIS

Spondylolisthesis was first described by Kilian in 1854 as a forward slipping of the last lumbar vertebra on the sacrum, without reference to any defects in the pars interarticularis.[15, 24] In the following year (1855), Robert of Coblenz, working with cadaver vertebrae, demonstrated the mechanism of forward slipping of the vertebrae with bilateral arch defects, and declared that such forward slipping was impossible in the presence of an intact vertebral arch.[15] Subsequent workers, however, soon discovered examples of spondylolisthesis both with and without intact vertebral arches.[15]

Controversy soon arose as to whether these abnormalities found at postmortem examination represented congenital or acquired lesions. As previously noted, a definite familial incidence of spondylolysis had been reported. Rambaud and Renault (1864) propounded a congenital theory of origin for spondylolysis, based on an erroneous observation in the fetal neural arch — a double ossification center, which failed to fuse in the normal manner. This theory of congenital origin has persisted down through the years, being ratified by numerous authorities, including Schmorl, before being definitively put to rest by the exhaustive research of Rowe and Roche,[18] who were unable to find a single example of double ossification center in a series of 509 fetal spines. True congenital spondylolysis present at birth has never been described. Borkow and Kleiger[1] noted roentgen findings of spondylolytic spondylolisthesis in an infant aged four months, in whom a lower back deformity was noted at birth; Wiltse[26] makes anecdotal reference to the same case, claiming that the spondylolisthesis was discovered at age six weeks. This is apparently the

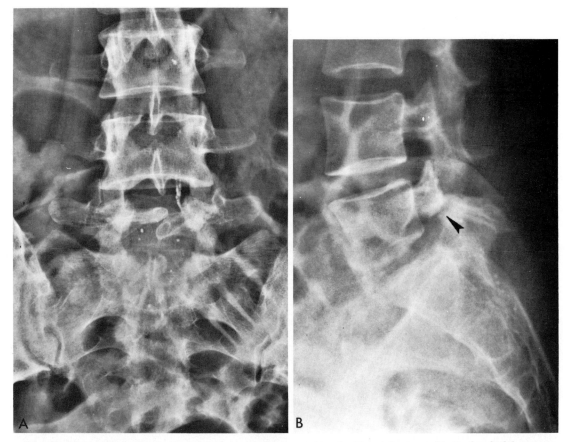

Figure 10–7. Spondylolysis with spina bifida occulta. *A,* Frontal view: Note the bifid spinous process of L-5 vertebra. *B,* Lateral view: Note the pars interarticularis defect at L-5 level (arrow) with adjacent bony sclerosis.

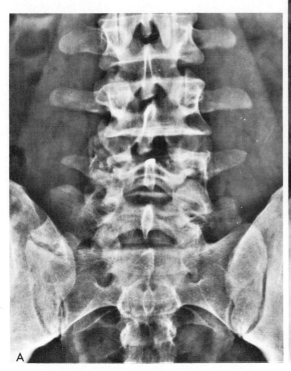
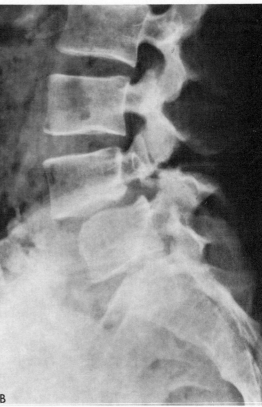

Figure 10–8. Spondylolisthesis occurring above a transitional vertebra. *A*, Frontal view. L-5 vertebra is transitional in nature, being tethered to the sacrum by an assimilation joint involving its right transverse process. Bilateral pars defects may be seen in L-4 vertebra above. *B*, Lateral view (same case as Fig. 10–3). Spondylolytic spondylolisthesis has occurred at the L-4 level. Were it not for the stabilizing influence of the transitional anomaly, spondylolisthesis might have occurred at the L-5 level instead.

youngest case of pars interarticularis defect on record. (Other types of spondylolisthesis, such as those resulting from malformed articular processes or from generalized bone disease, may more clearly represent congenital conditions, however.)

An acquired origin of spondylolisthesis was first proposed by Lane in 1893.[15, 24] Many observations support his concept of acquired spondylolisthesis, which may be summarized as follows:[15] 1. pars defects are unknown in fetuses or in stillborns; 2. they are hardly ever seen before the usual age of walking, that is, one year; 3. the incidence of pars defects increases with age; 4. slipping may occur with an elongated but intact pars before a break occurs; 5. the break sometimes heals; 6. the extent of vertebral slip has no relation to the width of the pars defect; and 7. the edges of the defect (as seen on the lateral radiograph) often appear irregular, and histologically resemble a pseudarthrosis, rather than being smooth

and rounded off, as might be expected with a congenital lesion.

In short, spondylolysis may be considered as a type of stress or fatigue fracture of the pars interarticularis resulting from repeated mechanical stress placed on the vertebral arch by walking erect, extending the lumbar vertebrae in lordosis.[15, 25–27]

If this is true, why does spondylolysis occur in only 5 per cent of the erect population, instead of in everyone? And how do we explain the familial incidence? Wiltse, building on the work of Brocher, Taillard, and Newman, proposes this answer: "The defect in the pars interarticularis is caused by two factors: First, an hereditary defect or dysplasia in the cartilage model of the arch of the affected vertebra, and usually present in several other vertebrae in the same individual; and second, the strain on the pars interarticularis in the lower lumbar spine consequent to the stance, and lumbar lordosis, characteristic of man. Stress or strain alone will not produce the lesion unless the dysplasia is present."[11, 25] Whether the underlying bony defect represents a hereditary dysplasia, as Wiltse suggests, or an aseptic necrosis or ischemic insult as suggested by others, remains unclear.

This double etiologic theory of congenital dysplasia plus the acquired effect of recurrent stress seems the most attractive explanation for spondylolysis offered to date. Still, some observations may remain unaccounted for. If the incidence of spondylolysis is truly increased in certain groups of athletes (weight lifters, football linemen) compared with the general population, as suggested by others,[2] then dysplasia of the vertebral arch cannot be the complete answer, unless we are to assume that such athletes have a greater incidence of dysplastic vertebral arches than does the population at large. Repeated stress of increased magnitude may be capable of dividing the normal pars interarticularis as well. In any case, it is difficult to prove or disprove the antecedent existence of bone dysplasia in any given patient who has developed spondylolysis.

MECHANISMS OF INJURY IN SPONDYLOLYSIS

The exact mechanism of injury responsible for spondylolysis in the lumbar spine remains unclear, although it is increasingly evident that the injury itself consists of a fatigue fracture resulting from repeated mechanical stresses brought to bear on the pars interarticularis. Stewart,[23] in attempting to explain the high incidence of spondylolysis in Alaskan Eskimos, noted that they were subject to repeated falls on the buttocks due to slipping on icy rock.[15, 23] In an allied observation, Newman and Stone[15] described the "toddling posture" assumed by a small child at the age when walking begins. The hips, not yet fully extended, cause hyperextension in the erect lumbar spine, placing excessive strain and forward thrust on the lower lumbar vertebrae. Unsteady on their feet at first, children are subject to falls at this age, often landing on their buttocks with the back erect and their legs extended in front. Interestingly, spondylolysis is first noted at about this age.[15]

It may be that as the spine develops with age and passes through the osteoid stage to one of denser cortical bone, the tendency to stretching or attenuation of the pars interarticularis under stress becomes less, and that to spondylolysis increases. This sequence is reflected in the age distribution of earlier "congenital" (Newman Type I) spondylolisthesis and later spondylolytic (Newman Type II) spondylolisthesis observed by Newman and Stone in their series. Included was a child who first exhibited stretching or elongation of the vertebral arch, and then subsequently a pars defect in the elongated arch at the age of six. Capener has described a similar case in a little girl of seven[15] and Wiltse alludes to the same phenomenon.[26]

The pars interarticularis, joining the articular processes to the pedicles, transverse processes, and laminae, may be considered the pivotal center of the vertebral arch. Bending forces are applied to the pars interarticularis and inferior articular process upon erect load-bearing with the lumbar spine extended. Although attempts to fracture the pars interarticularis by flexion of cadaver spines have all failed, when extension forces were exerted on isolated lumbar vertebrae some success was obtained in mechanically reproducing fractures of the pars interarticularis (spondylolytic fractures).[2, 18, 24] Schinz et al.[20] assert that in spondylolysis of L-5 the defect is exaggerated by increasing extension or lumbar lordosis, while spondylolytic defects in higher lumbar segments are more widely separated by spinal flexion. It may be that mechanisms of injury that produce spondylolysis in the upper lumbar spine differ from those in the lower.

MECHANISMS OF INJURY IN SPONDYLOLISTHESIS

Newman[15] described marked stretching or elongation of the L-4 and L-5 pedicles in the spine of a six year old girl afflicted with osteogenesis imperfecta. Pedicle elongation was moderate at the third lumbar level, slight at the second and first, and imperceptible above. He postulated that, in this patient with a generalized weakness of bone, the extent of spinal deformity mirrored the mechanical stress placed upon it by normal activity in the erect position, that is, she exhibited a "plastic" spine. He concluded that such stress or "thrust" was maximal in the lower lumbar spine.

Three factors oppose forward slipping in the normal lumbar spine, according to Newman: 1. adequate articular processes; 2. an intact vertebral arch; and 3. normal bone structure.

Defects in these three factors allow spondylolisthesis to occur. 1. Defective articular processes facilitate "congenital" spondylolisthesis, as we will see in Chapter 11. Degenerative changes in the apophyseal joints and intervertebral disks may also allow sliding to occur. 2. Vertebral arch defects constitute an integral part of spondylolytic spondylolisthesis. 3. Structural inadequacy of bone may permit spondylolisthesis to occur in the absence of defects of the articular processes or the vertebral arch, as in Newman's little girl with osteogenesis imperfecta.

TYPES OF SPONDYLOLISTHESIS

1. Spondylolytic (Newman Type II) spondylolisthesis, as we have seen, involves forward slipping of one vertebra upon another, usually L-5 on S-1, as a consequence of defects in the pars interarticularis, usually on both sides of the vertebral arch (Fig. 10–9).

An increased lumbosacral angle of Ferguson (Fig. 10–10) is often noted on the lateral radiograph of the lumbar spine in more advanced grades of spondylolisthesis. Normally measuring 34 degrees from the horizontal, this increase in the lumbosacral angle causes the sacral promontory to resemble an inclined plane, down which the vertebrae above may more easily slip. An increased lumbar lordosis usually accompanies this finding. Mechanically, such a posture might be expected to exert traction on the vertebral arches of L-4 and L-5, or to increase the degree of spondylolisthesis once defects had occurred.

The body of a vertebra with spondylolytic spondylolisthesis often becomes wedge-shaped on lateral view, with the apex of the wedge directed toward the vertebral arch (Fig. 10–11). The extent of wedging is proportional to the increase in the lumbosacral angle noted previously, and a statistically valid correlation exists between the extent

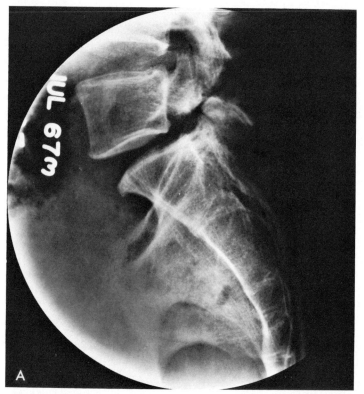

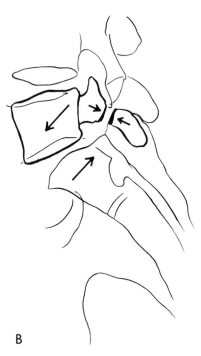

Figure 10–9. Spondylolytic spondylolisthesis. Spondylolytic (Newman Type II) spondylolisthesis involves forward slipping of one vertebra upon another, usually L-5 on S-1 (large arrows), as a consequence of pars interarticularis defects (small arrows), usually bilateral.

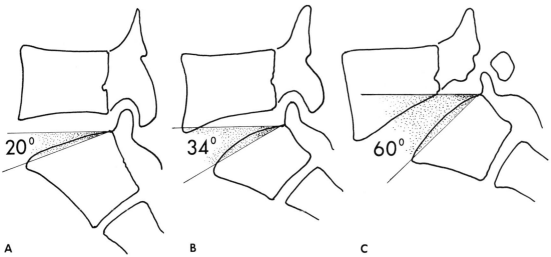

Figure 10–10. Comparison of spondylolytic and nonspondylolytic spondylolisthesis. *A,* Non-spondylolytic spondylolisthesis. When compared with *B* (normal spine), the lumbosacral angle of Ferguson is reduced. The sacrum is more nearly vertical in position, with the surface of the sacral promontory more nearly horizontal, and a diminished lumbar lordotic curve. The last lumbar vertebral body approaches the rectangular in shape. *B,* Normal spine. The lumbosacral angle of Ferguson measures 34°. The last lumbar vertebral body is midway between rectangular and wedged in shape. *C,* Spondylolytic spondylolisthesis: The lumbosacral angle of Ferguson is enlarged (in the vicinity of 60°) with an increase in lumbar lordosis and tilt of the sacral promontory. The last lumbar vertebral body has assumed a wedged shape, increasing with the extent of the slip. (Note spondylolytic defect outlined posteriorly.)

of vertebral wedge deformity in spondylolytic spondylolisthesis and its degree of slip.[22] Interestingly, in nonspondylolytic spondylolisthesis, the reverse occurs: the lumbosacral angle is decreased, the lumbar lordosis is diminished, and the bodies of L-4 and L-5 vertebrae are more rectangular than normal on lateral view, resulting in increased mechanical stability in the lumbar spine (Fig. 10–10).[15, 17]

In children at the age when spondylolisthesis is usually first discovered (six to seven years), the wedge-shaped deformity of the lower lumbar vertebral bodies is not

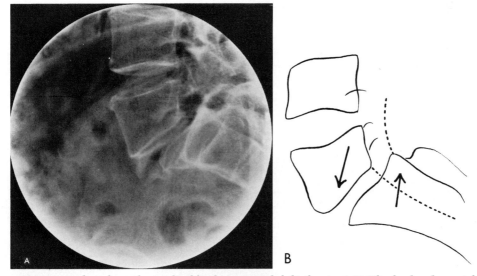

Figure 10–11. Wedge-shaped vertebral body in spondylolisthesis. *A,B,* The body of a vertebra with spondylolisthesis (here, L-5) often becomes wedge-shaped on lateral view, with the apex of the wedge directed toward the vertebral arch. A statistically valid correlation exists between the degree of vertebral wedge deformity and the extent of slip. (See also Figs. 10–31, 10–33*B*.)

yet apparent. Wiltse[26] believes that the presence of spondylolysis subsequently alters weight transmission through the lumbar spine to increase mechanical pressure on the posterior portion of the vertebral body, and thereby impedes its subsequent growth in height. He does not believe that the wedged configuration of the lower lumbar vertebral bodies or the increased tilt of the sacral promontory contributes mechanically to the extent of slippage, however.[11]

2. Unilateral spondylolysis (about 20 per cent of all spondylolysis) is frequently associated with reactive sclerosis about the opposite pars interarticularis and pedicle at the same level (Fig. 10–12). This is believed to be the result of increased mechanical stress on the intact pars and pedicle due to altered patterns of weight-bearing, as was noted with congenital hypoplasia of the pedicle in Chapter 8. The increased stress may, however, cause a fatigue fracture in the pars interarticularis opposite the defect; in this manner, unilateral spondylolysis may progress to bilateral involvement, especially if a predisposition to spondylolysis is considered to exist. In such cases, the wider or more clearly defined pars defect will appear on the side opposite the sclerotic pars and pedicle, and may be considered to represent the initial lesion.[10] (Fig. 10–13).

3. "Congenital" (Newman Type I) spondylolisthesis, or lumbosacral subluxation, results from structural abnormalities of the articular processes, allowing forward slipping to occur. This will be discussed in Chapter 11.

4. Nonspondylolytic, "degenerative" (Newman Type IV) spondylolisthesis may occur with degenerative changes in the apophyseal joints, intervertebral disks, and paraspinal soft tissues. It too will be discussed in Chapter 11.

5. Traumatic (Newman Type III) spondylolisthesis, spondyloschisis, or traumatic spondylolysis: Spondylolysis probably represents a fatigue or stress fracture of the pars interarticularis, the result of continual, repeated mechanical weight-bearing stress on the vertebral arch.[25-27] The role of acute injury in spondylolysis is unclear, but it is probably small. Although many patients with spondylolysis are able to relate their symptoms to an episode of back trauma, the injury is often of a relatively minor nature, and others give no history of any significant back injury at all.[15]

A number of cases of acute, traumatic fracture of the pars interarticularis have been reported in the literature, which have gone on to heal with immobilization of the spine.[12, 14, 16] Few of these cases have convincing radiologic proof that no spondyloly-

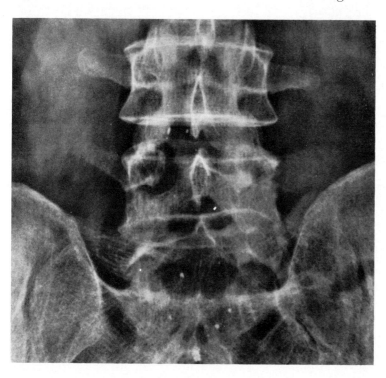

Figure 10–12. Unilateral spondylolysis. Unilateral spondylolysis is present on the right at L-4 (crescentic lucency on anteroposterior view). The opposite pars and pedicle of L-4 vertebra exhibit reactive sclerosis.

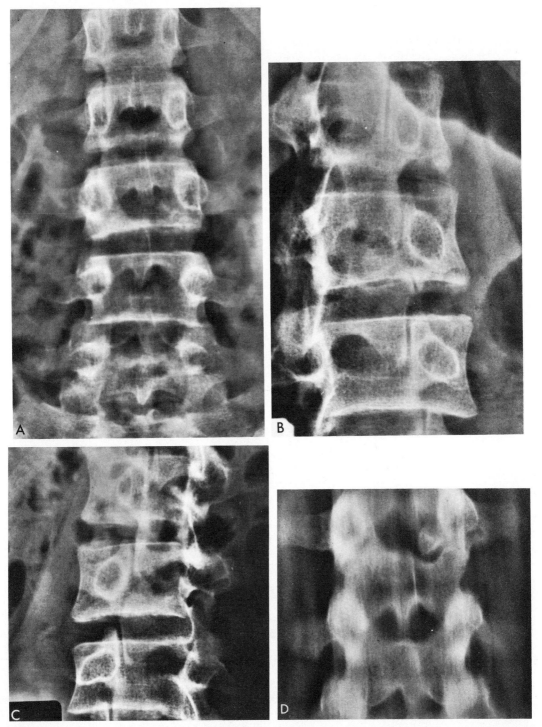

Figure 10–13. Unilateral spondylolysis. *A*, Frontal view. Spondylolysis involves the left pars interarticularis of L-3 vertebra. Reactive sclerosis has occurred in the opposite pedicle of L-3, on the right. *B*, Right anterior oblique view. A well-established pars defect is present on the left, with degenerative and proliferative changes about the vertebral arch fragments (see also tomogram, *D*). *C*, Left anterior oblique view. A fatigue fracture or recent pars defect has occurred on the right as well, so spondylolysis is now bilateral. Note the sclerosis about the right pedicle, indicating the left pars defect to have preceded the right in time. *D*, Tomographic section of the same case. Degenerative and proliferative changes have occurred about the left pars defect, with formation of a pseudarthrosis at this site between the vertebral arch fragments. The right pars defect is only faintly seen on this section. (Courtesy of R. H. Freiberger, M.D., Hospital for Special Surgery, New York, N.Y.)

sis existed prior to the trauma. Were these injuries in fact acute fractures, or did they represent examples of the more usual spondylolysis incidentally associated with back injuries? Lob was unable to find a single convincing case of isolated pars fracture resulting from spinal injury in his series of over 700 exhaustively analyzed cases of spinal injury. He observes that the normal pars interarticularis consists of such dense, stout bone that a force of injury sufficient to fracture it invariably produces a severe spinal fracture-dislocation easily distinguished from spondylolysis.[8] Moreover, the bone is normally densest and strongest at the lower lumbar levels where pars defects usually occur. Isolated fractures of the vertebral arch resulting from direct injury are extremely unusual, and involve the laminae rather than the pars interarticularis when they do occur.[15]

An episode of back trauma may complete the separation of a stressed pars interarticularis in a patient predisposed to a spondylolysis by fatigue changes in his vertebral arch. However, most patients with a history of recent injury and back pain who exhibit spondylolysis radiologically do not in fact have acute fractures of the pars interarticularis.[26, 27]

Healing of fractures occurring elsewhere in the vertebral arch proceeds to solid union with three to seven months' immobilization, and a dense mass of callus forms about the fracture site in the process.[8] This is only rarely the case with spondylolysis, however, which by and large heals poorly with immobilization and exhibits little or no callus formation in the process.[26] (Fig. 10–14).

6. Postoperative spondylolisthesis: Certain types of spondylolytic spondylolisthesis are clearly related to abnormal weight-bearing stresses, termed "spondylolisthesis acquisita." These may involve the uppermost or lowermost levels of a spinal fusion, where the spine is subject to increased bending stresses (Fig. 10–15). Another type of acquired spondylolytic spondylolisthesis

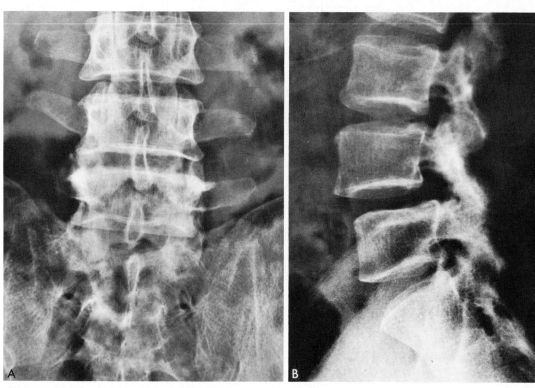

Figure 10–14. Healing in spondylolytic spondylolisthesis. Note proliferative changes (increase in bone density) about each pars interarticularis of L-4, associated with Grade II spondylolytic spondylolisthesis on lateral view. These changes represent attempted healing of the spondylolysis. (Courtesy of R. H. Freiberger, M.D., Hospital for Special Surgery, New York, N.Y.)

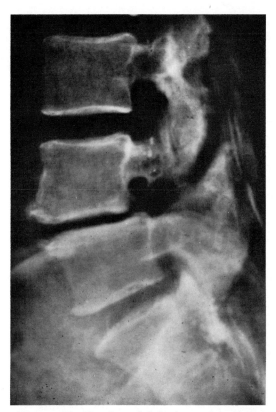

Figure 10–15. Spondylolisthesis acquisita (pseudarthrosis). This patient underwent posterior fusion from L-3 vertebra to the sacrum, and subsequently developed a pseudarthrosis at the L-4/5 level, with spondylolisthesis. (Note the alignment of the vertebral bodies.) In other cases, extensive degenerative change involving the lowermost or uppermost vertebrae of a fused segment may accomplish the same effect.

may result after extensive laminectomies have mechanically weakened the pars interarticularis on each side to the extent that forward slipping of a vertebral body becomes possible (Fig. 10–16).[26]

7. Spondylolisthesis and other bone diseases: Termed "pathological (Newman Type V) spondylolisthesis," this type of spondylolisthesis may arise in a spine already weakened by bone disease, presumably in response to mechanical "thrust" at the lower lumbar levels from the erect stance. Such diseases include osteogenesis imperfecta, achondroplasia, Paget's disease of bone, and localized disorders such as tuberculous spondylitis and deposits of metastatic malignancy occurring in the pedicles or pars interarticularis.[15] Four cases of osteopetrosis associated with spondylolysis were recently reported in a family of six siblings[19] in which the osteopetrosis and spondylolysis seemed to go together—that is, siblings unaffected by osteopetrosis showed no spondylolysis. Increased brittleness of bone in osteopetrosis apparently predisposed the vertebral arches to stress fracture, with reduced resilience. We have seen a similar case (Fig. 10–17).

CLINICAL FINDINGS

Patients with radiologically demonstrable pars defects commonly complain of low back pain, and may relate the pain to a recent injury, although major trauma is not a constant feature of the history. Disability on stooping and lifting and with hard labor is typical. Pain radiated into the hips and legs in 17 per cent of patients in Meyerding's cases of spondylolisthesis,[13] but less than 2 per cent of his patients complained of deformity, stiffness, or paralysis. Ten per cent with spondylolytic spondylolisthesis remained asymptomatic, the diagnosis being made incidentally during radiologic investigation for unrelated complaints. In children, over 50 per cent of all cases of spondylolysis are asymptomatic at the time of diagnosis.[11] Close attention should be paid to youngsters or adolescents with low back pain and spasm of the paraspinal muscles, as early diagnosis of developing spondylolisthesis improves the result of treatment.[25]

On physical examination lesser degrees of spondylolisthesis may go undetected save for some nonspecific muscle spasm in the paraspinal region. However, in more severe grades of spondylolisthesis, examination of the back will reveal a prominent lordosis with shortening of the lumbar spine, a prominent sacrum and spinous process at L-5 level, and a characteristic midline dimple or groove just above this due to depression of the spinous processes with slipping.[3, 13]

RADIOLOGIC FINDINGS

Radiologic evaluation of the lumbar spine for possible spondylolysis should include, in addition to the standard frontal and lateral views of the lumbosacral spine, 45 degree

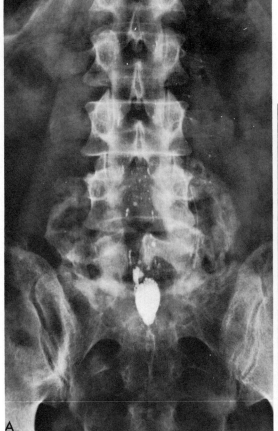

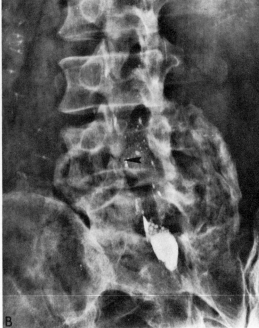

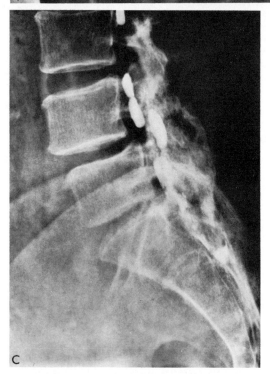

Figure 10–16. Spondylolisthesis acquisita following laminectomy. *A*, Frontal view: Extensive laminectomies, associated with posterolateral fusion, have severely weakened the L-4 vertebral arch. *B*, Left anterior oblique view: Spondylolysis has resulted at the L-4 level (arrow) as a result of mechanical undermining of the vertebral arch. *C*, Lateral view: Grade I spondylolisthesis has eventuated at the L-4 level in consequence of the spondylolysis.

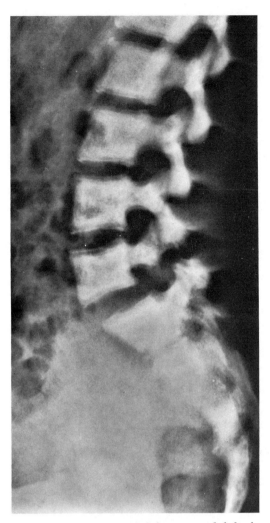

Figure 10–17. Spondylolytic spondylolisthesis with osteopetrosis. Increased brittleness of bone in this six-year-old patient with osteopetrosis has predisposed him to stress fractures of the vertebral arch, shown here at the L-5 level, with associated Grade I spondylolisthesis. Note the generalized increase in skeletal density and the "bone-within-a-bone" appearance of the vertebral bodies characteristic of this disorder.

oblique projections and a collimated "cone-down" lateral view of the lumbosacral joint. Although pars defects may be visualized on the lateral view as often as on the oblique views (and indeed more clearly in some), the oblique views often provide confirmation in questionable cases. An anteroposterior tilt view of the lower lumbar spine, with the central ray angled 30 degrees toward the head with the patient supine, may open up the defects clearly. When severe

osteophytic spurring and hypertrophic change obscure the anatomic detail in the lower lumbar spine, tomography may be required to make the diagnosis.[3]

The pars interarticularis forms the "neck" of the "Scottie dog" as it appears on radiographic views (Fig. 10–18). The classic appearance of spondylolysis on the oblique view is that of the "collar" or "broken neck" of the "Scottie dog" (Figs. 10–19 A, 10–20 C, D). The pars defect may be clearly shown on the lateral view (Fig. 10–20 A, B), lumbar tilt view (Fig. 10–19 B), or even the anteroposterior view (Fig. 10–20 E, F). The width of the pars defect may vary from a narrow or even incomplete fissure through the pars interarticularis to extensive bony defects including portions of the pedicle and superior articular process; such lesions become difficult to distinguish from congenital hypoplasias (see Chapter 9).

The margins of the defect are usually smooth (Fig. 10–21), although the degree of definition may vary, some appearing rather indistinct. Sclerosis of the affected pars interarticularis is also variable, and may be the earliest radiologic finding in spondylolysis, preceding the development of a stress or fatigue fracture in the pars interarticularis. These defects may develop insidiously, and may extend initially only partway through the thickness of the pars interarticularis, becoming complete as the condition progresses; in other cases, partial healing of a completed defect may present a similar appearance (Fig. 10–14). Extensive defects, however, may be accompanied by little or no sclerosis in the vicinity of the defect.

Unilateral spondylolysis often exhibits sclerotic changes in the pars and pedicle opposite the defect, as has been previously noted, in which bilateral spondylolysis may subsequently develop.[10] Lateral deflection of the spinous process above toward the affected pars interarticularis may be noted on anteroposterior view. Spreading of the pars defect allows anterior advancement of the related superior articular process. This in turn causes slight rotation of the affected vertebral arch above toward the defect, reflected by the change in spinous process alignment. This rotary malalignment is similar to that encountered in rotary fracture-dislocations (Chapter 7) and congenital pedicle defects (Chapter 8). It is exaggerated in the upright position; in milder cases, it may

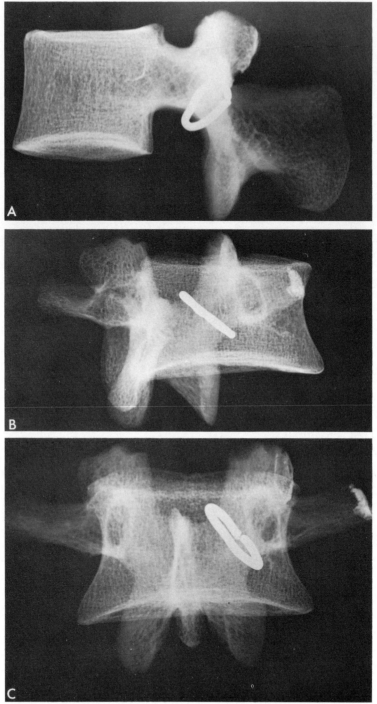

Figure 10–18. Radiographic identification of the pars interarticularis. *A*, Lateral view. A metal ring has been placed around the pars interarticularis of this disarticulated lumbar vertebra. Note the relation of the pars interarticularis to the articular processes above and below. *B*, Right anterior oblique view. Note the characteristic contour of the "Scottie dog." The left transverse process becomes his nose; the left pedicle, his eye; the left superior articular process, his ear; the left pars interarticularis, his neck (with the metal ring serving as a "collar"); the left inferior articular process, his foreleg; the left lamina, his trunk; the right inferior articular process, his hindleg; and the spinous process, his tail. *C*, Frontal view. Note the relationship of the pars interarticularis to the pedicle, lamina, and spinous process.

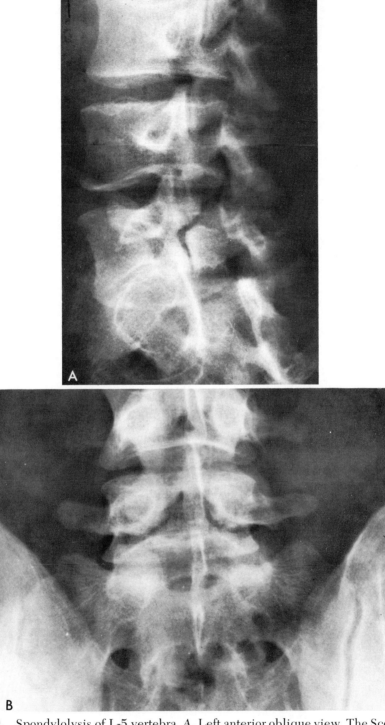

Figure 10–19. Spondylolysis of L-5 vertebra. *A,* Left anterior oblique view. The Scottie dog's neck appears "broken." *B,* Same case, 30° lumbar tilt view: When the central ray is angled 30° toward the head with the patient supine, spondylolytic defects of the vertebral arch are "opened up" and may be seen to advantage. (Defects here involve L-5 vertebra.)

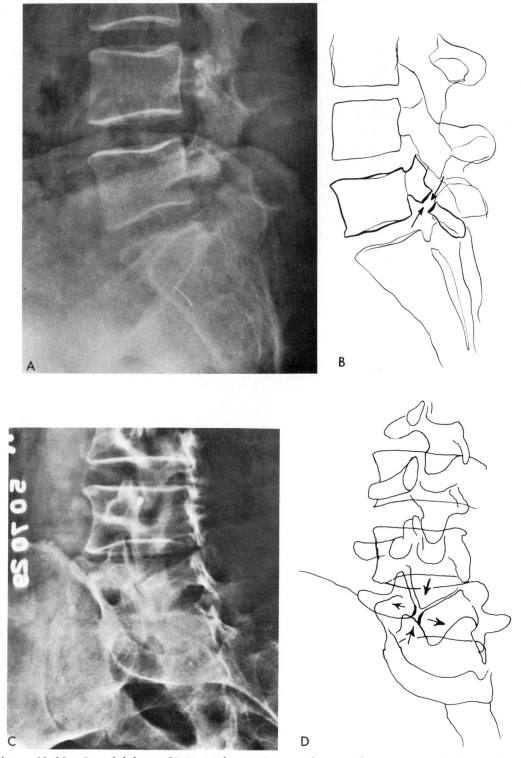

Figure 10–20. Spondylolysis of L-5 vertebra. *A, B*, Lateral view: The pars interarticularis defect at L-5 is clearly shown (arrow). *C,D*, Left anterior oblique view: The neck of the "Scottie dog" appears broken at the L-5 level, when compared with the levels above.

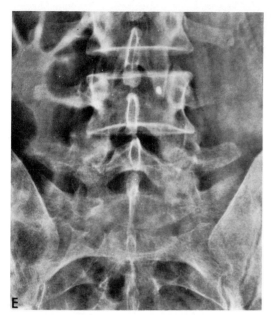
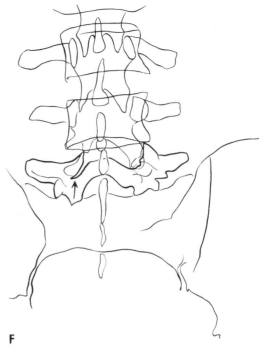

E **F**

Figure 10–20 Continued. E,F, Frontal view: The pars defect is well seen on the right at the L-5 level even on this view (arrow).

disappear altogether if the spine is not stressed in this way.[10]

Evaluation of the presence and degree of spondylolisthetic slippage is made on the lateral view, which should be taken erect to accentuate the deformity. Meyerding[13] was the first to propose a grading of spondylolisthesis based on the radiologic findings. His system, as now employed, divides the surface of the vertebral body beneath the slip into fourths; slippage between the bodies of up to one-fourth of their sagittal diameter constitutes a Grade I spondylolisthesis, of one-fourth to one-half Grade II, and so on. This is measured by noting the position of the posterior aspect of the vertebral body above relative to the body below (Figs. 10–22 through 10–28).

Gradual erosion of the anterior, and in some cases the posterior, aspects of the sacral promontory appear with higher grades of spondylolisthesis. This wearing down of the sacrum by the displaced vertebra above signifies abnormal mobility at the lumbosacral joint, and suggests a "rocking" or "teeter-totter" movement of the lumbar spine on the sacrum, most conspicuous in children with spondylolisthesis.[5]

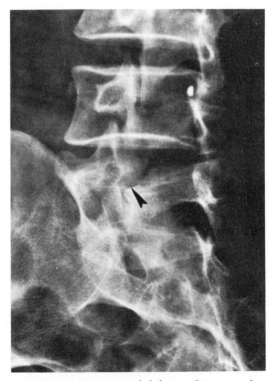

Figure 10–21. Spondylolysis of L-5 vertebra, left anterior oblique view. The margins of the defect (arrow) appear smooth, and the borders are relatively well defined, suggesting chronic bony change rather than an acute fracture of the pars interarticularis.

421

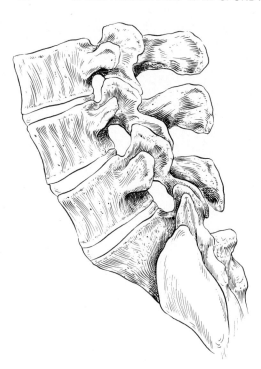

Figure 10–22 through 10–26 inclusive. Grading of spondylolisthesis.

Figure 10–22. Normal lumbosacral spine, for reference.

Figure 10–23. Grade I spondylolisthesis. L-5 vertebra has slipped forward on S-1 to the extent of one-quarter the sagittal diameter of the sacral promontory.

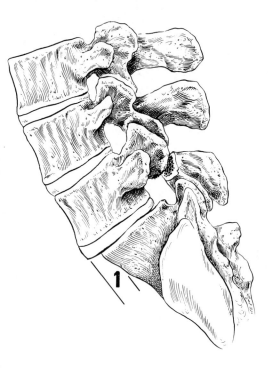

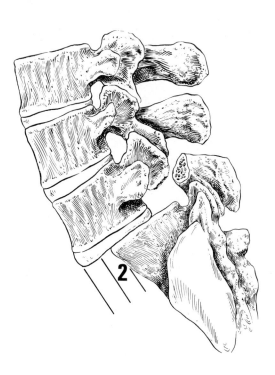

Figure 10–24. Grade II spondylolisthesis. Forward slipping of L-5 on S-1 has progressed to half the sagittal diameter of S-1 vertebra.

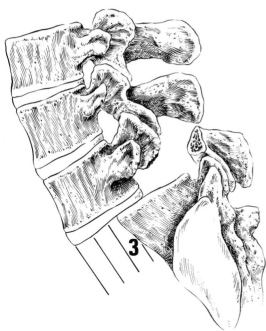

Figure 10–25. Grade III spondylolisthesis. Forward slipping has advanced to three-quarters of the S-1 diameter.

Degenerative changes almost always ensue in the intervertebral joints involved by spondylolisthesis in adults (Fig. 10–29), and may be recognized on the radiograph. Shearing stress is exerted on the fibers of the anulus fibrosus by forward displacement of the vertebral body above, deforming the intervertebral disk. With the passage of time and progressive disk degeneration, the changes of osteochondrosis supervene in both intervertebral disk and apophyseal joints at the level of spondylolisthesis. A loss of height of the disk space, subchondral sclerosis, a "vacuum sign," and osteophyte formation involving the adjoining vertebral body surfaces appear, with osteoarthrotic changes of the apophyseal joints.

In the more advanced grades of spondylolisthesis, a large shelving and supporting anterior osteophyte may grow from the lip of the vertebral body below, behaving as a mechanical buttress or strut to help stabilize the spine (Fig. 10–30). Alternatively, a "ball-and-socket" configuration of the vertebral bodies at the level of spondylolisthesis may serve the same purpose. This consists of a hemispheric convexity of the cranial end-plate of the body below, the so-called *torus promontoralis sustentaculum*, which

reciprocates with a concave impression in the caudal end-plate of the body above (Figs. 10–31, 10–32).[3] The wedge-shaped or trapezoidal appearance of the spondylolisthetic vertebral body has been noted previously (Figs. 10–11, 10–31, 10–33 B).[22, 26]

In cases of advanced spondylolisthesis, weight-bearing stresses may displace the anteriorly slipping vertebral body downward by the combined weight of the head, arms, and torso acting through the vertebral column. On the frontal view the lumbar spine may appear abnormally foreshortened. The contours of the caudally displaced vertebral body present an inverted curvilinear density below the plane of the affected joint. Brailsford described this finding as a *bow-line* (1929); other writers have likened it to an *inverted Napoleon's hat* or *gendarme's cap*[28] (Fig. 10–33 A). The forward slip and downward displacement become readily apparent on the lateral view (Fig. 10–33 B). Tilting of the sacral promontory and stretching of the spondylolytic defects promote mechanical instability at the lumbosacral joint and accelerate the spondylolisthetic deformity.

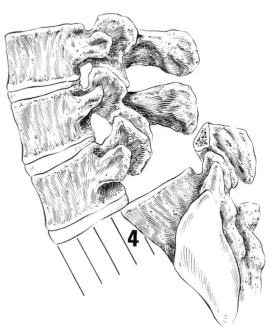

Figure 10–26. Grade IV spondylolisthesis. Further advance of L-5 on S-1 has occurred in excess of three-quarters of the S-1 diameter. Complete dislocation of the lumbosacral joint may occur. (These higher grades usually represent examples of "congenital" spondylolisthesis.)

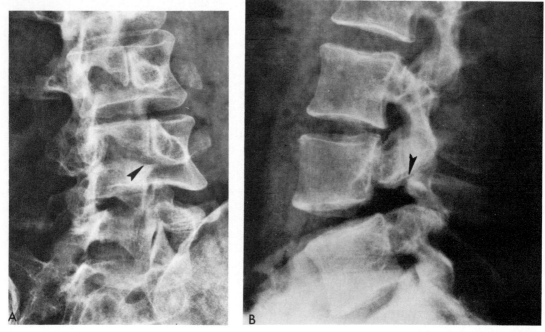

Figure 10–27. Grade I spondylolytic spondylolisthesis of L-4 vertebra. *A,* Right anterior oblique view. Note the pars defect at L-4 level (arrow). *B,* Lateral view. Grade I spondylolisthetic slip of L-4 vertebra on L-5 has resulted from the spondylolytic separation (arrow). Note the slight forward displacement of L-4 vertebral body relative to L-5.

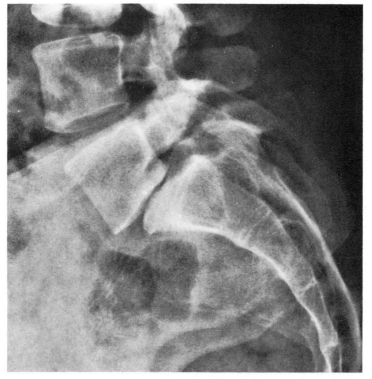

Figure 10–28. Grade II spondylolytic spondylolisthesis of L-5 vertebra. The vertebral body of L-5 has slipped between one-quarter to halfway off the sacral promontory. Degenerative change has occurred in the lumbosacral intervertebral disk as well.

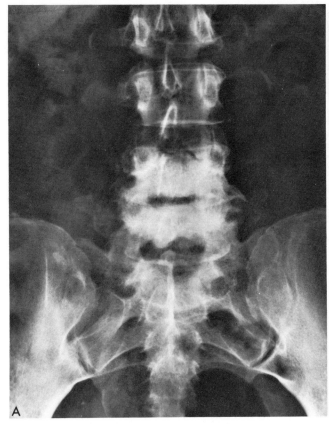

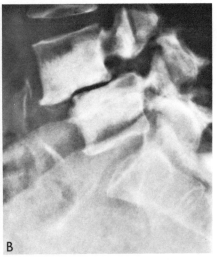

Figure 10–29. Intervertebral disk degeneration with spondylolisthesis. *A,* Frontal view. Marked reactive bony sclerosis has occurred in the L-4 and L-5 vertebral bodies adjacent to the degenerated intervertebral disk, and osteophyte formation may be noted to the left of the disk space. *B,* Lateral view. A Grade II spondylolytic spondylolisthesis has exerted shearing stress on the fibers of the anulus fibrosus. Note marked loss of height of the affected in-

tervertebral disk when compared with the disks above and below, the "vacuum sign" of gas within the degenerated disk, and severe subchondral sclerosis of the adjoining vertebral bodies. The L-4 pars defect can be clearly seen posteriorly.

Figure 10–30. Advanced spondylolisthesis. In the more advanced grades of spondylolisthesis, a large, shelving, supporting anterior osteophyte may grow from the lip of the vertebral body below, behaving as a mechanical buttress or strut to help stabilize the spine. (This case, representing a Grade III spondylolisthesis, and the examples of Grade IV spondylolisthesis which follow, are actually examples of "congenital" spondylolisthesis, the type most commonly represented in advanced grades of spondylolisthesis, which will be discussed in Chapter 11.) (Courtesy of R. H. Freiberger, M.D., Hospital for Special Surgery, New York, N.Y.)

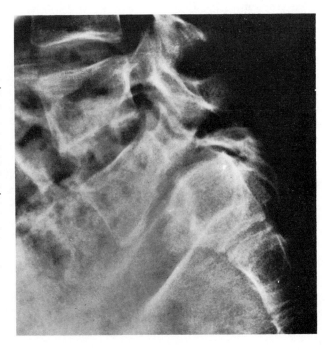

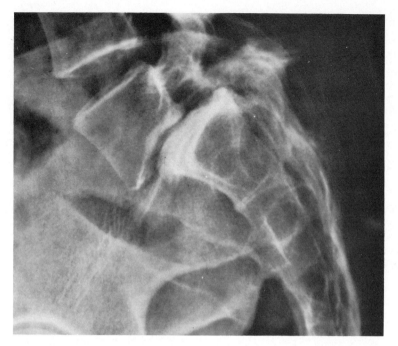

Figure 10–31. Grade II spondylolisthesis of L-5 vertebra. The vertebral body of L-5 has slipped halfway off the sacral promontory. The lumbosacral joint exhibits, in addition to severe disk degeneration, a "ball-and-socket" configuration, with formation of a hemispherical convexity of the sacral promontory or torus promontoralis sustentaculum, to help stabilize the joint. Note also the trapezoidal shape assumed by the body of L-5 vertebra.

DIFFERENTIAL DIAGNOSIS OF SPONDYLOLYSIS

1. Isolated fractures of the normal pars interarticularis, if they truly exist, are infrequent, as we have previously seen. Acute traumatic fracture of the normal pars interarticularis is almost always accompanied by severe spinal injury elsewhere.[8] An isolated pars fracture would exhibit sharp, irregular

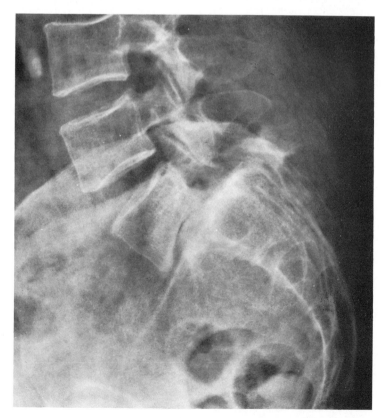

Figure 10–32. Grade III spondylolisthesis of L-5 vertebra. The vertebral body of L-5 has slipped between 50 per cent to 75 per cent off the sacral promontory. A prominent torus promontoralis sustentaculum has resulted, lending mechanical support to the unstable joint. A severe degree of degenerative change in the lumbosacral joint has occurred as well.

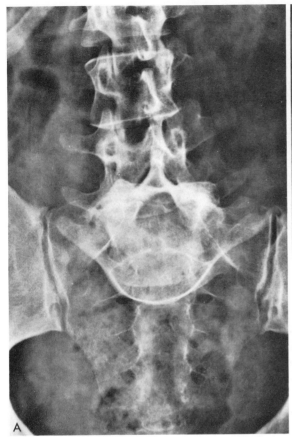

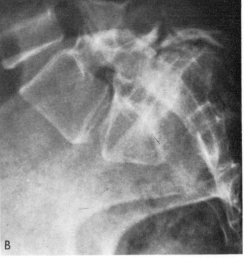

Figure 10–33. Advanced (Grade IV) spondylolisthesis. *A*, Frontal view. The lumbar spine appears abnormally foreshortened. The contours of the caudally displaced vertebral body present an inverted curvilinear density, or "bow-line," resembling an "inverted Napoleon's hat." *B*, Lateral view. The forward slip and downward displacement are readily apparent. In this patient, the lumbar spinal column has been completely displaced from the sacrum and has sunk down anterior to it. Note the marked wedge-shaped deformity of L-5 vertebral body.

Figure 10–34. Spondylolysis of L-5 vertebra, left anterior oblique view. The edges of the spondylolytic defect (arrow) appear rounded and well-defined. Considerable bony sclerosis has resulted below the inferior margin of the defect, in the vicinity of the arrow.

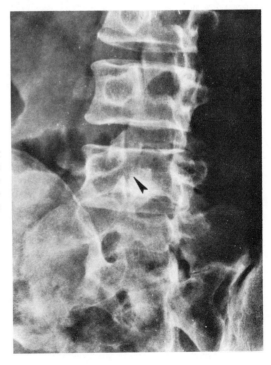

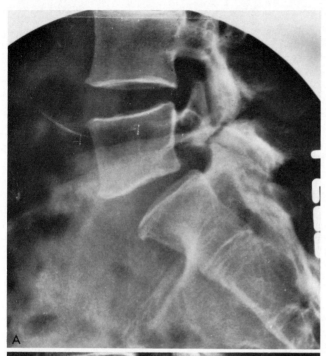

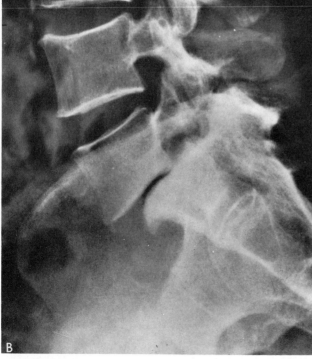

Figure 10–35. Progression of spondylolytic spondylolisthesis with time. *A,* Grade I spondylolytic spondylolisthesis of L-5 vertebra in a young man. *B,* Same patient, nineteen years later. Progression to Grade II has occurred. Note also the severe lumbosacral disk degeneration, which has been occasioned in the interval, with marked proliferative reaction of the sacral promontory and "vacuum" formation in the intervertebral disk. (Courtesy of R. H. Freiberger, M.D., Hospital for Special Surgery, New York, N. Y.)

margins between the fragments, and no loss of bone would be expected in the vertebral arch, nor sclerosis of the bone at the fracture site. Isolated unilateral pars fractures are mechanically difficult to explain, being analogous to breaking the handle of a tea-cup in only one place.[26] In suspected acute unilateral fracture, the opposite pars and pedicle would be of the same density as those above and below. Dense callus formation would be expected with healing of acute pars interarticularis fractures.

Spondylolysis, on the other hand, exhibits rounding of the defect edges, loss of bone in the vertebral arch proportionate to the width of the defect, and a variable degree of bony sclerosis about its margins (Fig. 10–34). Reactive sclerosis of the opposite pedicle and pars interarticularis indicates that a unilateral pars defect is not of recent origin.[10] Pars defects in general heal poorly, with scanty callus formation upon immobilization.[8, 26]

2. *Congenital clefts* of the vertebral arch may involve the pedicles or their roots in the vertebral body (retrosomic clefts), the laminae (retroisthmatic clefts), the articular processes, or the spinous process. Such clefts have not been found to originate in the pars interarticularis, however. The location of congenital clefts thus allows them to be distinguished from the more common pars defects in most instances, when appropriate views are obtained.

COMPLICATIONS OF SPONDYLOLYTIC SPONDYLOLISTHESIS

1. Progression of spondylolytic spondylolisthesis may occur with time, and has been radiologically documented (Fig. 10–35). Progression of more than one grade after the individual has reached adulthood is unusual, however.[3, 26]
2. Nerve root compression in patients with spondylolisthesis may arise by one of several mechanisms:
   a. Posterior herniation of the nucleus pulposus may occur as a sequel of disk degeneration resulting from spondylolisthesis, compressing the nerve roots of the cauda equina. Myelogra-

phy may help to provide the diagnosis.
   b. Degenerative osteophytes may form about the intervertebral foramina for the lumbar and sacral nerve roots, and may compress the nerves.
   c. In other cases, the nerve roots may be bound down by scar and fibrous adhesions forming about the pars defects, or caught between shifting bony fragments of the vertebral arch.
   d. In advanced cases of spondylolisthesis, the cauda equina may be subjected to shearing stress at the level of slippage, producing traction of the nerve roots over the posterior aspect of the vertebral body below the slip. This complication is proportional to the extent of slippage, although relatively uncommon overall (Fig. 10–36).[15]

FINDINGS AT SURGERY

At surgery, when the posterior aspect of the spine has been exposed, the characteristic feature of spondylolytic spondylolisthesis is looseness of the vertebral arch. The spinous process may be easily shifted back and forth with a surgical clamp when bilateral pars defects exist. This abnormal mobility may be increased by attendant tears or degeneration of the posterior ligament complex.[15]

HEALING

We have seen that an inability of the altered pars interarticularis to heal normally is characteristic of spondylolysis. Healing has been noted in some cases of spondylolytic spondylolisthesis, however, sometimes with elongation of the pars and persistence of spondylolisthetic slippage.[26] Such healing as does occur is slow, with little callus formation, in keeping with the concept of a disturbance in the underlying bone interfering with the process of repair. Rapid healing of a pars defect with abundant callus formation suggests a fracture or a more acute form of injury.[8, 26]

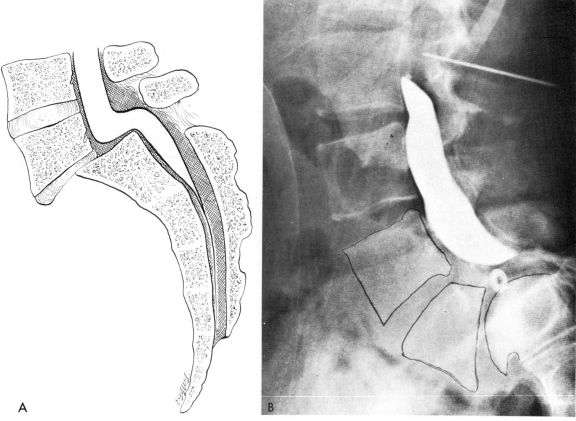

Figure 10–36. Nerve root traction in advanced spondylolisthesis. *A,* Diagram: Shearing stress has been exerted on the cauda equina at the lumbosacral level by the spondylolisthetic slip, resulting in traction of the nerve roots in the caudal sac over the posterior aspect of the sacral promontory. *B,* Myelographic demonstration of caudal sac and nerve root compression in a patient with advanced spondylolisthesis by the mechanism illustrated above. (The bony lumbosacral contours have been outlined.)

REFERENCES

1. Borkow, S. E. and Kleiger, B.: Spondylolisthesis in the newborn. Clin. Orthop., *81*:73, 1971.
2. Cyron, B. M., Hutton, W. C., and Troup, J. D. G.: Spondylolytic fractures. J. Bone & Jt. Surg., *58-B*:462, 1976.
3. Epstein, B. S.: The Spine, A Radiological Text and Atlas. 3rd ed. Philadelphia, Lea & Febiger, 1969.
4. Grantham, S. A., and Imbriglia, J. E.: Double-level spondylolysis and transitional vertebrae. J. Bone & Jt. Surg., *57-A*:713, 1975.
5. Hensinger, R. N., Lang, J. R., and MacEwen, G. D.: Surgical management of spondylolisthesis in children and adolescents. Spine, *1*:207, 1976.
6. Kettelkamp, D. B., and Wright, D. G.: Spondylolysis in the Alaskan Eskimo. J. Bone & Jt. Surg., *53-A*:563, 1971.
7. Lerner, H. H., and Gazin, A. I.: Interarticular isthmus hiatus (spondylolysis). Radiology, *46*:573, 1946.
8. Lob, A.: Die Wirbelsäulenverletzungen und ihre Ausheilung. 2nd ed. Stuttgart, Georg Thieme Verlag, 1954.
9. Macnab, I.: Spondylolisthesis with an intact neural arch—the so-called pseudo-spondylolisthesis. J. Bone & Jt. Surg., *32-B*:325, 1950.
10. Maldague, B. E., and Malghem, J. J.: Unilateral arch hypertrophy with spinous tilt: a sign of arch deficiency. Radiology, *121*:567, 1976.
11. McKee, B. W., Alexander, W. J., and Dunbar, J. S.: Spondylolysis and spondylolisthesis in children: a review. J. Canad. Assoc. Radiol., *22*:100, 1971.
12. Melamed, A.: Fracture of pars interarticularis of lumbar vertebra. Amer. J. Roentgenol. *94*:584, 1965.
13. Meyerding, H. W.: Spondylolisthesis as an etiologic factor in backache. JAMA, *111*:1971, 1938.
14. Moreton, R. D.: Spondylolysis. JAMA, *195*:671, 1966.
15. Newman, P. H., and Stone, K. H.: The etiology of

spondylolisthesis. J. Bone & Jt. Surg., 45-B:39, 1963.

16. Rabuschka, S. E., Apfelbach, H., and Love, L.: Spontaneous healing of spondylolysis of the fifth lumbar vertebra. Clin. Orthop., 93:256 1973.

17. Rosenberg, N. J.: Degenerative spondylolisthesis: Predisposing factors. J. Bone & Jt. Surg., 57-A:467, 1975.

18. Rowe, G. G., and Roche, M. B.: The etiology of separate neural arch. J. Bone & Jt. Surg., 35-A:102, 1953.

19. Saha, M. M., Bhardwaj, O. P., Srivastava, G., et al.: Osteopetrosis with spondylolysis — four cases in one family. Brit. J. Radiol., 43:738, 1970.

20. Schinz, H. R., Baensch, W. E., Friedl, L., and Uehlinger, E.: Roentgen Diagnostics, Vol. II, Skeleton. New York, Grune & Stratton, 1968.

21. Schmorl, G. and Junghanns, H.: The Human Spine in Health and Disease. 2nd American ed. by E. F. Besemann. New York, Grune & Stratton, 1971.

22. Sim, G. P. G.: Vertebral contour in spondylolisthesis. Brit. J. Radiol., 46:250, 1973.

23. Stewart, T. D.: The age incidence of neural arch defects in Alaskan natives, considered from the standpoint of etiology. J. Bone & Jt. Surg., 35-A:937, 1953.

24. Sullivan, C. R., and Bickell, W. H.: The problem of traumatic spondylolysis. Amer. J. Surg., 100:698, 1960.

25. Wiltse, L. L.: The Etiology of Spondylolisthesis. J. Bone & Jt. Surg., 44-A:539, 1962.

26. Wiltse, L. L.: Spondylolisthesis. In The A.A.O.S. Symposium on the Spine. St. Louis, C. V. Mosby Co., pp. 143–168, 1969.

27. Wiltse, L. L., Widell, E. H., and Jackson, D. W.: Fatigue fracture: the basic lesion in isthmic spondylolisthesis. J. Bone & Jt. Surg., 57-A: 17, 1975.

28. Zatzkin, H. R.: The Roentgen Diagnosis of Trauma. Chicago. Year Book Medical Publishers, 1965.

Chapter 11

SPONDYLOLISTHESIS WITHOUT SPONDYLOLYSIS

NONSPONDYLOLYTIC SPONDYLOLISTHESIS

Definitions

Nonspondylolytic spondylolisthesis is defined as forward slipping of one vertebral body upon another — as in spondylolytic spondylolisthesis — but with an intact vertebral arch. Synonyms include *articular spondylolisthesis, spondylolisthesis with an intact neural arch, degenerative spondylolisthesis, pseudospondylolisthesis,* and *Newman Type IV spondylolisthesis.*

Incidence

First described by Lane in 1893, nonspondylolytic spondylolisthesis is a disease of older age groups, rarely occurring before age 50 and never before age 40.[11, 15] The average age at the time of diagnosis was 65 in Newman's series.[10] Females show an increased incidence, ranging from 3:1 to 4:1 in different series.[10, 11] Blacks are involved three times as often as whites.[11] By far the most commonly affected intervertebral level is the L-4/L-5 joint (80 per cent of Rosenberg's series), followed by the lumbosacral joint (9 per cent) and the L-3/L-4 joint (7 per cent) (Figs. 11–1, 11–2). More than one joint was involved in 5 per cent of his patients.[10, 11] (The term "joint" here, although not strictly correct in anatomical terms, is used to refer to the soft tissue structures uniting two adjacent vertebrae, i.e., intervertebral disk, apophyseal joints, and supporting ligaments, and will be employed for the sake of simplicity.)

The extent of vertebral slippage in nonspondylolytic spondylolisthesis does not exceed one centimeter, or 25 per cent of the sagittal diameter of the vertebral body.[6, 14] The mean value in Rosenberg's series was 14 per cent of the vertebral diameter.[11] In evaluating sequential radiographs of patients with nonspondylolytic spondylolisthesis, Newman and Stone found that slipping occurred at an average rate of two millimeters per year during the period of progression.

Etiology and Mechanism of Injury

Junghanns described alterations in the apophyseal joints in nonspondylolytic spondylolisthesis, but was uncertain whether they were the cause or the result of the associated severe degenerative arthritis. These apophyseal alterations included an increase in the "pedicle-facet" angle of the affected vertebra, the angle subtended by the long axis of the pedicle or vertebral root at its intersection with the plane of the apophyseal joint (Fig. 11–3B).[12] An increase in this angle indicates a more horizontal alignment of the apophyseal joints seen on the lateral view, allowing overriding of the articular surfaces of the apophyseal joints, once the supporting soft tissue structures had been weakened by degenerative arthritis.[6, 11]

Newman and Stone were unable to document alterations in the "pedicle-facet" angle in their cases of nonspondylolytic spondylolisthesis, and did not find overriding of the apophyseal joints. They observed alignment of the lumbosacral apophyseal joints in a more coronal plane in their pa-

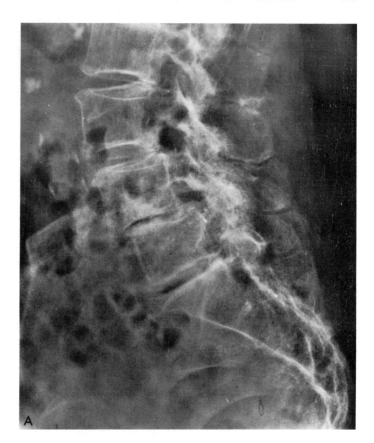

Figure 11–1. Nonspondylolytic spondylolisthesis. *A,B,* Forward slipping of L-4 vertebra upon L-5 has occurred (arrows), with the L-4 vertebral arch remaining intact. Note severe degenerative changes in the intervertebral joints of the L-4/L-5 and lumbosacral levels, both anteriorly and posteriorly. (Slight slipping of L-3 on L-4 has occurred as well.)

(Figure continued on next page.)

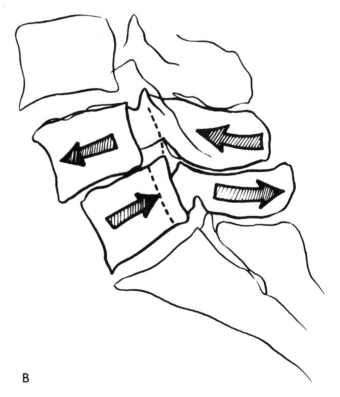

B

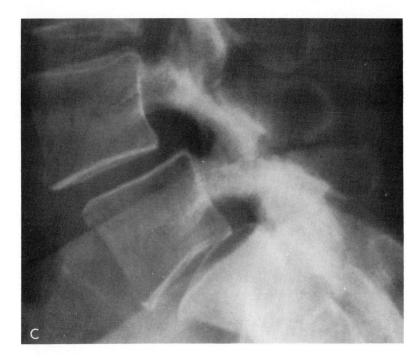

Figure 11–1 Continued. C, double forward slipping of L-4 L-5 and L-5 on S-1.

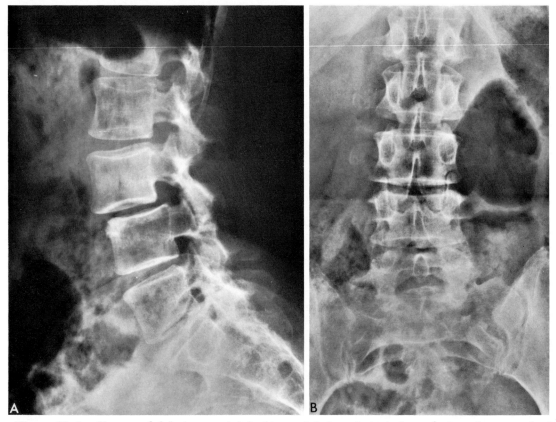

Figure 11–2. Nonspondylolytic spondylolisthesis of L-3 on L-4. *A,* Lateral view. Intervertebral disk degeneration at L-3/L-4 with reactive sclerosis of L-4 vertebral body accompany a non-spondylolytic spondylolisthesis at this level. *B,* Frontal view. Erosion and widening of the apophyseal joint surfaces at the level of spondylolisthesis have cast a prominent "W"-shaped shadow between the slipping vertebrae.

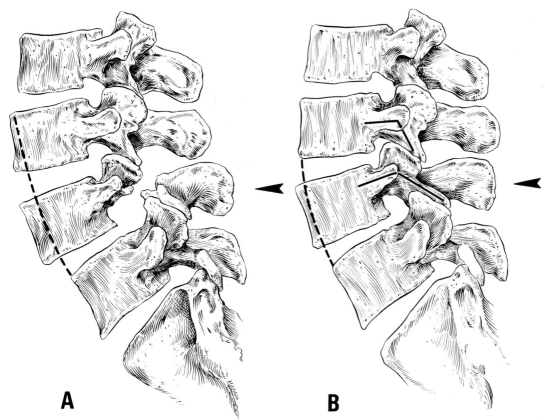

A   **B**

Figure 11–3. Comparison of spondylolytic with nonspondylolytic spondylolisthesis. *A,* Spondylolytic spondylolisthesis. Bilateral pars defects at L-4 level have allowed the body and anterior vertebral arch components of L-4 vertebra to slide forward on L-5. Note that while the body of L-4 advances, the spinous process and posterior part of the vertebral arch remain behind (arrow). As the spinous processes above L-4 move forward with the body of L-4, palpation of the back in spondylolytic spondylolisthesis will reveal prominence of the spinous process at the vertebral level affected. *B,* Nonspondylolytic spondylolisthesis. L-4 vertebra has maintained an intact arch while slipping forward in its entirety on L-5. Some observers have noted an increased "pedicle-facet angle" of the affected vertebra (drawn here on L-4) relative to adjacent vertebrae (drawn on L-3) in nonspondylolytic spondylolisthesis. As the arch of the slipping vertebra remains intact, its spinous process advances with it (arrow). Palpation of the back then reveals prominence of the spinous process below the level of the slipping vertebra.

tients with nonspondylolytic spondylolisthesis, affording greater stability to the lumbosacral joint. This placed relatively greater stress on the L-4/L-5 joint above, where the apophyseal joints were more obliquely disposed between the coronal and sagittal planes.[10, 11] At surgery, they found that the inferior articular processes of the slipping vertebra (usually L-4) had ground their way forward between the superior articular processes of the vertebra below (usually L-5), eventually being arrested by an anterior hook on the superior processes before the slipping could become too severe.[10]

Positional changes in the lumbar spine with nonspondylolytic spondylolisthesis are opposite to those seen in spondylolytic spondylolisthesis. The normal lumbar spine, unaffected by either form of spondylolisthesis, occupies the center of a spectrum of positional change that tends toward spondylolytic spondylolisthesis on one end, and nonspondylolytic spondylolisthesis on the other (Fig. 10–10). In spondylolytic spondylolisthesis, the lumbosacral angle is increased, the sacrum assumes a more horizontal position, lumbar lordosis is increased, and the vertebral body of L-5 is wedge-shaped (see Chapter 10). In nonspondylolytic spondylolisthesis, the lumbosacral angle is decreased, while the sacrum is more nearly vertical, lumbar lordosis is straightened, and the L-5 body approximates a rectangular shape (Fig. 10–10).[11] Rosenberg postulated that increased stability at the lumbosacral joint resulting from these

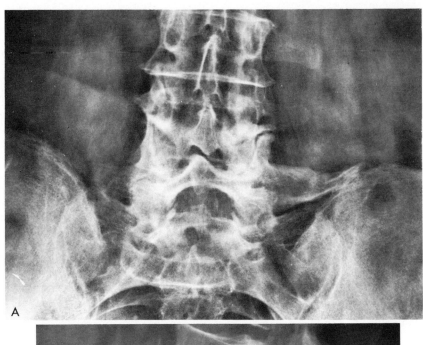

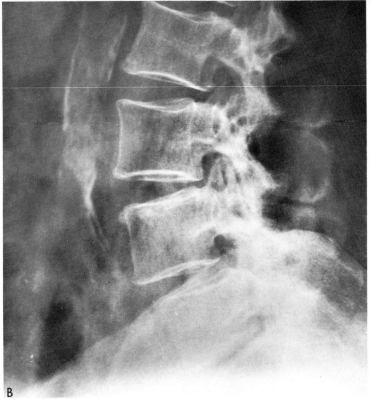

Figure 11–4. Nonspondylolytic spondylolisthesis with calcified iliolumbar ligaments. *A,* Frontal view. Calcification has occurred in the iliolumbar ligaments extending between the transverse processes of L-5 vertebra and the iliac crests on either side. This has fixed L-5 vertebra to the pelvis, thus inhibiting normal motion at the lumbosacral joint. (Sacralization of L-5 vertebra would have a similar effect.) *B,* Lateral view. Stabilization of L-5 vertebra has thrown abnormal stress on the L-4/L-5 joint above, resulting in nonspondylolytic spondylolisthesis of L-4 vertebra upon L-5. (Courtesy of R. H. Freiberger, M.D., Hospital for Special Surgery, New York, N.Y.)

changes threw abnormal stress on the L-4/L-5 joint above, with the subsequent development of nonspondylolytic spondylolisthesis. The increased incidence of sacralization of L-5 vertebra noted in his series lends further support to his theory, as such sacralized vertebrae exhibit very little motion at the lumbosacral joint (Fig. 11–4). Similarly, the reduced incidence of lumbosacral spina bifida occulta and other vertebral arch defects in patients with nonspondylolytic spondylolisthesis also argues for greater than normal stability at the lumbosacral joint, shifting excessive mechanical stress to the joint above.[10, 11]

Clinical Findings

Patients with nonspondylolytic spondylolisthesis most commonly complain of low back pain, sometimes extending into the buttock or thigh. A small proportion remain asymptomatic. In Rosenberg's series, symptoms in the leg or foot occurred in 30 per cent. The intensity of the pain was rarely severe, although involvement of higher lumbar levels (L-3) was associated with increased symptoms. Disturbances in gait were present in some, and genital or perineal numbness and urinary incontinence were noted in a few, although the correlation of these symptoms with herniated nuclear disks occurring in the series was not stated. No relation between the severity of symptoms and the extent of vertebral slip could be drawn.[11]

Many of Newman and Stone's patients gave a long history of backache extending back to the third or fourth decade. It was noted that radiologic changes of nonspondylolytic spondylolisthesis developed in several patients with initially normal radiographs who complained of low back pain; they concluded that a soft tissue lesion in these patients considerably antedated the vertebral displacement.

On physical examination, increased rigidity of the lumbar spine may be noted, with an inability to decrease the lumbar lordosis in flexion, and tenderness to deep palpation of the L-4 and L-5 spinous processes (Fig. 11–5).[6] Increased laxity of the pelvitrochanteric and hamstring muscles may be pres-

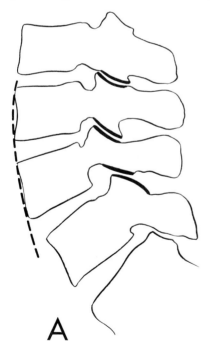
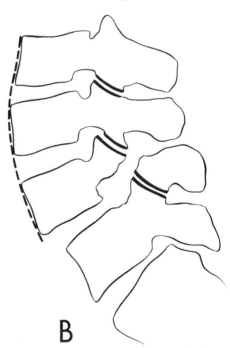

Figure 11–5. Spinous process changes in spondylolytic and nonspondylolytic spondylolisthesis. *A*, Nonspondylolytic spondylolisthesis. As the vertebral arch remains intact, the spinous process of the slipping vertebra advances, relative to the spinous process below. The spinous process prominent on physical examination therefore represents the vertebral level below the slip. *B*, Spondylolytic spondylolisthesis. Owing to the spondylolytic arch defect, the spinous process of the slipping vertebra remains behind as the body and pedicles slip forward, and may be easily palpated on physical examination at the level of spondylolisthesis, rather than the level below.

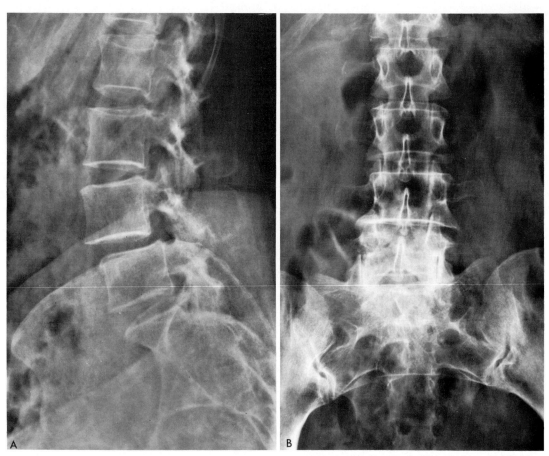

Figure 11–6. Nonspondylolytic spondylolisthesis. *A*, Lateral view. L-4 vertebra has slipped forward on L-5, with an intact vertebral arch. Note the osteophytic spurs in the angles between the pedicles and the superior articular processes affected by the spondylolisthesis, with a small anterior hook on the superior articular process of L-5 vertebra. The body of L-5 is more rectangular than normal, and the lumbar lordosis is straightened. *B*, Frontal view. The apophyseal joints exhibit proliferative change at both the L-4/5 and lumbosacral levels, with a "W"-shaped configuration of the apophyseal joint surfaces at the level of spondylolisthesis (L-4/5).

ent, allowing patients to touch their toes with ease, without bending their knees or straightening the lumbar lordosis.[11] Rosenberg found acute pain, muscle spasm, and a positive straight leg-raising test in 19 of his patients (10 per cent), seven of whom proved to have herniated disks on myelography.[11]

Neurologic deficits were documented in 50 per cent of Macnab's patients with nonspondylolytic spondylolisthesis and in 43 per cent of Rosenberg's; Newman and Stone found more nerve root injuries in nonspondylolytic spondylolisthesis than in any other type of spondylolisthesis. These injuries most often involved the fifth lumbar nerve root, less commonly the cauda equina. Diminished sensation to pin prick in the lateral aspect of the thigh was the most common finding. Decreased knee and ankle reflexes were present in 20 per cent of Rosenberg's patients.[6, 9, 10]

Radiologic Findings

In nonspondylolytic spondylolisthesis, forward slipping of a vertebra is noted on lateral view with an intact vertebral arch (Fig. 11–3). It is usually L-4 that slips forward on L-5 in an older patient (Figs. 11–6, 11–7). The apophyseal joints frequently show proliferative degeneration at the level of slippage, and oblique views are usually required to evaluate each pars interarticularis satisfactorily for stress fracture or spondylolysis. The articular facets are frequently eroded, so that wider surfaces of the articular processes are in contact at the joints than is normally the case (Fig. 11–7 B). On anteroposterior view, these widened apophyseal joint surfaces produce a prominent "W"-shaped shadow between the slipping vertebrae (Figs. 11–2 B, 11–6 B). Osteophytic spurs may grow in the angles between

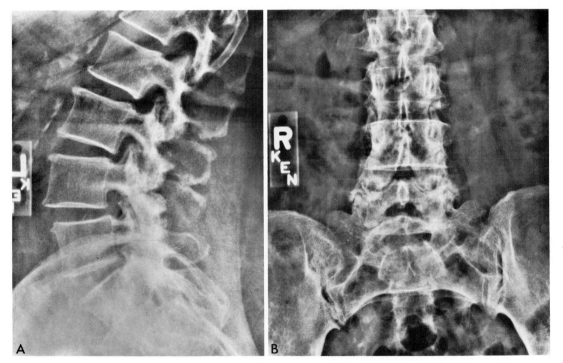

Figure 11–7. Nonspondylolytic spondylolisthesis of L-4 on L-5. *A,* Lateral view. L-4 vertebra has slipped forward on L-5, with an intact vertebral arch. A prominent anterior hook has arisen on the superior articular process of L-5, encroaching upon the intervertebral foramen between L-4 and L-5. *B,* Frontal view. The articular facets at the level of spondylolisthesis are eroded and rounded off, with wider surfaces of the articular processes in contact at the joints than is normally the case. The joint surfaces have been extended laterally by osteophyte formation on both sides.

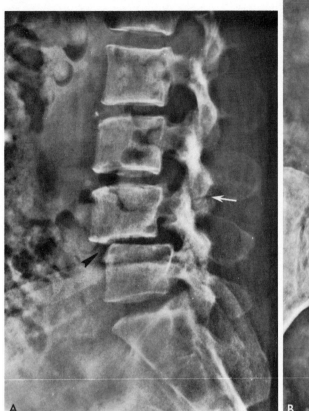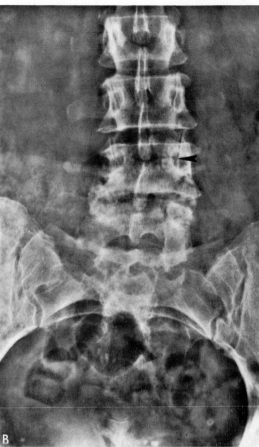

Figure 11–8. Degenerative changes in nonspondylolytic spondylolisthesis. *A*, Lateral view. Severe intervertebral disk degeneration accompanies nonspondylolytic spondylolisthesis at the L-4/5 level (black arrow), and anterior vertebral edge separations may be noted involving the L-3 and L-4 vertebral bodies as well. A horizontal lucency crossing one inferior articular process of L-3 (white arrow) indicates an unfused fracture or apophysis. *B*, Frontal view. The apophyseal joints exhibit proliferative and degenerative changes. An unfused fracture or apophysis of the left inferior articular process of L-3 vertebra is again seen (black arrow).

the pedicles and the superior articular processes affected by the spondylolisthesis, and they may encroach upon the spinal canal (Fig. 11–6 *A*).[10, 11] These correspond to the anterior hooks described by Newman and Stone that ultimately retard further forward slipping of the articular processes (Fig. 11–7 *A*).

Radiologic evidence of lower lumbar intervertebral disk degeneration is variable in nonspondylolytic spondylolisthesis, not exceeding 45 per cent of the patients in Rosenberg's series, and not necessarily confined to the level of spondylolisthesis (Fig. 11–8).[10]

The plane of the sacral promontory is more nearly horizontal on the lateral view, with the sacrum and L-5 in a more vertical position than normal. The lumbosacral angle is decreased, and the lumbar lordosis is diminished. In spondylolytic spondylolisthesis, the opposite is true (Fig. 10–10). The body of L-5 is more rectangular than normal on lateral view, whereas in spondylolytic spondylolisthesis in older patients it is more wedge-shaped than normal.[11]

Lumbar myelography in patients with nonspondylolytic spondylolisthesis may demonstrate an hourglass constriction of the thecal space at the level of the spondylolisthesis, due to compression by osteophytic outgrowths from the articular processes. Herniation of the nucleus pulposus was demonstrated in seven of Rosenberg's 29 patients with positive myelograms: at the L-4/L-5 level in three, at the lumbosacral level in three, and at the L-3/L-4 level in one.[11]

Operative Findings

At surgery, no instability of the vertebral arch is found, as is typically noted in spondylolytic spondylolisthesis. The vertebral canal is narrowed by proliferative bony changes about the apophyseal joints on either side. The fifth lumbar nerve root may be compressed beneath the anterior edge of the superior articular processes of L-5.[10]

CONGENITAL (NEWMAN TYPE I) SPONDYLOLISTHESIS

Definition

Congenital (Newman Type I) spondylolisthesis is a type of nonspondylolytic spondylolisthesis first appearing in young children, characterized by elongation of the vertebral arch of L-5 associated with congenital deficiencies of the sacrum (Fig. 11–9). The term "congenital" has been employed to distinguish this type of nonspondylolytic spondylolisthesis from the adult-onset, or "degenerative," form discussed above, which does not appear before age 40, and is not associated with defects of the sacrum or significant elongation of the vertebral arch. The term "congenital" in this sense does not imply the existence of spondylolisthesis at birth, as was discussed in Chapter 10, although the posterior sacral deficiency is truly congenital in origin. Synonyms for congenital spondylolisthesis include *lumbosacral subluxation* and *spondyloptosis.*

Incidence

Although the peak incidence in Newman's series was from 15 to 25 years of age

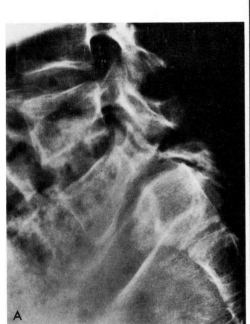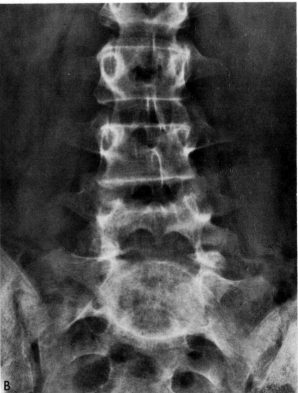

Figure 11–9.   Congenital spondylolisthesis. *A,* Lateral view: Deficient posteriorly, the sacrum lacks superior articular processes, allowing L-5 vertebra to slide forward. The vertebral arch of L-5 has been elongated and severely stretched over the sacrum, barely remaining intact. Anterior buttressing of the sacral promontory reflects lumbosacral disk degeneration, and appears to represent an attempt to stabilize the joint mechanically. *B,* Frontal view: The upper sacrum is posteriorly deficient, lacking arches and spinous processes. (Courtesy of R. H. Freiberger, M.D., Hospital for Special Surgery, New York, N.Y.)

at the time of diagnosis, radiologic changes in congenital spondylolisthesis may be noted in early childhood, and affected children may complain of back pain. A female predominance of greater than 2:1 has been noted.[10]

Etiology and Mechanism of Injury

Congenital spondylolisthesis often causes major displacement of the vertebrae above the sacrum, with complete "caving in" of the lumbosacral spine as a result. The condition originates with deficient development of the sacrum. Posterior defects occur in one or more of the sacral vertebral arches, especially at the first sacral level. Associated with this is a hypoplasia or complete absence of the articular processes of S-1, which normally articulate with the inferior articular processes of the last lumbar vertebra to block forward slipping. This allows the vertebra to slip forward and downward over the top of the sacrum, its articular processes slowly grooving the top of the sacrum

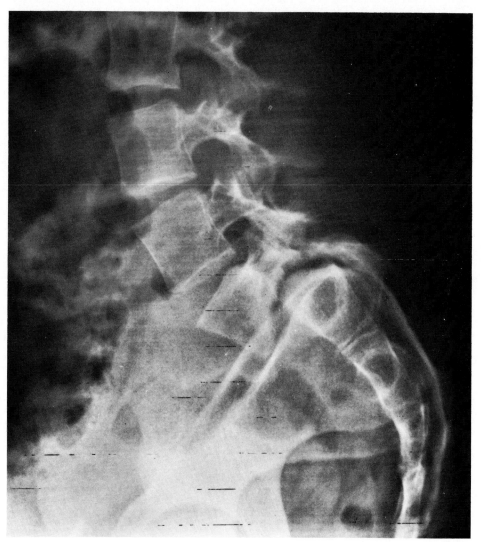

Figure 11–10. Congenital spondylolisthesis. The articular processes of S-1 are absent, reflecting deficient development of the posterior sacrum. Forward gliding of the last lumbar vertebra is marked on this lateral view, virtually amounting to 100 per cent; its body is wedge-shaped, and its vertebral arch severely stretched. Owing to tightness of the hamstring muscles, the long axis of the sacrum is more vertical, enhancing anterior displacement of the last lumbar vertebra.

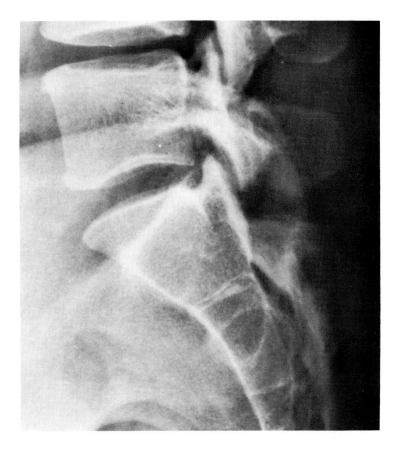

Figure 11–11. Normal upper sacrum. Compare the normal articular processes of this sacrum, as seen on lateral view, with those in Figure 11–10.

as it passes over. The anterior aspect of the last lumbar spinous process eventually abuts against the fibrous defect in the vertebral arch of S-1, arresting further forward motion. Stretching and elongation of the lower lumbar vertebral arches follows, in response to increased mechanical traction on the pedicle and pars interarticularis. The pars interarticularis generally remains intact, although it may occasionally break.[10]

Clinical Findings

In children with spondylolisthesis, the "congenital" type occurs earlier and produces more severe symptoms and deformity than does the spondylolytic type, as a rule. These symptoms may produce a "clinical crisis" in patients of age 10 to 20 who present with a rigid lumbar spine, spasticity of the hamstring muscles in the legs, and often lumbar scoliosis. The scoliosis may result from reflex muscle spasm, or from an unequal degree of forward slip on one side of the vertebral arch compared with the other.

The trunk may exhibit shortening, with anterior sagging or "caving in" of the lower lumbar spine. The pelvis may tilt backward, with flaring of the iliac crests and flattening of the buttocks, due to hamstring tightness. Signs of nerve root injury may be elicited, most often of the first sacral root, less often of the cauda equina.[7, 10]

Radiologic Findings

Deficient development of the posterior sacrum is characteristic of congenital spondylolisthesis, with spina bifida of the S-1 arch, and absent or rudimentary sacral articular processes (Figs. 11–10, 11–11). Forward gliding of the last lumbar vertebra is often marked on the lateral view, exceeding half the sagittal diameter of the vertebral bodies in 50 per cent of Newman and Stone's cases, and reaching 100 per cent in some. The most advanced grades of spondylolisthesis are usually all representative of this type (Fig. 11–12). Owing to tightness of the hamstring muscles in higher grades of

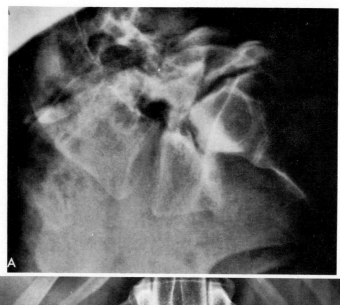

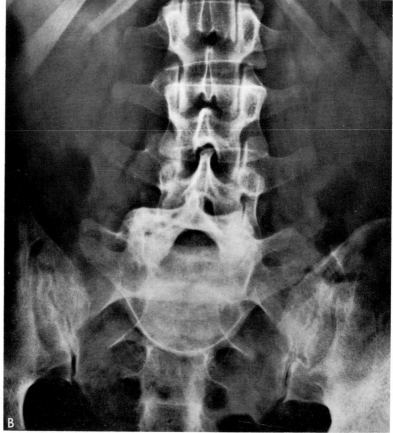

Figure 11–12. Congenital spondylolisthesis. *A,* Lateral view. An advanced grade of lumbosacral spondylolisthesis is present, attaining 100 per cent in this patient with congenital spondylolisthesis. Stretching of the pedicle and pars interarticularis of L-5 on both sides has effectively pulled them apart to produce bilateral pars defects. *B,* Frontal view. Marked forward and downward displacement of the last lumbar vertebra on the sacrum has shortened the lumbar spine. The anterior edge of the displaced lumbar vertebral body casts an "inverted Napoleon's hat" shadow over the upper sacrum. (Courtesy of R. H. Freiberger, M.D., Hospital for Special Surgery, New York, N.Y.)

"congenital" spondylolisthesis, the long axis of the sacrum is more vertical on lateral view, enhancing anterior displacement of the last lumbar vertebra (Fig. 11–10). Stretching and elongation of the pedicle and pars interarticularis may be seen bilaterally ("like a piece of taffy candy might do if pulled"[14]), but they usually remain intact (Fig. 11–9 A). (Stress fractures or pars defects have been described in these patients, however [Fig. 11–12]). In contrast to the "Scottie dog collar" or pars defect, on oblique view in "congenital" spondylolisthesis the affected pedicle and pars interarticularis resemble a "greyhound," being stretched out but intact. Degenerative changes in the lumbosacral disk are often extensive, and wearing away of both the anterior and the posterior aspects of the sacral promontory may be produced by the rocking or "teeter-totter" instability of the lumbosacral joint (Figs. 11–12 A, 11–13 A).[7, 10]

Lumbar myelography in congenital spondylolisthesis reveals an S-shaped stretching of the caudal sac between the two lowest lumbar vertebral arches and the posterior aspect of the sacral promontory, with constriction of the thecal space.

Another type of congenital spondylolis-thesis has been noted in young children with hypoplastic lower lumbar articular processes resulting in small, flat apophyseal joints mechanically incompetent to prevent forward gliding of the vertebrae. Posterior sacral deficiency is not a feature of these cases.[4]

Operative Findings

At surgery, no looseness of the last lumbar vertebral arch is encountered in congenital spondylolisthesis, such as is found in spondylolytic spondylolisthesis. Indeed, fibrous defects of one or more sacral arches are found, especially at the first sacral level, where the defect is indented by the anteriorly displaced last lumbar spinous process. The first sacral nerve roots and the cauda equina are stretched between the lower lumbar vertebral arches and the back of the sacral promontory.[10]

RETROSPONDYLOLISTHESIS

Definitions

Retrospondylolisthesis (retrolisthesis) denotes a backward displacement of one verte-

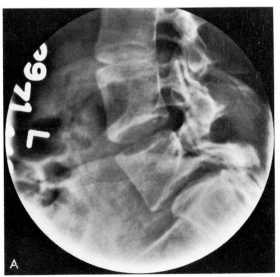
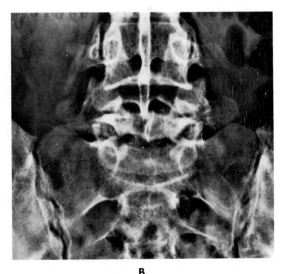

Figure 11–13. Congenital spondylolisthesis. *A*, Lateral view. Degenerative change in the lumbosacral intervertebral disk occurs early in congenital spondylolisthesis. A rocking or "teeter-totter" instability of the lumbosacral joint may be produced, with wearing away of both the anterior and posterior aspects of the sacral promontory. (See also Fig. 11–12.) *B*, Frontal view. The articular processes, laminae and spinous process of S-1 are deficient posteriorly. (Courtesy of David B. Levine, M.D., Hospital for Special Surgery, New York, N.Y.)

bra upon another, the opposite deformity to spondylolisthesis. Synonyms include *reverse spondylolisthesis, vertebral retroposition, spondylolisthesis posterior, retrodisplacement,* and *posterior displacement.*[5, 9, 12, 13, 14] Retrolisthesis was first recognized radiologically in 1929 by Brailsford, and by Hibbs and Swift in the same year.[9] As with nonspondylolytic spondylolisthesis, no defects of the vertebral arch are associated.

Incidence

Retrolisthesis has been observed in 4.7 per cent of autopsied lumbar vertebral columns overall.[12] It most frequently involves the cervical and lumbar spine, in which the greatest mobility occurs. Schmorl and Junghanns initially noted retrolisthesis to involve L-2 vertebra most often, and L-1 thereafter;[12] later authors have noted the frequency of L-5 involvement on S-1.[2, 5, 9, 14] No increased association of lumbosacral vertebral anomalies with retrolisthesis has been observed.[5]

Etiology

Retrospondylolisthesis is frequently associated with intervertebral disk degeneration, as has been widely noted.[2, 5, 9, 12, 13, 14] Disk degeneration was radiologically obvious in 86 per cent of Gillespie's cases of retrolisthesis, all of whom had sustained herniated disk nuclei at the lumbosacral joint level. Loss of normal thickness and turgor allows the body of L-5 to "sink" backward on the sacrum,[13] and permits "telescoping" of the associated apophyseal joints, as the inferior articular processes of the vertebra above slide downward and backward on the superior articular processes below (Fig. 11–14). Stretching or tearing of the apophyseal joint capsules allows the abnormal "telescoping" to occur. Degen-

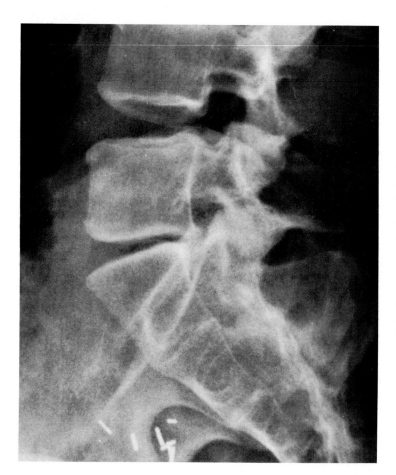

Figure 11–14. Retrospondylolisthesis of L-5 on S-1 vertebrae. Loss of normal intervertebral disk thickness and turgor allows the body of L-5 to "sink" backward on the sacrum, and permits "telescoping" of the apophyseal joints at this level, in which the L-5 inferior articular processes slide downward and backward on the S-1 superior articular processes. (Note the narrowing of the lumbosacral intervertebral foramen as a result.)

erative changes in the affected apophyseal joints may be absent or minimal, however, and the articular cartilage may be preserved.[14] Initially, this loosening of the intervertebral joints may be apparent only upon extension of the vertebral column in the upright lateral view; such "primary instability" indicates an early stage of intervertebral disk degeneration.[14]

The anatomic alignment of the apophyseal joints has been correlated with retrospondylolisthesis. Orientation of the apophyseal joint surfaces in the sagittal plane was believed by Hibbs and Swift to facilitate backward gliding;[9] alternatively, Ferguson postulated that alignment of the joint surfaces in the coronal plane would have the same effect.[5]

Melamed and Ansfield believed that retrolisthesis of the upper lumbar vertebrae occurred because the direction of vertebral slippage was "downhill" along the upper half of the lumbar lordotic curve in the erect position (Fig. 11–15). At the lumbosacral junction, a vertically oriented sacrum with a horizontal promontory and decreased lumbosacral angle would tilt the lumbar spine backward and predispose to backward slipping (Fig. 11–16).[9]

Spinal trauma may contribute to retrospondylolisthesis by soft tissue injuries to the intervertebral disk and apophyseal capsular attachments. Posterior displacement was noted in 70 per cent of cases in one series of vertebral fractures,[12] the injured vertebra sliding posteriorly upon the one beneath after injury to the sustaining soft tissues.

Congenital forms of retrospondylolisthesis may exist; examples in young children have been described. Similar deformities have been described in ankylosing spondylitis and in tuberculous and pyogenic spondylitis.[5, 9]

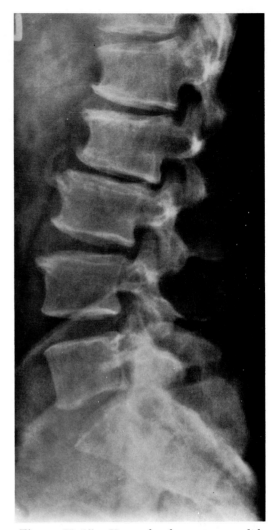

Figure 11–15. Upper lumbar retrospondylolisthesis. Degenerative disk disease in the upper lumbar spine has facilitated the development of retrolisthesis, with "downhill" slipping along the upper half of the lumbar lordotic curve in the erect position. The curves formed by the anterior and posterior surfaces of the vertebral bodies are out of alignment. The inferior articular processes of the displaced vertebrae project further posteriorly and inferiorly than normal. The normal upper lumbar lordosis has been effaced, with straightening out and even a slight kyphosis of this portion of the spine.

Radiologic Findings

The following criteria have been proposed by Melamed and Ansfield for the radiologic diagnosis of retrospondylolisthesis:[9]

1. Evidence of intervertebral disk degeneration (Figs. 11–15, 11–16, 11–17).
2. A break in the curves formed by both the anterior and the posterior surfaces of the vertebral bodies at the level of retrolisthesis (Figs. 11–15, 11–16, 11–17).
3. Anteroposterior narrowing of the intervertebral foramina at the level of retrolisthesis, often resulting in an "hourglass" or "figure eight" contour on lateral view (Figs. 11–17, 11–18).
4. "Telescoping," or abnormal widening, of the affected apophyseal joints. The in-

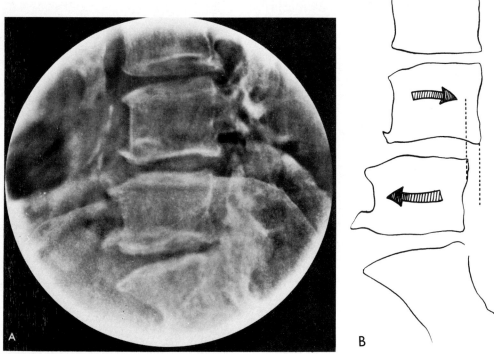

Figure 11–16. Retrospondylolisthesis of L-4 on L-5. *A,B,* A vertically oriented sacrum with a horizontal promontory and decreased lumbosacral angle tilts the lumbar spine backward, predisposing to backward slipping (arrows). Intervertebral disk degeneration is present. Both the anterior and posterior vertebral body surfaces are out of alignment at the level of retrolisthesis.

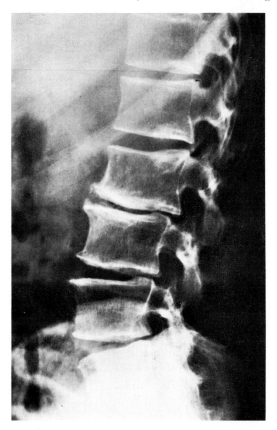

Figure 11–17. Lumbar retrospondylolisthesis. Although the lumbar spine exhibits intervertebral disk degeneration from L-2 down, retrolisthesis is most prominent along the upper half of the lumbar lordotic curve, being maximal at L-2/3, and reducing the normal lumbar lordosis. Note the narrowing of the intervertebral foramina affected by the retrolisthesis, and increased widening or separation of the involved apophyseal joints on lateral view, indicating loosening and degenerative change in the apophyseal joint capsules as well.

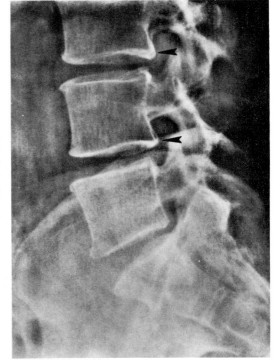

Figure 11–18. Lumbar retrospondylolisthesis. The curves formed by both the anterior and posterior vertebral body surfaces are out of alignment at the levels of retrolisthesis (arrows). Anteroposterior narrowing of the intervertebral foramina between the displaced vertebrae has resulted in an "hourglass" or "figure-of-eight" contour of the foramina on lateral view.

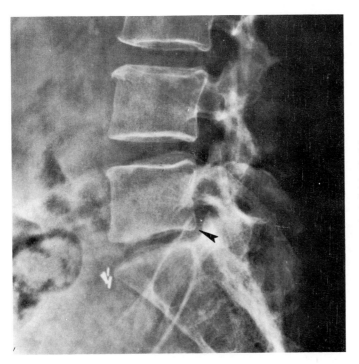

Figure 11–19. "Pseudo-retrospondylolisthesis" of L-5 on S-1. The body of L-5 protrudes posteriorly behind the sacral promontory (arrow), producing a "step" in the posterior contour formed by these surfaces. In this case the anterior vertebral contour between L-5 vertebral body and the sacrum remains intact.

ferior articular processes of the displaced vertebra may project further posteriorly and inferiorly than do others above and below (Figs. 11–15, 11–17).

5. Relative prominence of the spinous process of the posteriorly displaced vertebra.

6. Alteration of the normal lumbar lordosis — straightening of the spine above the retrolisthesis often occurs (Figs. 11–15, 11–17).

7. Failure to eliminate radiologic signs of retrolisthesis upon obtaining a true lateral projection without spinal rotation (see below).

DIFFERENTIAL DIAGNOSIS OF RETROSPONDYLOLISTHESIS

In some normal subjects the sagittal diameter of the body of L-5 exceeds that of the sacral promontory. In others, the body of L-5 is kidney-shaped on transverse section, causing it to protrude posteriorly behind the sacral promontory. This produces a "step" in the contour of the posterior surfaces of the L-5 body and the sacrum, which may be suggestive of retrospondylolisthesis, as was noted by Willis (Fig. 11–19).[13] Slight degrees of rotation departing from the true lateral projection will enhance this "pseudo-

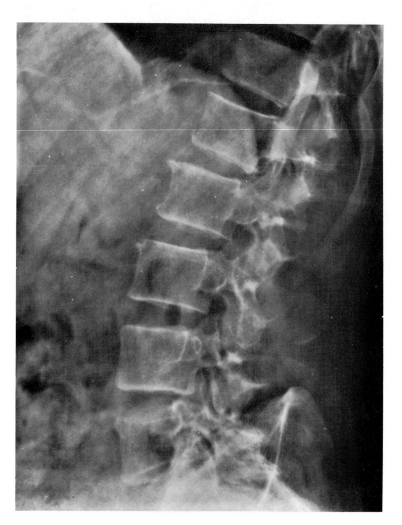

Figure 11–20. "Staircase" effect. A lateral view of the spine with the patient improperly positioned, so that the torso is rotated, has produced a "staircase" effect in the posterior contour of the upper lumbar body surfaces suggestive of retrospondylolisthesis. (Note that the articular processes and posterior body surfaces of the involved vertebrae are out of alignment, indicating the presence of rotation artifact.)

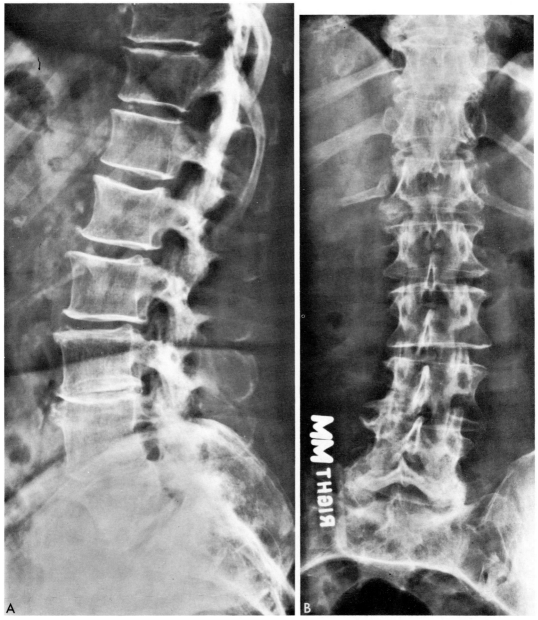

Figure 11–21. "Staircase" effect due to scoliosis. *A*, Lateral view. A "staircase" effect simulating retrospondylolisthesis involves the upper lumbar spine on lateral view. Is this case due to improper positioning? *B*, Frontal view: Rotoscoliosis of the spine is demonstrated, accounting for the "staircase" effect seen on lateral view. This is not the fault of the technician!

retrospondylolisthesis" effect if the L-5 vertebral body is kidney-shaped. In these cases, the anterior vertebral contour-lines will remain intact, and the other criteria for retrospondylolisthesis noted above will not be present.

A "staircase" effect may be produced in the posterior contour of the upper lumbar vertebral bodies by rotation of the lumbar spine on lateral view. This constitutes another technical artifact that should not be confused with true retrospondylolisthesis.[9] Improper positioning of the patient on the lateral projection may be the fault in some cases (Fig. 11–20); in others, a rotoscoliosis of the thoracolumbar spine may be responsible, which may be confirmed on anteroposterior views of the spine (Fig. 11–21).

REFERENCES

1. Epstein, B. S.: The Spine, A Radiologic Text and Atlas. 3rd ed. Philadelphia, Lea & Febiger, 1969.
2. Fletcher, G. H.: Backward displacement of the fifth lumbar vertebra in degenerative disc disease. J. Bone & Jt. Surg., 29:1019, 1947.
3. Freiberger, R. H.: Personal communication, 1976.
4. Freiberger, R. H.: Personal communication, 1976.
5. Gillespie, H. W.: Vertebral retroposition (reversed spondylolisthesis). Brit. J. Radiol., 24:193, 1951.
6. Macnab, I.: Spondylolisthesis with an intact neural arch—the so-called pseudo-spondylolisthesis. J. Bone & Jt. Surg., 32-B:325, 1950.
7. Hensinger, R. N., Lang, J. R., and MacEwen, G. D.: Surgical management of spondylolisthesis in children and adolescents. Spine, 1:207, 1976.
8. McKee, B. W., Alexander, W. J., and Dunbar, J. S.: Spondylolysis and spondylolisthesis in children: a review. J. Canad. Assoc. Radiol., 22:100, 1971.
9. Melamed, A., and Ansfield, D. J.: Posterior displacement of lumbar vertebrae. Amer J. Roentgenol. 58:307, 1947.
10. Newman, P. H., and Stone, K. H.: The etiology of spondylolisthesis. J. Bone & Jt. Surg., 45-B: 39, 1963.
11. Rosenberg, N. J.: Degenerative spondylolisthesis: predisposing factors. J. Bone & Jt. Surg., 57-A:467, 1975.
12. Schmorl, G., and Junghanns, H.: The Human Spine in Health and Disease. 2nd American ed. by E. F. Besemann. New York, Grune & Stratton, 1971.
13. Willis, T. A.: Retrodisplacement. Amer. J. Roentgenol. 90:1263, 1963.
14. Wiltse, L. L.: Spondylolisthesis. In The A.A.O.S. Symposium on the Spine. St. Louis, C. V. Mosby Co., 1967.
15. Wiltse, L. L., Widell, E. H., and Jackson, D. W.: Fatigue fracture: the basic lesion in isthmic spondylolisthesis. J. Bone & Jt. Surg., 57-A:17, 1975.

INDEX

Note: In this index, page numbers in *italics* refer to illustrations; page numbers followed by (t) refer to tables.